YOUR LIFE IN YOUR HANDS

Understand, Prevent and Overcome Breast Cancer and Ovarian Cancer

Professor Jane A. Plant

www.janeplant.com

03809388

For my children Mark, Emma
and Thomas

20 19 18 17 16 15 14 13 12 11 10 9 8 7 6

This edition published in Great Britain in 2007 by
Virgin Books, an imprint of Ebury Publishing,
a Random House Group Company

First published in hardback in 2000 and in paperback in 2001
by Virgin Publishing Ltd

Updated edition published in paperback in 2003 by Virgin Books Ltd

The Random House Group Limited supports The Forest Stewardship Council
(FSC®), the leading international forest certification organisation. Our books
carrying the FSC label are printed on FSC® certified paper. FSC is the only forest
certification scheme endorsed by the leading environmental organisations,
including Greenpeace. Our paper procurement policy can be found at
www.randomhouse.co.uk/environment

MIX
Paper from
responsible sources
FSC® C016897

A catalogue record for this book is available from the British Library.

ISBN: 978 0 7535 1204 3

Typeset by TW Typesetting, Plymouth, Devon
Printed and bound by CPI Group (UK) Ltd, Croydon, CR0 4YY

Contents

Author's Note

The diagnosis and treatment of medical conditions is a responsibility shared between you and your medical advisors. All diets should begin with a medical check-up to make certain that no special health problems exist and to confirm that there are no medical reasons why you should not undertake a change of diet.

The diagram of a breast on page 29 is reprinted from *Basic Anatomy and Physiology* by H.G.Q. Rowett, by kind permission of John Murray (Publishers) Ltd.

The painting on page 111 is reprinted by kind permission of Réunion des Musées Nationaux.

Cancer Support

I recommend people requiring individual supervision or personal help to contact Cancer Support by telephone 020 8439 8818, or by e-mail: info@cancersupportinternational.com

For further information on this book, please e-mail or visit:

info@yourlifeinyourhands.co.uk
www.plantprogramme.com
www.janeplant.com
www.cancersupportinternational.com

Acknowledgements

I should like to acknowledge the help and support of my family, friends and colleagues. I should like to thank my daughter, Emma, for reading the manuscript and making helpful suggestions that have improved it. I should also like to thank my youngest son, Tom, now a doctor, for the many interesting discussions we have had which have improved my knowledge of the subject. The initial manuscript was typed by Kathe Fairhurst. I thank Dr Margaret Sprackling FRCP for her help in the search for truth and I am most grateful to Henry Haslam for his help with the book.

Preface to the Fourth Edition

It is now 2007, and it is 14 years since my breast-cancer secondaries disappeared following a fundamental change in my diet and lifestyle. My cancer had spread to the lymph nodes in my neck, in spite of radical mastectomy, three further operations, 35 radiotherapy treatments, irradiation of my ovaries to induce the menopause and several chemotherapy treatments. Despite all this treatment, my doctors had given me only months to live. I then recalled that people in rural China, where I had worked as a scientist, had a very low incidence of breast cancer. At that point I changed my diet and lifestyle, and to everyone's amazement, including, I have to admit, my own, the large cancerous lump in my neck disappeared within weeks.

Since that time I have not even had a scare, and my annual check-ups at Charing Cross Hospital have tended to focus more on my diet and lifestyle than on my cancer.

I have talked to senior doctors who have said that they personally have not met anyone who has survived such serious illness and had been very sceptical about my books until they had talked to me.

My experience, and that of many other women who had followed my diet and lifestyle, led me to write *Your Life in Your Hands*, which was published in 2000. This was followed in 2001 by *The Plant Programme* and in 2005 by *Eating for Better Health*, written with Gill Tidey, cookbooks which complement the dietary advice in *Your Life in Your Hands*.[1] From the many communications I have received from people all over the world I have become aware of the beneficial effects of my diet and lifestyle in treating other cancers such as ovarian cancer, endometrial cancer and oesophageal and colorectal cancer; information on ovarian cancer is included in this new edition of *Your Life in Your Hands*.

In my research for this book I became aware that the same factors implicated in breast cancer were also implicated in prostate cancer, and in 2004 I wrote *Prostate Cancer: understand, prevent and overcome,* now in its second edition.

Information on other cancers is now available on the website, www.cancersupportinternational.com. This website provides up-to-date science-based information and support to cancer sufferers, and includes a forum for people to discuss their experiences of their illness, treatments, diet and lifestyle. I receive many communications from men and women who have complemented their conventional medical treatment with the diet and lifestyle that I recommend, and I know from these communications that many of them are now healthy and cancer-free.

Since the first edition of this book was published, seven years ago, more and more scientific evidence has appeared to support its findings and recommendations. It is perhaps worth noting that, despite the press seizing on one or two of the most sensational recommendations of the book – eliminating dairy produce and reducing exposure to hormone-disrupting and hormone-mimicking chemicals – there were originally seven food factors and five lifestyle factors to be addressed – there are now ten for each.

Examples of new supporting evidence include the results of studies conducted by eminent researchers that show the link between breast cancer and high dairy and calcium intake. There is also more and more evidence that the disease is associated with high circulating levels of a chemical messenger in the body called IGF-I and that this is linked to food factors identified in this book, especially high dietary intakes of dairy produce, trans fatty acids and refined carbohydrate and low dietary intakes of vegetables and fruit. There is also much evidence that a high-oestrogen diet is linked to breast cancer, and this book identifies the main dietary sources of dangerous animal oestrogens. It also debunks the propaganda against soya, which is high in protective phyto-oestrogens.

There is, in addition, further evidence of the importance of the correct balance of oils in the diet, as well as increasing evidence against consuming man-made vitamins and minerals, including megadoses of vitamin C or calcium to fight cancer. Evidence of the association of breast cancer and carcinogenic chemicals such as those in pesticides also continues to mount.

The reason all the recently published science has confirmed the findings and recommendations in my books and shown them to be so soundly based is not because I am clairvoyant or indeed particularly clever. It is simply because my books are based on research into the peer-reviewed scientific literature. Because of my scientific training, I am able to read information in publications written in the sort of scientific shorthand that all scientists tend to use to communicate with other specialists in their field, and translate it into simple straightforward English to make it accessible to a wider readership. I am also able to recognise biased studies funded by vested-interest groups such as the dairy or pharmaceutical industries. The extent to which medical practice is influenced by vested-interest groups is something that many others, including the *British Medical Journal* (*BMJ*), now take very seriously. The *BMJ* now requires that authors of any paper published by them should declare the funding sources of their study or other potential conflicts of interest. For this reason, many of the references in this book are from the *BMJ*. There is also concern about bias and misinformation in relation to our food. In *Save yourself from breast cancer*,[2] Robert D. Kradjian, head of the breast-surgery division at the Seton Medical Centre, Daly City, California, states the problem as follows:

The issue is clear. Much of our highly varied, desired, and profitable food supply has been found to be dangerous. The people who furnish this food and who are enriched by its sale do not want you to know this. They have generously contributed to scientists who have supported, and are willing to continue to support, their products. If those scientists suddenly have a change of heart, and seriously challenge the safety of that food, you may be certain that the bulk of the food-industry financial support will promptly disappear.

Whom are you going to believe? Those with no financial gain from the sale of food and with the backing of the world's scientific literature? Or are you going to follow those who have at times devised flawed studies and reaped millions of dollars in support of the industries that they fail to seriously criticise? You must decide, and your health will be substantially determined by your decision.

Happily, many medical professionals and scientists have been supportive of my work, and in 2005 I was given Life Fellowship of the Royal Society of Medicine. I am aware that many doctors are now recommending my books to their breast-cancer and prostate-cancer patients and to sufferers of other types of cancer including colorectal cancer. Increasingly, I am invited to address medical societies and cancer support groups, and I obtain very positive feedback from these occasions.

Perhaps it's worth mentioning that the diet will NOT cause osteoporosis. Quite the reverse. The book *Understanding, Preventing and Overcoming Osteoporosis*,[3] which I wrote with Gill Tidey, provides the scientific evidence that this disease, like breast cancer and prostate cancer, is strongly linked to the Western diet and has an extremely low incidence in countries such as China. The osteoporosis book contains many more delicious, healthy recipes which complement those in *The Plant Programme* and *Eating for Better Health*, and it is particularly helpful to those concerned about cancer spreading to their bones or who are taking medication that can cause bone thinning.

This fourth edition of *Your Life in Your Hands* aims to bring you the most up-to-date scientific information on treatment. I look first at new developments in the conventional medical diagnosis and treatment of breast cancer and ovarian cancer. I then describe what cancer is, in simple, unscary language, and show that, instead of it involving some terrifying invasion of our bodies, it is simply our own cells behaving badly in conditions that encourage them to lose control.

I go on to describe some of the latest research findings into growth factors and hormone-disrupting and hormone-mimicking substances in our food, drink and environment, which I believe are responsible for the dramatic increase in breast cancer and ovarian cancer throughout the West. I take forward the debate on chemopreventive substances in our diet and I provide simple, practical advice on how to reduce your risk of suffering from breast or ovarian cancer – advice that will also help to treat the disease in those already affected. I look again at the politics of the problem, such as links between the pharmaceutical industry and medical clinicians, and the failure of the press to root out bias and flawed science funded by vested interest groups such as the dairy industry.

Perhaps I should explain that I have left the main body of the first edition largely unaltered. This means that readers who are familiar with the first edition will not have to search the whole book for new material: the new text is all gathered together in the Updates to each chapter, in the second half of the book. This is the pattern that was adopted in the second edition. The third edition added the case histories that are now found at the end of the book. In this edition, the Updates have been revised to incorporate the latest developments.

In each Update I explain fully all the science and its implications, and at the end of the Updates to Chapters Two to Six I summarise the main points 'in a nutshell' to help to make the arguments easier to follow. The scientific references on which the book is based are also included, should you or your doctor wish to follow them up.

Finally, I should like to reassure readers that I wrote this book in my own time, with no funding or influence from any vested-interest group, and that I have tried to ensure that the science on which it is based is, to the best of my knowledge, objective, authoritative and as free as possible from commercial, political or other such influences.

Welcome

This book has come about as a result of many hundreds of conversations I have had with women who want answers.

Breast cancer is a puzzling, and frightening, subject. As someone who has suffered five times from progressively more advanced breast cancer, which eventually spread to my lymph system before it was finally defeated, I know from first-hand experience just how terrifying it can be. But although breast cancer is a subject that frightens many women, this is *not* a frightening book. Quite the opposite, in fact: it is empowering and optimistic. It is a story of hope.

Over the past century, Western women have achieved extraordinary progress in a great many areas. We now have the power to vote for our governance, the methods to plan our families and to ensure that a high proportion of our children survive, and we can be educated alongside men in any subject we choose. Despite all these impressive and valuable gains, today's 'epidemic' of breast cancer now jeopardises our well-being, assaults the very symbols of our femininity and motherhood and indeed menaces our lives as few other threats do.

The facts are stark and shocking. For adult women (aged between 25 and 75) the leading cause of death is cancer[1]: and the type of cancer that kills most women is breast cancer.[2] Out of about every ten women you know, one of them (I hope not you) is likely to contract breast cancer.[3] These dry statistics actually understate the severity of the situation, because breast cancer affects the lives of far more people than that: when you include all the spouses, sons, daughters, mothers, fathers, friends, colleagues and loved ones whose lives are blighted by this disease, then you begin to realise just what a modern-day scourge we are dealing with. Almost no one in the Western world can consider themselves immune from its impact. Indeed, our increasing affluence appears to make matters worse.

Most diseases affect the poorer rather than the wealthier, more-educated members of society, but breast and prostate cancer are different. They mainly affect the higher socio-economic groups.[4] Indeed, the slang name for breast cancer in China translates as 'Rich Woman's Disease' as it mainly attacks women who follow a Western middle-class lifestyle.

For too long women have unquestioningly accepted that a proportion of us will be affected by breast cancer. We have been persuaded to be too passive about prevention and agreed that there is little or nothing we can do ourselves to prevent a disease that, quite literally, decimates the female population. And the overwhelming majority of our medical, scientific, political and financial efforts are directed towards detecting and treating, rather than preventing, this awful disease.

The message you'll read in these pages is very different.

I believe that all women have the right to the best available information so that they can make informed decisions for themselves. My aim in this book is to set before you, clearly and plainly, vital information that can help you to drastically cut your risk of contracting – and dying from – breast cancer. One of the frustrations for most women is not knowing how to help themselves. We know that if we smoke we increase our risk of lung cancer and if we sunbathe too much, we increase our risk of skin cancer, so we can choose whether to take these risks. But in the case of breast cancer, we are too often made to feel helpless because we are rarely told about anything we can actually do to protect ourselves. Although we are told of many risk factors for breast cancer, they do not translate into anything we can actually do. This makes us feel powerless.

For the first time, this book makes available to all women a compelling body of new evidence which points to the under-lying causes of breast cancer. It is my hope that women will use this information to prevent or treat this disease in themselves or those close to them. There is also much useful information gleaned from my own personal experience on the very practical aspects of dealing with the disease, including diagnosis and treatment. In addition, I have observed in my research that much of the data and information about prostate cancer leads to conclusions similar to those regarding the cause and treat-ment of breast cancer. Anticipating the care that the women who read this will extend to the men in their lives, I have included much about prostate cancer. You will also find suggestions on how, by changing values and behaviour patterns aimed at improving the environment, we can reduce our exposure as a society to some of the factors which may contribute to these diseases.

This book chronicles, in part, my journey through five progressively worse episodes of breast cancer and describes how I used my training as a scientist to cope with both the disease and the treatments I was given for it. That scientific training had taught me to observe and record everything, to root out every fragment of information and to sift the relevant from the irrelevant, the rational from the irrational, and to keep asking those two key questions that are at the very heart of science: why and how? This book contains what I believe to be the answers to those two questions regarding breast cancer.

If this book had been around even two years before my first diagnosis of breast cancer, I am sure that I would never have had the disease. I hope very much that you can put the information it contains to the best possible use in your own life.

Sincerely,

Jane A. Plant, CBE, D Univ, DSc, FRSM, FRSE,
FRSA, FRGS, FIMM, FGS, C Eng, C Geol
London

1 The Hat, The Boa Constrictor and The Scientist

In this chapter I explain to you why, as a natural scientist, my approach to the problem of breast cancer is so different from that of doctors and orthodox medical researchers. I then go on to explain how I used my training and experience to cope with all of the orthodox types of treatment a breast cancer patient is likely to undergo, including surgery, radiotherapy and chemotherapy. I explain the treatments clearly and simply and give lots of practical tips to help you cope, for example, to avoid or minimise hair loss during chemotherapy. In this chapter I have tried to make you feel as if you have a good and caring friend guiding you towards the light at the end of the tunnel.

Scientists can often seem to be rather strange people.

The truth is, scientists are different – we're trained to be. Let me explain what I mean by using the story I tell when I first lecture to new students at one of the universities I visit. It comes from a wonderful children's story you may already be familiar with: *The Little Prince* by Antoine de Saint-Exupéry. In this magical book the little prince draws a picture of a boa constrictor digesting an elephant. But when he shows his masterpiece to grown-ups and asks them whether they are frightened by the picture, they ask why they should be frightened by a picture of a hat. It is the ability to see that the hat is a boa constrictor digesting an elephant that distinguishes the best scientists.

I pondered deeply, then, over the adventures of the jungle. And after some work with a coloured pencil I succeeded in making my first drawing. My drawing Number One. It looked like this:

Let me give you a well-known example to show you what I mean. What sort of person sees an apple fall from a tree, wonders what force is drawing it down towards the earth – and then goes on to develop the whole concept of gravity?

Here's another example. What sort of person leaves a plate of glass coated with photographic emulsion next to a piece of granite in a drawer and, when he notices that the emulsion appears to have been damaged by 'emanations' coming from the granite, does not simply curse and throw it away? Instead, he deduces that previously unknown particles and rays have been emitted from the rock – and discovers radioactivity.

And one more. What sort of person attempts to culture bacteria in a petri dish, finds the experiment has gone 'mouldy', yet does not simply throw it away? Instead he looks carefully and observes that something in the fungus has killed the bacteria and discovers penicillin – thereby establishing the basis for the development of modern antibiotics.

All three people – Sir Isaac Newton, Henri Bequerel and Sir Alexander Fleming – saw things a little bit differently. It is this ability to see a familiar situation from a different viewpoint or angle which probably makes scientists seem rather odd to other people. But sometimes it results in a major leap forward in our understanding of the natural world.

Thinking like a creative scientist is more a state of mind than anything to do with training or education (although increasingly, we need to know and understand more and more facts before we can contribute new ideas).

This book sees things a little bit differently. For many decades, women have lived in the shadow of a devastating disease that continues to kill a high proportion of sufferers and which is associated in many women's minds with treatments that involve mutilating surgery and being subjected to irradiation or chemicals with frightening side effects. The disease is, of course, breast cancer. The only hope we are given is that with enough expenditure on research, we might one day find a truly effective treatment. Sadly, that day has been a very long time coming.

In these pages, I want to take you on a journey. Partly, it is the story of my own learning experiences with breast cancer, which I have suffered from five times and eventually conquered. But mainly, it is the story of a new and rather different way of seeing, understanding and treating this disease.

It is my hope that this book will serve two purposes. First, I want it to be directly useful to you, the reader. The straight-forward advice and simple lifestyle suggestions it contains will be of practical benefit to *every woman* in significantly reducing the risk of developing breast cancer. If you happen to be that one woman in ten who has developed breast cancer, then you will also find much additional information here which will give you a better chance of survival overall and help you to cope with rigorous treatment methods.

Secondly, it is vitally important that this book ignites a debate within the scientific and medical communities. Science is, at heart, an adversarial process. Progress is made by vigorous cross-questioning of your own and others' work. This book puts forward a new perspective on breast and prostate cancer and backs it up with compelling evidence from the scientific literature. The inescapable conclusion is that relatively small augmentations to the orthodox medical therapies currently being used in clinics and hospitals would result in major improvements in patient survival. For example, providing breast cancer patients with sound dietary advice as is common in the case of heart disease or diabetes, could greatly increase survival rates. So much suffering could be prevented, and so many lives could be saved, that the evidence must be heard – and acted upon – with the very greatest urgency.

HOW MY STORY BEGAN

I didn't choose to study breast cancer – it chose me. This is how it happened.

I first stumbled into science because I was an instinctive feminist. The boys at my local grammar school could choose between Latin, art and physics as GCE options, whilst at the Girls' School we could choose from only Latin, art or cookery. Although Latin was my best subject, I did not like it and resented the time spent on something that, as a teenager, I could see little point in. So I led a campaign for the girls to be offered the same choices as the boys and, for my efforts, became hoist with my own petard when I was obliged to study physics just as the boys did. Without quite realising it, I had started on the road to becoming 'a Scientist'.

At school I occasionally regretted what I had done, but at university I literally fell in love with the scientific subject I had chosen to do – geochemistry. I was the only woman to pursue the subject in Honours year; however, I was so dedicated and such a perfectionist that I had some problems. For example, after my final year examinations I ran away because I believed I had failed my exams. In fact, when my professor finally tracked me down it was to tell me that I had gained a first class honours degree.

After leaving university I married a young doctor who subsequently trained as an army psychiatrist, and had a son, named Mark. Our marriage failed and, in a protracted and painful custody battle, I lost my son to my ex-husband and his new wife, a psychologist. This has been a source of intense and chronic stress for the last thirty years of my life. Four years after I separated, I married my present husband Peter who, like me, is an earth scientist. We have two children, Emma, now twenty-six and Tom, now nineteen. You will read about them later.

I was lucky to be employed by the British Geological Survey as only the second woman scientist in its history. (Women had previously been employed only in a technical capacity.) I am now the Chief Scientist of the organisation and hopefully I am helping to encourage other women to progress in what in the past has been a very male-dominated subject.

Geochemistry is about the chemistry of the earth. My speciality is in understanding the chemistry of the surface of the earth, especially concentrations of chemicals where these occur either as natural concentrations in ore deposits or as a result of man's activity, for example, where there are landfill sites or contaminated land. I have frequently worked with biochemists, veterinarians, epidemiologists and medical geographers looking at the impact of chemicals in the environment on the health of humans, animals and crops. Early in my career, between 1975 and 1977, I served on a Royal Society committee concerned with geochemistry and health.[1] Since that time, my team of scientists at the British Geological Survey has been concerned with a wide range of human health problems related to the environment. Some of the methods we have developed allow us to make highly reproducible, high resolution maps showing the distribution of chemicals over the surface of the earth. We are able to look on our computer screens at the distribution of, say, arsenic and uranium (as potentially toxic elements) or zinc or iron (trace elements essential to animal and human health) in the same way people can look at the Earth's physiography – using remotely sensed photographs from space.[2] Almost from the beginning, these images, although intended for geologists, created a lot of interest from veterinarians, who found them helpful in diagnosing environmental and nutritional animal diseases in Britain. It was by working with them that I first began to learn of some of the amazing connections between geochemistry and biochemistry. I also learned when I was ill, that veterinary rather than medical literature provided the most fundamental answers based on biochemistry. Eventually, I established a team that is regarded as the best in the world in tackling health problems related to the levels of trace elements in the environment – some such as arsenic and fluoride can occur at levels so high that they cause disease; others such as selenium, iodine, zinc and cobalt can occur at such low levels they cause ill health in both man and animals. This is a particular problem in many developing countries.

Very recent work that the BGS team has conducted, which has received wide publicity, dealt with the problem of arsenic contamination in water from wells in Bangladesh. There the levels of arsenic in water can be so high that many people develop skin lesions where their skin becomes black and thickened and which, in a significant proportion of sufferers, becomes cancerous.

What I had learned as a result of this type of environmental detective work time and time again was that until you identified the *fundamental cause* of such problems, there was little or nothing that could be done to help the affected individuals. And until you've found the cause (whether it's of breast cancer or any other disease) and effectively neutralised it, then you can never, ever claim to have 'cured' the problem.

Until 1987, I had no interest in cancer because, like most people, I never imagined that it could happen to me. I had never smoked or sunbathed, rarely drank alcohol and ate what most experts would consider to be a healthy diet. I even wore and used cosmetics that I had checked contained no harmful chemicals. My lifestyle was hectic, certainly (it still is!), but no more stressful than many other women's.

Then, one Friday evening in September of that year, my life changed for ever.

I was in northern Canada examining gold deposits ahead of a major scientific conference in Toronto. I was working on a project aimed at understanding how gold, which is the rarest element on earth, could become concentrated by factors of up to about 10,000-times by natural geological processes to form economic ore deposits. I was feeling pleased because I had begun to see clues that would lead to new theories and models, which subsequently I published in peer-reviewed papers (*see* p. 19) and in a textbook I wrote over the next few years. It had been a gruelling day working down the gold mine. It was hot, sweaty and dirty work, not to mention noisy and dusty and I couldn't wait to get back to my hotel and the luxury of soap, hot water and fresh towels.

Finally back in my room, I dried myself and returned to my bedroom to search for a bra. As I was walking around topless hunting for my underwear, I suddenly saw in the low angle, late afternoon sunlight, a lump about the size of a large pea just under the skin of my left breast. I felt it and was immediately overwhelmed with fear and panic; my mouth went dry and I felt sick. I knew without a doubt that I had breast cancer. Over the next week or so, I was to become very familiar with the feel of the cancer. I was surprised by how hard it felt – like a compressed rubber ball surrounding one of the ducts in my left breast. I was angry with myself for not having examined my breasts before but, somehow, I had never thought the advice applied to me. I was only 42 – surely too young to get cancer? My family and loved ones, my developing career, the many happy and productive years I had always imagined to be ahead of me ... In one heart-stopping moment, everything came crashing to a very full stop.

After the initial shock had subsided somewhat, I tried to think what to do. My husband was working in Jamaica and I had no contact telephone number (this is common among geologists), and my children were both staying with their grandmother. In any case, I saw no point in upsetting them. The first thing I did was to telephone one of my oldest and dearest friends. Dr John Camac had been my doctor throughout my childhood and was still my mother's doctor. Despite the fact that it must have been about midnight in Britain, he was wonderful to me. He guided me through a careful self-examination. He knew me well enough not to give me false reassurances and we agreed that the lump that I had found probably was cancer but that it appeared to be very localised and could probably be treated by lumpectomy on my return to Britain. With his advice and the help of a friend in Canada, I decided to stay for the conference until I had honoured my commitments, but also to go to the famous Princess Margaret hospital in Toronto for an examination and diagnosis.

I thus spent the next week alternately being a professional scientist chairing sessions or giving lectures in front of an audience of about 800 people; attending a specialist breast clinic for examinations and biopsies finally to be given the diagnosis of cancer; and sitting alone or with friends feeling like a terrified five-year-old worrying what the future held. Most people have some attractive feature – for example long legs, beautiful hair or eyes, and so on. In my case, it had been my boobs. I had a small waist and shapely breasts. Before I was married, my surname was Lunn and this led to two of my teenage nicknames – busty Lunn or lusty bun! The thought of losing one of my breasts terrified me. Would it mean that people would treat me as an object of pity? Would my colleagues joke about me?

By the time I returned to London my local doctor had already managed to get me an appointment with the breast cancer clinic in a leading London teaching hospital, the Charing Cross Hospital. I shall never forget the scene that greeted me on my first visit. The waiting room was full to bursting with strained-looking women and their supporters; the atmosphere was thick with fear and anxiety; there was no conversation and, mostly, we avoided even making eye contact with each other. Even then, I noted that most of the women appeared well groomed but they were of different ages, different shapes and builds and with different breast sizes. There were two black women, one woman of Indian appearance, one woman of Middle Eastern appearance, but no Oriental women. Looking back I realise that I was already searching for clues about the cause of breast cancer by looking for common factors among the women affected. Of course, if it were that easy someone would have identified the factors long ago but it was impossible for me to suppress my instincts as a scientist. Seeing those scared faces – and knowing how scared I felt too – was the first time I fully understood what a common disease breast cancer is, and how dreadful and widespread is the damage it causes to women, their families and friends.

Over the months and years that followed my first visit to that clinic, I made it my business to learn as much as I could about this devastating disease. In times of great personal crisis, people usually fall back on the fundamental things they know best and trust most. For some, it may be their religious faith. For others, it could be close friends and loved ones. In my case, when disaster struck, I fell back on what I trusted most: my scientific training.

And that's what saved my life.

HOW SCIENCE SERVES US – AND WHY IT SOMETIMES DOESN'T

A good scientist will see things a little bit differently. As a science 'insider', I'd like to tell you something about the way that science works, which will help you to make sense of the differing approaches that scientists have adopted towards breast cancer.

When I lecture to my students, I like to ask them to visualise science as a mighty oak tree – a tree of knowledge, if you like. Start deep down under the earth, at the very tips of the ever-probing roots. This is where lots of discoveries are constantly being made and new facts found. Then some of these are brought together to form larger roots, and finally, the whole knowledge can be assembled to give a total or holistic trunk to the tree. This last function – the assembling of disparate bits of information to give a new insight or theory or sometimes a major breakthrough – has often been achieved by one individual with a grasp of many or all of the different aspects of a problem, who has the good fortune to be in the right place at the right time to make all the necessary connections. Finally, this newly acquired knowledge flows to the branches and leaves, as the information is communicated to the world at large – who may use it for good or ill.

This is, of course, a simplification of a complex and dynamic subject, but it is a useful way of understanding the way in which science has always functioned to deliver the fruits of its labours to society. In recent years, however, things have changed significantly, and not for the better. Today, the overwhelming trend is to devote maximum attention and resources (money, people, equipment and facilities) to scientists working at the root tips; often using very expensive, high-technology methods. Sometimes, this approach is called 'bottom-up' science (as opposed to 'top-down'). The great natural scientist James E. Lovelock lucidly explains the problem in his book *Gaia: the practical science of planetary medicine*: 'To understand the physiology of the earth requires a "top-down" view of the earth as a whole system. We need science, but it must grow from the top down as well as the bottom up!'

Science that exclusively and narrowly focuses on the extreme root tips at the expense of everything else can be bad science. My friend, Professor John Dewey FRS, of Oxford University, made this point recently in a thoughtful and thought-provoking article in the science journal *Geoscientist* (John is a modern scientific hero, being one of the pioneers of plate tectonic theory which explains how the Earth's surface has evolved over time). He wrote:

> In our ambitious scramble for funds and recognition, we have forgotten the traditional values of scholarship, the seamless integration of research and teaching to generate knowledge and science. Scholarship includes intense library research and reading literature more than five years old.[3]

There is a word to describe what has happened to many branches of science in recent decades, which is increasingly used pejoratively: reductionism.

The current emphasis on high-technology reductionist science means, to put it candidly, that we are spending more and more, to learn more and more about less and less. Let me try to illustrate the problem using an old Indian folk tale about six blind men and an elephant. A long time ago in the valley of the Brahmaputra Valley in India there lived six men who had been blind since birth but who were inclined to boast to each other of their learning. For some reason they became interested in elephants and they hired a guide called Dookiram to take them to visit one. As they neared the elephant the first man fell against its side. He examined all he could feel of the animal and declared the elephant to be like a great wall; the second reached out and felt one of its tusks and declared it to be exactly like a spear; while a third, grasping its trunk, declared it to be like a serpent and so on and so forth. Each blind sage thus developed his own opinion of what the elephant was really like, firmly based on his own experience, and they subsequently argued long and hard about the true nature of the elephant. The story concludes that 'each blind man was partly right though all of them were wrong'.

And that's the problem with too great a reliance on reductionism: a classic case of not being able to see the wood for the trees. As far as cancer research is concerned it means that we are studying ever smaller parts of the total process involved in the development of the disease, such as some aspect of cell biology or molecular chemistry – in some cases just one gene, or the protein it encodes for. But this increasing specialisation and compartmentalisation of cancer research, each subdivision with its own jargon (which other researchers may not understand), simply isn't producing the results that society is entitled to. In commercial terms, the return on our huge investment has been feeble: if cancer research had been a business, the shareholders would have sacked the management and changed the strategy long ago.

Reductionist science produces masses and masses of data. This is, in fact, a chronic problem with science today: too many people are providing too much information, yet too few people have time to read and digest it. I suspect that in some cases scientists are repeating the same work without knowing about it. Too many people talking – too few people reading, digesting, analysing and synthesising. What happens to all the data this work generates? Well, it gets published in learned journals, helping to create scientists' reputations, and wins more funding for yet more research. But how much of this work is directly beneficial to cancer patients? Disappointingly little, I suspect.

There's another problem caused by the emphasis on reductionist science, too. Its all-pervading influence has made any other type of scientific endeavour more difficult to pursue. In particular, I'm talking about the sort of science which takes place further up the tree trunk – the sort of science that involves analysing, synthesising or reviewing the work of others. This is now highly unfashionable. It is thought not to be creative and not to provide the original cutting-edge ideas that 'bottom-up' science produces. Hence there are few prizes or distinctions for scientists carrying out such tasks and it is difficult to find sources of funding for this type of work. Also, review papers are generally not welcomed by the most prestigious research journals and they count for little on the Curriculum Vitae of individual scientists.

The implied aim of reductionist science, in the case of cancer research, is to find the single 'magic bullet', that one missing piece of the jigsaw, the ultimate answer, the Holy Grail. Hence modern medical research in general, and especially in the case of cancer research, is aimed at trying to find a pure form of a chemical compound which has a clearly defined (stoichiometric) chemical formula which can be administered in quantitative doses and shown in statistically designed clinical studies to significantly and reproducibly affect the outcome of the disease.

But what if it doesn't exist?

What if our belief in 'magic bullets' is just that – magical, illusory, not based in reality? In that case, no amount of scientific research and no amount of expenditure will ever find it. We will have wasted many fortunes, many decades and many women's lives for virtually nothing.

In the meantime, we are left with surgery, radiotherapy and chemotherapy – albeit improved and refined – as the main front-line treatments against breast cancer, as they have been since the 1950s, together with hormone based methods such as the drug Tamoxifen. True, there have been small, incremental improvements, but little that is having much impact on the incidence of breast cancer or affecting the long-term survival of many sufferers (*see* Figure 1, page 82).

A reductionist approach towards breast cancer research also, sooner or later, runs into the law of diminishing returns, whereby we have to spend more and more economic resources in order to achieve less and less. That's why all the cancer charities you know seem to have an inexhaustible appetite for money and why many of them are the best-funded charities in existence. The only message we all seem to receive loud and clear is: 'Give us another billion or so, and give us another decade . . . and then, at last, we may finally have a cure that works.'

Maybe. But even if a cure were identified would we be able to afford to prescribe it to all breast cancer sufferers? The National Health Service in the UK is already in difficulty because of the cost of prescribing expensive new drugs which have cost a lot of money to develop. In a lead article in the *Independent on Sunday* newspaper on 14 November 1999, it was claimed that, at a recent conference, leading oncologists (cancer specialists) warned that they simply didn't have enough money in their budgets to enable them to prescribe the latest medicines and that they were forced to keep this vital fact from patients.[4] The same article also described how a patient managed to persuade a charity to pay for her treatment using a new drug called Docetaxel.

The high-technology approach to developing drugs for cancer is leading to many new drugs which are extremely expensive – which are then strongly marketed, often directly to patients via the World Wide Web – although they may prolong life for only a few weeks or months. Hence there are increasingly highly charged emotional debates between individual patients and their families who, understandably, wish to have the latest treatment, and health authorities and organisations that find it difficult to justify the large aggregated bills for groups of patients for marginal benefit. Is this approach really helpful to breast cancer sufferers except in the very short term?

The high-technology approach to finding a cure for cancer was discussed in an article by Andrew Tyler in the *New Statesman* of 12 June 1992. In the article, it was claimed that 'medical charities are overly dazzled by the search for miracle cures . . .' Tyler argues that 'It is more thrilling to invest in biomiracles than in commonplace strategies of healthy living and eating, even though an objective analysis of the record shows that industrial medicine's war against what have been called the "diseases of affluence" – cancer, heart disease, emphysema, diabetes, bronchitis – has been lost. Yet the public exalts the technodocs as never before.' Later in the article, he asserts that '. . . there has been no real progress in the past twenty years in extending the survival rates of patients with the most common solid malignant tumours – the ones that kill the majority of people – despite a massive and ceaseless flow of research funds.'

According to Tyler, 'The two major UK cancer research charities, the Imperial Cancer Research Fund and the Cancer Research Campaign, are clearly persuaded by the evidence linking high oestrogen levels with breast cancer. But the method they favour for reducing oestrogen is not dietary, but the administration of a powerful drug known as Tamoxifen. The plan is to give the product to 15,000 healthy women who are identified as high risk, to see if the incidence of breast cancer can be reduced. Giving drugs to people who show no sign of illness is a novel and lucrative way of doing business.'

I'm always suspicious when cancer charities hold out their hands, yet again, promising to supply us with a cure for cancer – if only we'll just give them one more handout. The truth is that science is curiosity-driven, not money-driven. You cannot 'buy' good science no matter how much money you spend; no more than a millionaire with advanced lung cancer can 'buy' back his good health. Science is not a commodity; it is a way of life, a way of thinking. Great scientists such as Newton and Darwin did not demand vast fees to be paid before they would do any work: they were able to take their time, largely free of financial constraints or political intervention (other than from the church) to discover scientific theories from first principles.

The modern era in cancer research really began in America when President Richard Nixon proclaimed 'war' on cancer in his State of the Union address in 1971. And right from the beginning, it was dominated by reductionist scientific thinking, with its requirement for large-scale funding, extracted with the beguiling promise of a cure 'just round the corner'. 'Many people anticipated swift victory' recounts the news magazine *US News & World Report*, 'with the taming of the dread disease likened to a moon landing. Even as recently as 1984, the National Cancer Institute's director predicted that cancer deaths could be halved by the year 2000 in America.'

Such optimism was, of course, unjustified. Despite massive expenditure – $2 billion in the USA in 1996 alone – by 1992 the cancer death rate had risen by more than 6 per cent.[5] Adopting the battlefield metaphor so beloved of cancer scientists some critics have called Nixon's war on cancer a 'medical Vietnam.'

Certainly, there have been some significant medical success stories: for example, childhood cancers, particularly some leukaemias, can now be treated and cured quite effectively: between 75 and 80 per cent of children diagnosed with acute lymphocytic leukaemia can now be cured. But these bright spots are too few and far between.

So what, you may be wondering, is the alternative to relying so heavily on reductionist science? And is it any more effective in delivering tangible benefits to ordinary people?

Let me give you a couple of examples to explain how truly significant medical breakthroughs have been made in the past with minimal resources but with great intellect and flair and a large measure of common sense. Most doctors would agree that the greatest contribution to all mankind in overcoming infectious diseases came not from the use of antibiotics but from improvements to public health: a clean water supply, improved sanitation, better nutrition and proper housing. These improvements came about as we gradually increased our understanding of why and how infectious diseases were transmitted. An early example of this type of work was carried out by Dr John Snow, who showed the value of studying the pattern of occurrence of disease. He made the famous dot map that showed the location of deaths from the epidemic of cholera which occurred in central London in September 1854. Deaths were marked by dots and, in addition, the area's eleven water pumps were located by crosses. Examining the scatter over the surface of the map, Snow observed that cholera occurred almost entirely among those who lived near (and drank from) the Broad Street water pump. He had the handle of the contaminated pump removed, ending the neighbourhood epidemic which had taken more than 500 lives. This 'scientific detective work' is called epidemiology – literally the study of epidemics – and it has been used successfully many times to identify the cause of disease and, through public health medicine, to correct the things society was doing wrong.

In the case of cancer, Professor Sir Richard Doll's epidemiological study of lung cancer in the 1950s was one of the most significant advances in understanding cancer this century. Sir Richard Doll demonstrated beyond any shadow of a doubt the relationship between lung cancer and smoking tobacco. Lung cancer was shown not to be a curse visited on us by a wrathful God, nor to occur because of bad or faulty genes, but rather to be caused by something human beings were doing to themselves. For the first time we had a modern rationale and scientific understanding of the cause of a common type of cancer. Following Doll's work, we can now choose whether to smoke or not in the knowledge that by doing so we shall significantly increase our risk of getting lung cancer. Moreover, identifying the cause of lung cancer has led to people quitting the habit and approximately halved the death rate from the disease.[6] Since that time, rational explanations have been found for many other types of cancers. For example, mesothelioma – a type of chest wall cancer – is now known to be caused by exposure to asbestos dust, skin cancer to be caused by exposure to ultraviolet light or arsenic poisoning, and cervical cancer is known to be caused by infection by the sexually transmitted human papilloma (wart) virus, to give but a few examples.

All this background information suddenly becomes much more than an academic discussion when you've just had a diagnosis of breast cancer.

The first thing I did after my initial diagnosis was to fill out a questionnaire, which established that I was at low risk of contracting breast cancer! According to The Breast Cancer Society of Canada and Statistics Canada some of the main risk factors are:

- Family history of breast cancer, especially in mothers, daughters and sisters as well as relatives such as aunts, cousins and grandmothers. There is a six-times-greater risk if a mother or sister had breast cancer prior to menopause and up to ten-times-greater risk if the cancer was in both breasts for a mother or sister.
- A *slightly* higher risk for women who have never carried a full-term pregnancy or whose first pregnancy was after age 30.
- A higher risk with the early onset of menstruation or late onset of menopause.
- Other suggested risk factors include the prolonged use of the contraceptive pill before the first child, a history of benign breast lumps, the use of HRT, a high consumption of alcohol, obesity, and increased age.

In fact, most of these risk factors translate into indicators of a western middle-class lifestyle and may not mean very much. Let me explain. Before Professor Doll's work which showed that lung cancer was associated with tobacco smoking, a similar set of risk factors to those quoted for breast cancer could have been developed for lung cancer. In the 1950s, before Professor Doll reported his findings, these would probably have included: being male (at the time few women smoked); being working class, consuming alcohol, increasing age, coming from a family where others had had lung cancer (smokers tend to have parents who smoke), and so on. None of the risk factors *caused* lung cancer – they were simply features of the population who smoked. I believe that the situation with breast cancer risk factors is the same: they are *descriptions* of the population that contracts breast cancer.

Many doctors tend to see non-communicable diseases, especially breast and prostate cancer, as simply an inevitable result of ageing. For example, a recent article in the British Medical Journal spoke of '. . . the growing burden of non-communicable disease – in both developed and developing countries – as a consequence of population ageing. Cardio-vascular disease, cancer, neuropsychiatric conditions, and injury are fast becoming the leading causes of disability and premature death in most regions.'[7] There is no mention in the article of the influence of 'western diet and lifestyle' or other possible underlying causes of non-communicable diseases. According to this line of reasoning, age is a primary cause of cancer. I, for one, don't believe it.

In the period that followed my initial diagnosis, a grim sort of race ensued. As I suffered five times from progressively more advanced breast cancer, which eventually spread to my lymph system, I was simultaneously searching for greater scientific understanding of my disease, what might have caused it, and what might effectively make it disappear.

At the start I was very, very frightened. I kept questioning the basis of the therapy I was prescribed, investigating the data on outcomes myself and, as far as I could, evaluating all possible alternative therapies and theories. None of this made life easy for the cancer specialists treating me, but it made all the difference in the world to me. I felt less of a victim and looking back I realise that this approach saved my life.

Sometimes I became very confused indeed. At the time there were seriously conflicting views among medical professionals on the value of mastectomy versus lumpectomy just as, recently, there is a major controversy about the value of expenditure on mammography compared to improving chemotherapy. Then there is the undeclared state of war that seems to exist between orthodox and complementary medicine about what to do for the best, so that you can quickly and easily become entirely bewildered.

What was I to do? The only course of action that made any sense to me and gave me any feeling of security was to fall back on my scientific training.

Customarily, scientists approach a new problem in five stages:

1. **Gather Existing Information** Previous facts and theories are reviewed as objectively and impartially, but as critically, as possible.

2. **Produce New Information** This is collected by experiment or observations, without emotional involvement. In some cases new ideas are produced by analysis and synthesis of information produced by other scientists. To be a good scientist you must be prepared to admit you are wrong: arriving at the truth is what is important, not personal prestige. If you raise a question, even if you arrive at the wrong answer, you will be respected if you work with honesty and openness. At the beginning of my science career, I learned a saying that has always stayed with me and guided my work: 'the person who asks the questions solves the problem'.

3. **Evaluate** The new results are evaluated in relation to existing theories and new insights or ideas are identified.

4. **A New Hypothesis Is Proposed** Speculation must be identified as such and clearly separated from facts.

5. **Test The Hypothesis** If the hypothesis works, submit it for further testing and validation until you have a new theory. If it doesn't work, begin again.

In a recently published paper, Dr D E Packham of the University of Bath listed the characteristic values to which scientists have traditionally aspired:[8]

- Honest experimentation
- Meticulous respect for evidence
- Candid admission of mistakes or error
- Pursuit of truth
- Moral and intellectual independence of all political authority and economic power

- Openness to the public scrutiny of research by one's peers. (You will see that throughout the book I use the term 'peer reviewed' to indicate science published after it has been critically reviewed by other scientists. This type of information is distinguished from newspaper reports and other sources of information.)

This logical and ethical framework has been successfully used by scientists (whether they realised it or not) for centuries. And it is precisely how I began to approach the challenge of my own breast cancer.

What I discovered in the months and years that followed the diagnosis of my breast cancer is the subject of the rest of this book. There is indeed a great accumulated wealth of research – some of which goes back many decades – on the factors involved in breast and prostate cancer. As you read the chapters that follow, I am sure you will be just as astonished as I was initially to learn precisely how much has been discovered already but has not filtered through to the public. While it is true that some of the risk factors for breast cancer – such as increasing age, early age of onset of menstruation, late age of onset of the menopause and family history of breast cancer – are completely outside our control, there are many other risk factors which we can control – easily. These 'controllable' risk factors readily translate into simple changes that we can all make in our day-to-day lives to help prevent or treat breast cancer.

My message is: even advanced breast cancer can be overcome.

I know, because I've done it.

HOW MY STORY CONTINUED

What follows is what happened to me after that first fateful diagnosis: what I did wrong, what I did right and what I'd do differently if I knew then what I know today. I shall also explain the reasoning and rationale for current cancer therapy, and describe exactly how I felt to be a cancer patient.

One of the first questions I asked, one that many women with experience of breast cancer will understand, is 'Why me? Why has this awful thing happened to me?' Eventually, I found the answer to this question and it was very disquieting, because it brought home to me the high risk I had been running, despite what I'd thought was a healthy lifestyle. However, as I was to learn, a Western woman's lifestyle increases her risk of developing breast cancer; the risk increasing more and more every year.

Throughout the West, breast cancer is the most commonly occurring cancer affecting women.[9] In the European Union, for example, three times more women will be affected by breast cancer than by the second-in-line killer, bowel cancer. Breast cancer is relatively rare in women under age 25, and more than four out of five women affected are older than 50. Breast cancer remains the leading cause of cancer death in women between the ages of 40 and 55 in many Western countries. A small number of men also develop breast cancer.

Looked at another way, in the West, the risk of any woman developing breast cancer during her lifetime varies from about 1 in 8 in parts of the USA, to about 1 in 20 in parts of southern Europe. For women in the UK, the risk is about 1 in 12. Disturbingly, the risk has increased quite considerably in recent decades. For example, breast cancer attacked 1 woman in 20 in the USA in 1960, but by 1991 the rate was 1 in 9 (and it is even higher there now).[10] Between 1979 and 1987 the rates in the UK increased at approximately 2 per cent per annum but between 1988 and 1992 the annual rate of increase rose to nearly 4.5 per cent.[11]

So I should not have been so surprised to be one of those affected. The odds were high. However, what struck me very forcibly when I first became aware of these figures was the contrast between the comparatively high risk Western women run of contracting breast cancer, compared with the much lower risk of women living in the East (see Chapter Three). This was the first suspicion that there might be a cause for breast cancer, just as there is a specific cause for the high risk of lung cancer that smokers run. In the following chapters, I will tell you what I think that is: but first, let us go along the orthodox path of treatment that most breast cancer sufferers will follow to a greater or lesser extent, depending on the type of cancer they are suffering from and the stage that it has reached.

HOLDING YOUR GROUND

The typical route through cancer treatment is surgery, radiotherapy and chemotherapy. My therapy was typical: rad-

ical mastectomy, 3 further operations, 35 radiotherapy treatments, 5 irradiations of my ovaries to induce the menopause and
eliminate my own oestrogen and 12 chemotherapy treatments.
This all sounds like a barrage of therapies; and indeed, some
alternative therapists use the analogy of breast cancer treatment
as a battle between the disease and the treatments – with the
patient as the battlefield. Although this analogy is not popular
with cancer charities or doctors, one of the things you must
realise from the outset is the heavy toll that surgery, anaesthesia,
radiotherapy and chemotherapy will take on your body. Many
people have to take breaks or give up treatments, especially
chemotherapy courses, because they become too ill – for
example, if their blood cell counts fall to too low a level.
Treatment can be particularly distressing for men with the
disease, especially if the only clinics and literature available are
aimed at women. To cope with treatment you need to ensure you
are equipped physically, emotionally and practically. Dietary
and other methods to keep my body as well nourished as possible
helped me cope physically. Using my scientific knowledge I
developed other coping strategies to ensure that radioactive
substances (used for diagnosis) or chemotherapeutic substances
(used for treatment) were removed from my body as soon as
possible after they had done their job. I outline these coping
strategies in a tips section at the end of this chapter. I have found
that other breast cancer sufferers find such tips very helpful.

A VICTIM NO MORE

Cancer patients often feel as if the disease is their 'fault' – either
a genetic defect, something to do with 'blocked emotions'
(research shows that there's no such thing as a 'cancer personality' – see Chapter Six) or the result of some other personal
failing. This isn't true. Additionally, conventional cancer therapy can 'process' patients to the extent that they no longer
understand what is really being done to them. A cancer patient
is a vulnerable person and the relentless procedures may
induce a feeling of loss of control. But it is vitally important to
retain control and develop a constructive working partnership
with your doctor. Let me show you how I stopped being a
victim, refused to hand over control to my doctors, and set out
to discover more about the 'big C' force that appeared to be
driving me relentlessly towards death.

In the case of breast cancer it is important to understand the different roles of research scientists including medical researchers and the role of clinical doctors. Doctors are professional human biologists who have taken an oath – the Hippocratic oath – which requires that they follow a strict code of ethical and professional behaviour. They tend to use only orthodox procedures that have been established by clinical trials usually based on pure chemical substances or standardised technical procedures validated by well-controlled, statistically based experiments using cell cultures or laboratory animals and, finally, patients. The growing threat of litigation against medical practitioners is making it more and more difficult for them to depart from orthodox medicine (although a recent series of articles about alternative medicine in the *British Medical Journal* shows the increasing acceptance of some of these methods by a profession that is necessarily conservative). Such ideas as using diet to treat illness go back to the Hippocratic School of Medicine that originated in Greece in about 400 BC. Hippocrates scorned the belief that disease is caused by magical or supernatural forces, and said that everything had a rational origin. He suggested that the causes of disease lay in air, water and food and noted the body's ability to heal itself given the right conditions related to these natural factors. Indeed there is an argument that modern Western medicine's departure from these traditional roots began with the use of surgery during the American Civil War. We all know the old maxim 'you are what you eat', to which perhaps should be added drink and breathe – in recognition of Hippocrates. Indeed, natural substances have been used in Chinese medicine for more than 3,000 years. As the World Health Organisation has pointed out, most of the people on Earth still rely on herbal treatments.

Like most groups of professionals, doctors range in their ability from excellent to poor. My experience with medical doctors encompasses both and is probably typical. I was fortunate, in some ways, because right from the beginning, I was not in awe of them as many patients are. Even before I embarked on a career in science, I had developed something of a questioning approach towards medical custom and convention, which probably stemmed from my father's treatment at the hands of psychiatrists. He was an extremely clever man – I still have many of his school prizes – but looking back, I realise that sadly he was a manic depressive and was on occasions pursued by what Sir Winston Churchill graphically described as 'the black dog'.[12] My father was treated privately and expensively in the 1950s and early 1960s by consultant psychiatrists whom my mother worked hard to pay. My recollection is of individuals using pseudo-science and an authoritarian manner to make money out of other people's distress. I remember to this day how my father was treated with the drug LSD and also with electro-convulsive therapy (ECT) – with machines that, at the time, were so poorly calibrated that no one knew the current or voltage that the patient's brain was subjected to. Tragically, his personality and intellect were permanently shattered so that he became almost childlike in his behaviour. Even now I can remember him begging not to be taken to the clinic for his treatments. Yet at the time, the far more gentle treatment for manic depression based on lithium was available. Had these doctors even heard of the value of lithium for manic depression before they stepped in with their 'heroic' solutions? I doubt it. I have since often discussed depression with medical doctors, but none has ever given me what I felt was a rational scientific explanation to justify ECT; indeed, one scientist specialising in brain chemistry likened its use to that of kicking a television to make it work. On the other hand, there is a rational explanation for how lithium helps the brain's 'water pump system' to help clear the brain of 'bad' chemicals, thereby helping to lift depression.

At the other end of the scale, the most brilliant, wise and sensible GP I have ever met was the doctor I've already mentioned (the one I telephoned in the middle of the night from Canada when I first felt a lump in my breast), John Camac. When my mother was first widowed and very lonely and upset, instead of dishing out anti-depressants, he bought her a beautiful little dog and he visited her every day until she felt able to cope. With his help and support she recovered very quickly. I wonder how many patients would actually be better off with poodles, rather than pills? It would certainly make for an unusual prescription!

According to the UK-based Patients' Association, British cancer patients are 'dying of politeness' because they do not press hard enough for the best treatment.[13] The Association has suggested that cancer survival in Britain is worse than many other Western countries because of the 'Yes, doctor' syndrome. Without being rude or aggressive, a woman with breast cancer can involve herself in informed and constructive discussion with her doctors provided she knows the treatment options. That is part of what I aim to do with this book.

Your relationship with your doctor, be it your GP or cancer specialist is crucial to how well you manage the disease. Although it is only natural to be anxious and afraid (and believe me, I was terrified), try to show your doctors that you will work with them to recover your health and that you wish to be fully involved in decisions. It is important that you establish a good relationship with your consultant. You will see later how my unjustified doubts and panic on one occasion probably cost me my breast.

How can you quickly tell whether your doctor is going to be a good bet? Here's a quick-and-easy ready reckoner I've produced for you to use: it makes no claim to be scientific,

A CHECK-UP FOR YOUR DOCTOR	
Possesses lots of common sense and explains things clearly and effectively	Treats you arrogantly or impatiently and falls back on confusing jargon if questioned
Follows his or her chosen vocation because s/he obviously cares about people	Authoritarian – gets a kick out of telling you what to do, gets angry when you ask questions or suggest what is wrong with you
Demonstrates s/he is up to date in their knowledge	Indicates s/he is ignorant of subjects that they should understand
Technically skilful e.g. knows how to carry out a thorough physical examination	Fails to give thorough examination or to come up with a meaningful diagnosis

Prepared to discuss your health with you on a partnership basis and to recommend dietary, lifestyle or other factors you can change yourself	Uninterested in underlying cause and displays a clear preference for empirical (suck it and see) methods to suppress symptoms; reaches for the prescription pad almost before you have started your second sentence

but it will help you focus your mind on the most important issues.

A frequent problem that patients encounter is the use by the medical profession of language which seems calculated to be obscure. In fact, more than two thousand years ago, the Greek physician Hippocrates warned doctors: 'Those things which are sacred are to be imparted only to sacred persons; and it is not lawful to impart them to the profane until they have been initiated in the mysteries of the science.' Today, too many doctors still seem to be following his advice. Before a medical student can become a doctor, s/he must be initiated into the secrets of a language which, it has been estimated, contains 10,000 new words – words which, to most of us, seem just as extinct as the Greek or Latin from which they originated.[14] Why, for example, should itching be called 'pruritis', a runny nose 'rhinorrhea', sneezing 'sternutation', or a headache 'cephalagia'? These are extreme examples, it is true, but they make a useful point: always insist on fully understanding what your doctor is saying to you, and if s/he starts to use new and alarming-sounding words, make sure you ask them to explain precisely what they are trying to tell you in simpler language. Once you understand the language your doctor is using, clarify any details by asking that they draw you a diagram, for instance. Then you will be in a much stronger position to evaluate, influence and, if necessary, query your diagnosis and treatment. Once my doctors realised I was a government scientist, they tolerated my questions and tried hard to answer and reassure me. But even then I felt I didn't know enough. It wasn't that they were holding anything back. It's just that their approach seemed so different from mine.

BREAST SELF-EXAMINATION AND AWARENESS

I was angry with myself for not having examined my breasts before. Why had I not followed advice and examined them regularly or had mammography? What should I have done and what can you do to help yourself?

There is controversy among health professionals about the value of breast screening and early detection, including self-examination. On the one hand there is the view that early detection significantly improves a woman's chances of survival. On the other hand, some senior doctors point out that by the time a tumour is detected, it may have been developing for several years and that it will already comprise many thousands of cells and the outcome will depend on the type and stage of cancer. According to the Breast Cancer Society of Canada (BCSC), the smallest lump usually felt by self-examination is about one centimetre across and contains about one billion cells.

In my own case, however, it was self-examination that saved my life. I had learned what cancer feels like and I know how to examine my breasts, lymph nodes and liver and I continue to do this regularly. Each time I had cancer, I was the one who found it, and I sought medical help immediately. Moreover, sometimes my cancer reappeared on a timescale of weeks, so waiting for mammograms or routine check-ups would not have helped me. Breast cancer in younger women generally tends to grow faster, which is one of the reasons why more frequent screening would be required to cut mortality rates in women less than 50 years of age, and that of course would increase the radiation dose the breasts receive.

The common-sense thing to do is to learn about your body and maintain a regular check on yourself so that you can identify problems as soon as possible and get early medical attention. According to the BCSC, patients with small tumours less than 2cm have 5-year survival rates of more than 90 per cent, compared with 60 per cent for patients with tumours over 5cm. Also, the sooner cancer is found the better are the chances for treatment using less drastic methods. If you need help in understanding how to examine your breasts, or other parts of your body, nurses attached to GP's surgeries are generally very knowledgeable and helpful. If their attitude is that you should leave examinations to medically trained professionals and your GP supports this view, then find another practice.

I have annual physical examinations of my breasts, armpits, lungs and liver at London's Charing Cross Hospital and these are available at most GP's surgeries that have Well-Women clinics. I recommend all women over 40 attend a Well-Women clinic at least once a year. Most breast cancers are found by women themselves (in Canada it has been estimated by the BCSC that nine out of ten breast cancers are found in this way), and teaching self-examination would be far more cost effective and would expose people to far less radiation than the repeated use of mammograms. In addition, by examining your breasts regularly you learn how they feel normally and you will be able to recognise significant changes and go to your doctor for advice. Initially this may involve doctors in more consultations but in the long term helping people to understand their bodies and take charge of their own health would save time. In the UK a helpful 'Breast Awareness Guide' has been produced by Boots the Chemists and the charity 'Breast Cancer Care'.[15] Breast awareness is described as follows. 'Every woman should remain aware of her breasts throughout her lifetime. Breast size and shape vary considerably from woman to woman, and so do nipple size and shape. Breast awareness means knowing what is normal for you at all times in your monthly cycle and therefore being able to detect any change which might be unusual for you. Detecting a change early means that any treatments necessary may have a better outcome.'

Breast self-examination should start as young as possible so that you learn how your body feels normally but it becomes more important after the age of 40. It should be done each month at the same time (a few days after your period has ended), continuing even after the menopause. The first thing to remember is that most lumps in the breast are *not* cancer.

Looking at this simplified drawing of a breast (above), you will see that each breast consists of fifteen to twenty lobes or segments, each with a duct that opens on to the nipple. Tumours usually develop in the milk sacs or the ducts and, more rarely, in the supporting structures. Most breast cancers are hard and painless although occasionally they are soft. In carrying out your self-examination try to keep a balanced approach. Prepare to notice changes that may require medical follow-up but remember that they are not necessarily a sign of

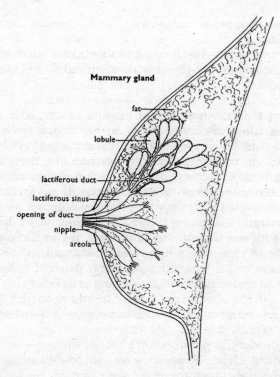

Mammary gland

fat

lobule

lactiferous duct

lactiferous sinus

opening of duct

nipple

areola

illness. Nine out of ten breast lumps turn out to be benign or harmless. Here are some useful tips on self-examination:

1. Look at your breasts in a mirror and note any changes in the differences between them. Do this first with your arms by your side, then with your arms raised and your hands cupped at the back of your head. Be alert to any changes in the size or shape of your breasts, any change in the colour of the skin, any drawing in of a nipple or pulling in of the skin that looks like a dimple and of course any lumps. Lean forward and look at the shape of your breasts from as many angles as possible.

2. Lie down on your back and closely and systematically examine your breast tissue and the tissues in your armpit using the pads of the fingers of your opposite hand. Roll and press the breast area gently but firmly against the chest wall and note any changes especially hard lumps you

have not felt before. Also check for lumps just above the collar bone.

3. Be aware of any bleeding or blood-stained fluid leaking from the nipple. Gently squeeze each nipple to check for discharge.

Remember that although any of these signs can indicate an early cancer, they are more likely to be caused by a non-cancerous disease. In any case, if you find any of the symptoms listed above, see your doctor as soon as possible. Even if you are reassured that nothing is wrong, monitor changes and return to the doctor and press for a referral if you think there is a problem. On two occasions I used quantitative measurements to monitor lumps so I knew what they were doing. I made four tiny marks with indelible black ink at the top and bottom and two sides of the lump and I used callipers to make measurements which I recorded on graph paper. I found this very useful on one occasion in convincing my doctor that I had a problem (more about this later). In order to do this, I borrowed the callipers from a colleague who is an expert on fossils.

I am always surprised now when I hear of women – including the late, brave Helen Rollason who recently died of colon cancer – who have tumours in the liver that are so advanced that the doctor can feel them by simple physical examination, although the women themselves have no idea that they are there. The front lobes of the liver are near the surface on the body just below the rib cage and can be examined easily for obvious lumps. We should all learn the basics of our anatomy and how our body feels normally and we should examine ourselves regularly to find out when things are wrong – especially when they are seriously wrong. (Indeed, I believe we should be taught self-examination as part of biology lessons at school – not only would it involve us in making a positive commitment to our own health at an early age, it would make the lessons much more useful and relevant.)

Unfortunately we have all been persuaded to rely on high-technology methods which consume lots of resources that some senior doctors believe could be better used elsewhere. In the UK, NHS breast screening costs more than £35 million a year. If we used breast self-examination more effectively with annual examinations carried out by nurses attached to GP practices the resources freed up could be used elsewhere for better cancer treatment. For example, it has been argued that the money could be better spent in identifying the susceptibility of cancer cell cultures from patients to different chemical therapeutic agents before they are administered to the patient. This would have the potential for improving the effectiveness of the treatment and reducing unnecessary distress to many breast cancer sufferers.

A TESTING TIME

Charing Cross Hospital has a specialist breast cancer unit with a team that includes radiotherapists and chemotherapists, and before any treatment could be recommended, I underwent a series of tests to establish what sort of breast cancer I had and the stage it had reached. Doctors who specialise in breast cancer treatment categorise solid tumours according to the stage they have progressed to. In general, small tumours that have not spread to the lymph nodes or other more distant sites of the body are called stage one tumours; stage two and stage three tumours are more advanced, being larger and involving more lymph nodes. Stage four tumours have progressed to the point of establishing readily detectable secondary cancers (or metastases) elsewhere in the body. The organs breast cancer most commonly spreads to are the lungs, liver, bones and, more rarely, the brain.

Apart from a thorough physical examination and simple tests which indicated that my blood pressure and urine were normal, I had a mammogram, a needle biopsy, a chest X-ray, a liver scan and a bone scan.

Mammography, which involves X-raying the breast, is by now fairly familiar to most women. In the UK, it is offered on a three-yearly basis as a screening programme to women aged 50–64. Studies are underway to determine the benefits of screening for women aged from 65 to 69 years.

There is much debate about the value of mammography for early detection. Doctors who are opposed to expenditure on it believe that the outcome depends on the nature of the tumour and how aggressive it is rather than the stage at which it is detected. Mammography works best by detecting small grains of minerals comprising calcium oxalate and/or calcium phosphate which form around cancer cells. The main problem with it is that it depends on using X-rays on soft tissues (not broken bones) and in pre-menopausal women breast density is high. Also, benign 'lumps' may come and go through the monthly cycle and the overall texture of the breast may change making results difficult to interpret. Mammography therefore throws up some false positives and a smaller number of false negatives. Moreover, some doctors have expressed concern about the safety of repeated irradiation of the breasts because the effects of irradiation are thought to be cumulative. There is no good evidence in women younger than 50 that mammography saves lives or alters the course of cancer. Mammography is considered most effective in detecting breast cancer in women between the ages of 50 and 69. In Canada, for example, which has one of the highest rates of breast cancer in the world, it has been estimated that mammography has reduced mortality in the screened population of this age group by 30 per cent.

The mammography I underwent was painless although occasionally uncomfortable. The chest X-ray was also a painless test to examine my lungs for secondary cancer and, while the liver scan is slightly more complicated, again, it was completely painless. Liver scans are based on ultrasound and are similar to the tests used on pregnant women to obtain information about their unborn babies.

The bone scan was more involved and in my case had some entertaining aspects to it. I was first injected with a radioactive substance called technetium in a phosphate compound designed to 'stick' to the bones. The radioactive rays given off by the technetium can be detected and a picture of the skeleton, including irregularities such as tumours, can be built up on a computer screen. I had failed to read the instructions carefully and between being injected and having the scan I had been to the hospital cafeteria for a cup of tea with the friend who was with me. I did not go to 'empty my bladder' as I should have done. During the course of the scan I was struggling to look at the images as they appeared. When the scanner moved to my pelvic area there appeared to be an enormous large luminous mass near to what I thought was the base of my spine. Immediately my mind created a fearful image of being in a wheelchair crippled by cancer, until the radiographer's voice said, 'You didn't go for a pee did you?' My bladder was by now full of urine in which the radioactive isotope was concentrated. I was despatched to the loo and by the time I returned the cancer in my spine had disappeared! After the test I drank several glasses of a well-known cola which contains phosphoric acid to try to encourage my body to exchange the radioactive phosphates for the non-radioactive phosphate compounds in the cola as soon as possible. (Otherwise as discussed later, I never drink such products).

Doctors classify breast cancer into more than a dozen main types including lobular carcinoma which originates in the milk-producing glands and ductal carcinoma which is one of the commonest types of breast cancer. The results of all the tests established that I had stage one non-invasive ductal carcinoma.

MASTECTOMY OR LUMPECTOMY?

I was finally seen by the surgeon to be given the results of all these tests. Kindly but clearly he described the stage my cancer had reached and reassured me that a lumpectomy followed by radiotherapy would probably clear up the whole problem. He explained that this treatment, which he favoured, could increase my chances of a recurrence of breast cancer but did not affect the overall death rate. Put another way, in early breast cancer long-term survival following lumpectomy and radiotherapy is the same as for mastectomy. Hence, I stood a chance of keeping my breast but would not be risking my life by doing so.

One of the mistakes I made at this time was to go to the clinic alone. I was so distracted by the bad news that I lost several personal possessions. And I was confused about what had been said. The best advice is to take a partner or friend equipped with a notepad and pen.

The surgeon and the other consultants I have seen at Charing Cross Hospital have always been compassionate but honest, and I prefer this to being given false reassurances.

The mainstays of breast cancer treatment continue to be surgery – lumpectomy (removal of the lump); mastectomy (removal of the breast); radiotherapy (the use of radioactive rays – usually high energy X-rays to destroy cancer cells); chemotherapy (the use of chemicals to disrupt the physiology of the cancer cells), or hormone treatments such as Tamoxifen which, in certain types of breast cancer (classed as oestrogen-dependent), is thought to work by preventing the hormone oestrogen from reaching the receptor cells in the cancer or breast tissue cells generally. The problem with some of these treatments (mainly radiotherapy and chemotherapy) is that they can give rise to side effects so harmful that they compromise the benefits of the treatment (in some extreme cases causing other different types of cancer such as leukaemia to arise). Also, they can, for reasons which are not understood, fail in a significant proportion of cases. Hence doctors can only quote survival statistics to their patients. They cannot offer any assurance of a cure to an individual.

The tests that were carried out on me were used to decide the best treatment, or combination of treatments, for the type and stage of cancer I had. Since that time, I have talked to many other women who have had breast cancer and I have realised how lucky I was to have been treated at a centre of research and teaching excellence such as Charing Cross Hospital. Many women, including some who have been treated privately and expensively, have been treated by doctors who were general surgeons using an approach which can only be described as in the best tradition of 'muddling through'. There has been no attempt to assess the nature and scale of the problem at the outset. It is very important that you are treated by a specialist team such as that at Charing Cross Hospital. Ensure your GP knows your views and refuse to be fobbed off with anything less than treatment at a specialist centre of excellence. Your life, quite literally, may depend on it. In the case of surgery, for example, ensure you are treated by a surgeon who carries out at least thirty such operations a year, and ask about his or her success rates compared to the national average. Also ask about survival rates generally at the centre at which you are being treated. (Asking for such information is particularly important for men having prostate operations because this operation is more complicated than carrying out a mastectomy.) Such statistics need to be treated with caution however because some doctors will treat patients whom others regard as incurable. I remember asking senior doctors at Charing Cross at what point did they give up – was it when patients had less than a 50:50 chance of survival? I found their reply very moving. They said that, providing the patient wanted to try to survive, they would never give up.

It was on a Sunday afternoon during the period of waiting for radiotherapy that I made another and perhaps most regrettable of all my mistakes. I was suffering badly from pre-menstrual tension and both of my breasts felt sore and lumpy. The more I poked and prodded them, the more I began to imagine I could find tumours everywhere. Finally in desperation I rang the hospital. I couldn't see my usual surgeon at such short notice, so I was seen by another doctor. At the time, I did not know that the lumpectomy and radiotherapy versus mastectomy controversy was raging within the medical profession. Nor did I realise that doctors in the same team could hold radically different views (although I knew that scientists often do). Anyway, the man who saw me, unlike my usual surgeon, was clearly a mastectomy man. He told me absolutely and un-equivocally that my cancer, being non-invasive ductal carci-noma, must be treated by mastectomy. Otherwise, he claimed, I would be dead within three months. He maintained this position under strong pressure and cross-questioning from my husband, who like me is also a scientist. The doctor had, he claimed, recently completed his studies for a PhD on breast cancer classification and his recommendations to have a mastectomy were based on his findings. (I have always been suspicious of scientists who spend their lives describing and classifying things. I prefer scientists concerned with understanding fundamental processes and I should have remembered this.) My husband found the doctor totally unconvincing and tried to persuade me to ignore him. I left the consultation stunned and frightened, and feeling that for my youngest children's sake (they were six and thirteen at the time) I had to choose mastectomy.

When I saw my regular surgeon on the next appointment, I was adamant that I must have a mastectomy, although I felt I could not tell him why I had changed my mind. I will never understand why I believed his associate rather than him. Fear and panic induce reactions that can change people's behaviour, so the usually rational behave like frightened children. The thing I should have done was to ask for more time to reflect. I do not know, and will always wonder whether, if I had followed the treatment that my own surgeon had recommended, my cancer problems would at that point have been at an end.

Mastectomy is the traditional treatment for breast cancer and the thought of losing a breast is one of the biggest fears associated with the disease. Incidents of breast cancer have been documented back to the early Egyptians when the principle treatment was cautery or burning of the diseased tissue. Mastectomy was developed during the Renaissance by Andreas Vesalius, a Flemish anatomist. During the 1800s, surgeons began to keep detailed records of breast cancer patients. Their data showed that even those treated by mastectomy had a high rate of recurrence within eight years, especially when the lymph nodes under the arm were affected. (The importance of observing these lymph nodes was first recognised by a French physician Dr LeDran at the end of the eighteenth century.)

In the nineteenth century surgeons were committed to radical surgery. The Halsted operation developed in the USA in 1890 was particularly mutilating and involved removal of the breast, armpit and major chest muscles. When the first practitioners realised this was not improving patients' chances they began to remove parts of the shoulder as well. It was not until 1927 that the British surgeon Geoffrey Keynes (brother of the famous economist John Maynard Keynes) first suggested that radical surgery was both cruel and a waste of time. He had deduced that breast cancer, by the time it was detected, had often shed minute cells into the blood supply which could have travelled into the rest of the body. Hence, if the cancer had not already become disseminated (metastasised) such mutilations were pointless – and if it had, they were equally pointless.

The debate was still raging in the 1980s when I was treated, although the mastectomy operation used at the time generally involved removal of fewer chest muscles and was less mutilating. One reason for the dominance of mastectomy over lumpectomy in the UK was the relatively poor image of radiotherapy compared to surgery, although in France it had long been one of the preferred methods of treatment (perhaps part of Marie Curie's legacy). International clinical trials had already shown that in early breast cancer, lumpectomy followed by radiotherapy has the same life-saving value as mastectomy. My surgeon clearly knew this, but his colleague at the time was giving out contrary advice based only, it seems to me now, on his own PhD!

Mastectomy still has an important role if the tumour is large in proportion to the breast, in situations where there is more than one primary tumour, or when the breast has many tiny tumours throughout. But none of these situations applied to me.

I think the lesson of this experience is for patients to understand that medical procedures can often be the subject of far more controversy within the medical profession than the public usually realises. Different specialists may well take opposing views. Quite recently, for example, it became fashionable to prescribe cyclotron (machines used for speeding up sub-atomic particles) treatment for certain cancers (to kill cancer cells by bombarding them with neutrons). Millions of pounds were raised by charities to buy cyclotrons, and even the then British Prime Minister supported the appeal. Then serious side effects started to be reported. Eventually, the Medical Research Council and a number of cancer specialists called for the treatment to be abandoned.[16] Before agreeing to an important procedure, it would be wise to ask these questions:

- What is the overall success rate for the procedure? (and how is 'success' defined?)
- What is the likely outcome in my own situation?
- What other therapies are available, and how do they compare?
- What is the individual success rate of the specialist/surgeon involved?
- How does this compare to other specialists in the same field?
- What are the side effects (both common and rare)?
- What is the quality of my life going to be after the procedure?

A good doctor will take the time to answer these questions for you.

I had the mastectomy approximately two weeks later. Physically the operation is not difficult. I talked to my surgeon and my anaesthetist well ahead of the operation (standard practice at Charing Cross Hospital) and felt confident in their care for me. Just one thing: at Charing Cross it was standard practice for the surgeon to mark the breast or lump to be removed with a black felt-tip pen while you were fully awake. Although this is disturbing, especially in the case of your breast, just think how much more distressing it would be to come round from anaesthesia and find the wrong bit had been removed. Marking up prior to operations is not standard practice in all hospitals so, if necessary, insist that this is carried out *before* you are given your 'pre-med' or tranquilliser. Before my operation I was given a pre-med to relieve anxiety and after counting to ten for the anaesthetist I awoke in the recovery room.

Back on the ward I found I had a long line of stitches holding together a scar where my left breast had been and a tube draining from the scar into a bottle which had to accompany me wherever I went; the bottle contained some clear liquid and a trace of blood. The drain is used to prevent massive bruising around the scar. There was relatively little physical discomfort except for my left arm and the back of my left hand where the drip had been during my operation. After about three days the bottle and drain were removed (this was painless) and after about ten days the stitches were also removed (again this was painless). My surgeon visited me daily and, after a few days, told me that the pathology report on the breast tissue that had been removed showed no further cancer and that all my lymph nodes were clear. Lymph nodes in the armpit are the body's first line of defence against cancer spreading. Their condition is regarded as the most reliable indicator of the extent to which cancer cells have spread from the primary tumour. This is useful in assessing the stage cancer has reached. More modern methods of assessing lymph node involvement reduces the possibility of a condition known as lymphoedema – painful swellings of the inside of the arm. The condition can be helped but once it develops it is often incurable.

I was told that on the basis of the pathology report, I should have no further problems and no further treatment was recommended. In the late 1980s when I was treated, preventative or adjuvant chemotherapy, to treat undetected cancer, was rarely used in the UK. This is used more widely now and is thought to be partly responsible for some recent reduction in death rates from breast cancer in the UK. Research at Oxford University in the 1980s showed that five-year survival rates for women over 50 treated with adjuvant chemotherapy and Tamoxifen increased by 25 per cent. Such treatments had been introduced about ten years earlier in the USA. Recently, more effective tests have become available to identify those patients who may have undetected cancer and are most likely to benefit from further chemotherapy treatment.

I attended one or two physiotherapy sessions to improve movement in my left arm but then decided to do the exercises myself at my own pace and to suit my own schedule. Others may need the discipline of formal physiotherapy sessions.

DEALING WITH PAIN

I refused, and continue to refuse as far as possible, to take medication prescribed by doctors (including Tamoxifen) or available over the counter from pharmacists. Steroids are sometimes given to suppress various types of discomfort associated with cancer or its treatment, but since they depress immune function, I have always refused them. I also try to minimise my use of antibiotics and I cannot remember when I last used painkillers. None of these types of drugs is known to cause cancer, but I just do not like taking man-made chemicals if I can avoid doing so.

I was lucky to have suffered very little pain after surgery. If I had I would have tried acupuncture rather than chemical painkillers, especially morphine. Acupuncture is said to have originated in China over 4,000 years ago, when it was realised that arrow-wounded soldiers often made surprising recoveries from long-standing illnesses. In 220 BC, a proclamation was made by the Emperor Houang-Ti (the 'Yellow Emperor') which read in part:

I am disturbed by the amounts in taxes and dues that do not reach me on account of illness amongst the people. My wish is that we should no longer use medicine which poisons them, or out-of-date methods. I want those mysterious metal needles which direct energy, to be used instead.

Acupuncture for pain relief is one of the most widely accepted of all complementary medical disciplines. Indeed, the British Medical Association published a report on 'Alternative Therapy' in 1986, in which it accepted that there is a scientific basis for claims that acupuncture is effective as an analgesic (pain-reliever).[17] Some veterinary surgeons routinely use it for chronic pain relief for animals.[18] Overall, evidence from randomised controlled trials supports the use of acupuncture in pain conditions including post-operative pain. Such trials also provide evidence of an effect on nausea, hence acupuncture is a potentially valuable method of contributing to relieving some of the effects of cancer and cancer treatments and it does not add to the chemical burden of the body or cause other side effects.[19]

Acupuncture works by stimulating special nerve fibres which inhibit the transmission of other pain impulses to the brain and by stimulating production of the brain's natural painkillers, endorphins – which are capable of closing off pain for long periods of time – and other neurotransmitters such as serotonin. However, some aspects of acupuncture cannot be explained by conventional medicine. For example, changes in the electrical conductivity of acupuncture points associated with a particular organ have been recorded in patients with corresponding conventional diseases. There are no known anatomical or physiological explanations for these observations. Traditional acupuncturists supplement a detailed case history with observations that are said to give information about the patient's state of health. These include examination of the shape, coating and colour of the tongue; the colour of the face; and the strength, rhythm and quality of the pulse. Both Western and traditional practitioners may palpate to identify points at which pressure causes tenderness or pain. Acupuncture needles are extremely fine and do not hurt in the same way as, say, an injection; patients may even be unaware that a needle has been inserted. Many patients say they find acupuncture relaxing and sedating, though the method does not work well on everybody. If you use acupuncture it is essential to use only a fully qualified member of the British Acupuncture Council (or equivalent).

Variations include acupressure, where pressure is applied using studs on elasticated bands to the points traditionally used for acupuncture, and electroacupuncture (EAP), which uses an electrical pulse instead of inserting a needle in the acupuncture point. Lasers are sometimes used now instead of needles. Transcutaneous nerve stimulation or TENS does not use acupuncture points but stimulates nerves which block pain messages and it can be used at home. Hypnosis is another option for pain relief which is also thought to work by increasing endorphin production in the brain.*

---

* For further information on controlling the pain of cancer, including advanced cancer, see the paper by Kathleen M. Foley, *Scientific American*, September 1996.

BREAST REPLACEMENT

Initially I was given a soft piece of nylon filled with plastic wool to serve as a false breast. After about six weeks when the scar had healed significantly, I attended as an outpatient and was fitted with a well-designed silicone-gel-filled false boob or prosthesis by a caring helpful woman who specialises in this work. (The earliest prostheses comprised a cotton bag of birdseed!) Many people are now offered plastic surgery immediately or a short time after mastectomy. I have been offered this several times by Charing Cross Hospital but somehow I have never found the time. If I do find the time, I shall ask for the operation that uses a muscle from the back rather than the use of silicone or other breast implants. My silicone gel false breast starts leaking after about two years and the idea that such sticky material could get into my body is unthinkable. In the meantime, I have come to terms with my false breast. I wear relatively normal bras from Marks & Spencer and the only special things I buy for my wardrobe are swimsuits which have an inbuilt pouch for my false boob. Wearing the false boob can be uncomfortable in hot, humid weather conditions – especially working in field conditions as a geologist – although having clean cotton-backed covers helps. But my main problem is losing it! I even left it at Charing Cross Hospital after one of my routine examinations and it had to be posted back to me. The nurses in the breast clinic still tease me about this!

People vary in their openness about breast cancer and mastectomy. I decided to be open but relatively factual and low key about my situation (most people do not want to be 'confronted' or overwhelmed by other people's problems). Other breast cancer patients find different ways of coping and many women do not wish others to know that they have had a mastectomy. They often do not even want people to know they have had breast cancer, in case people assume they have had a mastectomy. These are matters that only individuals and their partners and families can decide for themselves.

THE HALF-TIME SCORE

At this early, crucial stage of treatment, it is worth examining what I did right and what I did wrong, because it may help others in making decisions which are right for them.

What I did right:

- Found the strength deep inside – and admitted to myself that there was a problem.
- Sought medical advice as soon as possible and obtained information to calm my fears.
- Ensured my GP sent me to a specialist hospital, not to a general surgeon.
- Involved my friends and family who were prepared to help, but understood that some were too scared or anxious or frightened to help me at the time (*see* Chapter Six).
- Attended for all the tests and followed instructions.
- Listened to people with a positive supportive approach.
- Tried to remove old wives' tales from my mind and develop a more rational, less scary concept of breast cancer based on scientific understanding (*see* Chapter Two).

What I did wrong:

- Panicked and scared myself by thinking of all the awful things that could happen.
- Listened to people with scary stories.
- Went alone to be given the breast cancer diagnosis. (Take a partner or friend equipped with a notepad and pen.)
- Was too much influenced by a doctor who was not the consultant in charge of my case.
- If I could revisit this stage in my illness, the one question I would ask would be 'Is mastectomy likely to be better than lumpectomy and radiotherapy?' This time I would believe my surgeon, not his colleague.

AN UNWELCOME RETURN

While I was in hospital I repeatedly asked the doctors and nurses what *caused* breast cancer and was there any way in which I could cut my risk of it recurring? Since they kept talking about oestrogen (more about this later) I asked if I could be given a diet to help to avoid taking extra oestrogen in my food or to reduce my own oestrogen levels. They seemed to find difficulty with this type of questioning, although I was allowed to talk to a dietician.

The dietician seemed completely bemused by my questions and, although promising to look into the matter, never came back to me and never responded to my phone calls. Overall, the advice was that I should try to forget breast cancer, put the situation behind me and think positively. The medical professionals at the time appeared to hold the view that they were the experts 'in charge' of me and I should not keep worrying myself. I believe that they did this with the best of intentions and with the prevailing wisdom that simply by thinking positively it would help me. (I'm pleased to say that the whole approach seems to be changing for the better now, with increasing efforts made, at least at Charing Cross, to fully inform and involve the patient in their treatment.)

But I felt unable to accept the advice. All my training meant that I must have a rational understanding of problems in order to deal with them, and simply trying to put things out of my mind and 'think positively' was not something I could do. So I began to read both orthodox and complementary medical texts on the subject and soon discovered references to the work of Dr Max Gerson and Dr Alec Forbes (medical doctors) both of whom had produced anti-cancer diets.[20] Of all the methods available at the time for treating cancer, the idea of changing my diet appeared to make the most sense, so I altered my diet and lifestyle to fit with the recommendations of the Bristol diet book. The Bristol diet is a general anti-cancer diet written by Dr Forbes (please see Author's Note, page viii). It describes the elements of good nutrition and recommends eating lots of unprocessed, unrefined foods such as pulses, cereals, sprouting seeds, with food cooked in ghee (purified butter). Some yoghurt and boiled milk is allowed. I told everyone who would listen to me, including my doctors at Charing Cross Hospital, how good this approach was and, despite their scepticism, I believed that I would never have any further problems with breast cancer.

For the next five years, I attended regularly for check-ups. But despite maintaining an optimistic attitude, I began to feel uneasy – as if something nasty was bubbling away just under the surface.

I can't say precisely when it first happened, but I began to be increasingly aware of a large, hard lump developing in the scar tissue under my left arm. This was where the drain had been. But whenever I mentioned it to the doctors carrying out my check-ups, they reassured me that it was just extra thick scar tissue. I accepted this, partly because I thought that I was living such a healthy lifestyle and following the Bristol diet so religiously that the lump could not possibly be cancer.

But it was.

After my check-up in 1992, I decided to measure the lump and plot its size to decide whether or not I was imagining that it was growing. I used indelible black ink which I renewed as it wore off and the sort of callipers that palaeontologists use to measure fossils. Early in 1993 when I attended Charing Cross for my check-up I took my plot with me. The lump had grown: although by less than two millimetres in a year. I showed the plot to the young doctor carrying out my routine check-up. I told her my concerns and about the reassurances I had been given. She decided to carry out a needle biopsy. Within days I had been recalled for surgery to remove the lump and two weeks later to remove yet another lump which was also cancerous which again I found in the scar tissue. This was the third time I had detected cancer.

There followed a series of tests after surgery, similar to those I had when first diagnosed with cancer in 1987. There were no signs that the cancer had spread and I was recommended to have a course of radiotherapy. I agreed, believing that this would clear what I described to my doctors as my mushroom field for cancer – my left chest wall where my breast had been.

Many people are afraid of radioactivity, and rightly so. It is used a great deal in diagnostic medicine, including mammography, X-rays and bone scans and in radiotherapy. It is worth remembering that in the UK, according to the independent authoritative National Radiological Protection Board, about twelve per cent of the average dose of ionising radiation (a particularly damaging type of radiation) received by UK citizens is from such medical sources, while less than one per cent is from the nuclear industry. In fact, most (about 60 per cent) of the ionising radiation dose we receive is as gamma rays or alpha particles from radon gas emitted from rocks, soils and the buildings in which we live and work.

Radiotherapy owes its origins to the first separation of the naturally occurring radioactive isotope radium — 226 from a type of uranium ore known as pitchblende, by Marie Curie, who was a student of Henri Bequerel, the person who first discovered radioactivity. Sadly, Marie Curie died of cancer: probably as a result of her exposure to radioactivity during her long years of research at a time when the dangers of uncontrolled exposure to radioactivity were not appreciated and when safeguards and precautions had not even been thought of, let alone put in place.

Radiotherapy now relies on irradiating cancer with powerful X-rays (invisible but very powerful electromagnetic waves of energy) delivered using an externally applied beam, or in some cases by implanting radioactive sources which emit gamma rays (even higher energy rays). The exact method by which radiation destroys cancer cells is not known, but it is thought either to inflict genetic damage sufficient to kill cells directly, or to induce the cells to commit suicide by the process doctors call apoptosis. It relies on the fact that healthy tissues can repair the damage from radiation exposure more readily than cancer cells.

One of the main benefits of radiation therapy is that it can preserve the anatomical structure around the cancer so it is less mutilating and disfiguring than surgery. Radiation can also destroy microscopic extensions of cancers that surgery can miss and is a safer option for older, frailer patients. Nevertheless, it sometimes fails to eradicate all the cancer cells in tumours and, like surgery, it is primarily a local treatment. It does not help in cases of stage 3–4 (metastatic) cancer, except to relieve symptoms. Whole body radiation exposure sufficient to kill all dispersed cancer cells would destroy tissues vital to life.

In my own case I was treated by powerful X-rays created and delivered by a machine called a linear accelerator. When I was referred for radiotherapy at Charing Cross Hospital, I was seen by an excellent consultant radiotherapist who immediately won my confidence because of his meticulous attention to detail in taking my case history and his excellent knowledge of surface anatomy. (I am amazed by how often I have to tell doctors where my lymph nodes are!) He explained clearly and patiently what would happen to me and answered all my questions fully – another sign of a good doctor.

After that I was taken to the treatment room where the angles and intensities for the X-ray beam to be delivered were calculated. The room looked very high tech – like something out of a James Bond movie – but any fear was dispelled by the kind and professional attitude of the radiographers. Tiny black tattoos were made on my skin as reference points. I still have them, but they seem to be unnoticeable unless I specially point them out to people. It was also explained to me that lung tissue is badly affected by radiotherapy and that I would lose approximately fifteen per cent of my lung capacity as a result of the treatment. (I wonder if smokers realise how limited the options for treating lung cancer are?) About a week later I began treatment. Every day I would check in and sit for a short time chatting to other patients in the waiting room. I would then be asked to change and a clean white smock would be waiting for me in a cubicle. All clothing and metallic objects must be removed from the area to be irradiated. Finally, I would go into the treatment room. I had to lie flat while a bag of saline was placed where my left breast would have been (I realised that this was done to reproduce the conditions for irradiation following lumpectomy). The machine was then moved into the first position by the radiographer who left the room but kept talking to me kindly and reassuringly as the beam was delivered. Each time I was treated my left chest wall area was irradiated using three different positions which had been designed to remove cancer cells from my chest wall while minimising radiation damage to my lungs.

Initially, the treatment had little or no effect on me, but gradually my skin looked and felt as if I had been very badly sunburned. One is warned against sunbathing after having radiation. To this day, if any sunlight reaches my chest, the edges of the square where I was irradiated reappear. There are many different recommendations for treating the soreness caused by radiotherapy especially from alternative practitioners, but even herbal remedies contain preservatives which I thought could aggravate my symptoms. In my own case I decided not to use any creams or potions but to maintain a good diet (which was still the Bristol diet) and increase my consumption of foods that contain chemicals similar to those used in anti-radiation pills given to astronauts (more about this later). Also, although I used simple soap on the rest of my body, I washed the burned area in plain water using a low energy shower. The doctors at Charing Cross were pleased that my skin recovered so well and so quickly after irradiation.

Many people confuse radiotherapy and chemotherapy. They have different side effects. In my own case, apart from the burn in the immediate irradiated area, I had no other problems. I know of no one treated by radiotherapy for breast cancer who lost their hair or felt nauseated (although irradiation of the head or digestive tract for other types of cancer can cause such symptoms). Throughout the radiotherapy I was given blood tests to ensure that I could continue with the treatment. I noticed the regularity with which the equipment was serviced and checked. This is very important, because poorly maintained radiotherapy equipment can be extremely dangerous. I was given 35 radiotherapy treatments over a period of 7 weeks. At the end of the treatment I was given a thorough physical check-up, repeated six weeks later, which indicated that I was free of cancer. I held a celebration lunch with some of my friends and felt relaxed and happy. This time, we'd really got it beaten.

But then, about six weeks later, on a Friday morning in July, I was chatting to one of my senior colleagues at the British Geological Survey. Idly, I put my right hand on my neck just above my collarbone.

There it was again – a small hard lump in what I knew to be one of my lymph nodes. I knew immediately that the cancer was back.

I can't begin to tell you how I felt. Perhaps you've seen those horror movies in which some supernatural evil killer keeps on returning from the dead to slay his victims. That's an underestimate of what I experienced. Why wouldn't this monster leave me alone? Surely I'd fought it, and defeated it, enough times? But it had come back again – unmistakably cancer. The chill realisation hit me that it wasn't going to let me go until it had claimed my life.

I rushed to the telephone and called the consultant radiotherapist's secretary. He returned my call in less than half an hour and explained that even if he saw me immediately there was little he could do because he needed the equipment available at the breast clinic. I was given an appointment for the following Tuesday afternoon. I am sure he knew by examining my neck that it was cancer again but another needle biopsy was carried out. He reassured me that even if it *was* cancer there were still treatment options available. It certainly didn't feel that way to me.

The lump was subsequently removed at a day surgery at Charing Cross because, although the operation was to remove cancer, it involved only minor surgery. By now I was so emotionally drained that I felt numb about it.

Afterwards, I was recommended to take Tamoxifen, but I declined on the basis that I knew that it had been linked to increased risk of other types of cancer, such as endometrial (lining of the womb) cancer.[21] Also I knew several women on Tamoxifen who, although putting up with unpleasant side effects, had nevertheless died of their cancer. And at times like that, it is personal perceptions not statistical data that we all respond to. I was therefore advised to have my menopause induced by irradiation of my ovaries to remove oestrogen and other hormones from my body.

'Ovarian ablation' can be carried out surgically or by using radiotherapy which is more common now. Mine was to be carried out using radiotherapy. I was more terrified of this than the radiotherapy I had had for my chest wall. I was particularly worried about having such a rapid menopause and imagined that, within a short time, I would look much older, with thin skin and grey hair and that I would develop frail bones. Also, I knew that after menopause most Western women change shape – by a process commonly referred to as 'middle-aged spread'. This reflects the change in hormone status to one more like that of men, in whom any added weight goes to the waist rather than the boobs or bum so that post-menopausal women can lose their typical feminine shape. I did begin to experience some hot flushes but after I started my new diet these stopped. Apparently I do not look post-menopausal because women colleagues at conferences frequently ask me if I have tampons they can borrow, while nurses and doctors doing smear tests or other routine medicals always ask me about my periods. My hair, skin and nails have actually improved and my shape is the same as it has been for the past twenty years. I am absolutely convinced that the dietary changes I describe later are responsible for this rejuvenating effect (a clue: most Eastern women manage to stay looking younger for longer).

About two weeks after the lump's removal, I attended Charing Cross as an outpatient to have the stitches removed. I remember the surgeon confirming casually that the lump had been made up of breast cancer cells, but then he asked me to go over to the mirror in the consulting room. Had he not made a good job? he asked me. Certainly, there was hardly a scar to be seen. However, I was not in the mood to congratulate him on his technical skill; instead I was furious at his insensitivity.

Did he not realise how devastated I was to know that I had cancer again. Since then, however, I have indeed admired how well the surgeon operated and been grateful that he used cosmetic surgery methods to conceal what could otherwise have been an ugly scar on my neck. I realise in retrospect that he was trying to be kind. Again he gave me a thorough physical examination and declared he could find no trace of cancer.

So that was it, then. No more cancer. By now, every cancerous cell in my body must surely have been cut out or irradiated into nothingness and my oestrogen – supposedly one of the BIG RISK FACTORS – must have been reduced if not removed.

If only that had been true.

About two weeks after the stitches had been removed, and a few days after the treatment to induce my menopause had been completed, I became aware of a larger, itchy swelling in the scar. This lump had appeared *in just a few days*. There was pain around it but the lump itself did not hurt, although it was very obvious. Indeed, it looked like half of a small boiled egg sticking out of the base of my neck. At first, I thought it was an infection and was given another appointment with the consultant radiotherapist. When he examined my neck and told me, as kindly and gently as he could, that it was cancer again, I was overwhelmed with foreboding.

Surely there was no hope now. I just wanted to give up. And die immediately. What was the point of going on?

For some reason I thought of the film *Butch Cassidy and the Sundance Kid*. Towards the end of the film, the two outlaws are pursued relentlessly by a posse of men. Whatever they do to escape, their pursuers just ride on mercilessly in pursuit. That is how I felt: whatever I did to fight my cancer *there was no escape*.

But yet again, the consultant radiotherapist was wonderful. He picked up my mood and spent time persuading me to undergo chemotherapy, despite my protestations that there was no point. (In retrospect I feel guilty for taking up so much of his valuable time.) Finally, I agreed that it was worth a try, if only to give me more time with my family, and he arranged that the treatment would begin three days later.

I was very worried about the idea of chemotherapy. I had a mental image of bald, thin people suffering from the side effects of their chemotherapy treatment, which I knew included severe nausea and vomiting. It was the idea of losing all my hair that worried me most. I decided to deal with this by treating myself to a really good wig from a reputable company. One thing I did, which is a simple tip that many people facing chemotherapy find helpful, was to involve my normal hairdresser. He helped me to choose a wig of the right colour and texture and trimmed it so that it looked almost identical to my normal hairstyle. As it happened, apart from the visit to my hairdresser to have the wig trimmed, I have never worn it because I did not lose any of my hair.

Charing Cross Hospital is famous for the excellence of its chemotherapy department. Chemotherapy involves the administration of anti-cancer drugs that travel throughout the whole body via the blood circulation system. Hence it is a systemic anti-cancer treatment. Many chemical compounds are currently in use and new ones are constantly being screened and tested. Chemotherapeutic drugs act by preventing cells from multiplying by interfering with their ability to replicate their DNA. In at least some cases, anti-cancer drugs (as in the case of radiotherapy) are thought to induce suicide or apoptosis of cancer cells. Unfortunately, while the chemotherapeutic agents are in the body they attack all cells undergoing cell division (mitosis). This is why they particularly affect tissues which have a fast turnover of cells such as the lining of the digestive tract, hair follicles and bone marrow. This is the reason for the common side effects of chemotherapy, which include nausea and vomiting, loss of hair and anaemia. Damage to the fast-growing cells of the bone marrow can be particularly problematic because, as well as causing anaemia, it reduces the ability to fight infections and can increase the potential for internal bleeding because too few red and white blood cells and platelets (the cells responsible for clotting) are produced.

The first chemotherapeutic drugs were developed during the 1940s and were a spin-off of the work carried out by the Nazis to develop methods of chemical warfare. Initially, chemotherapeutic drugs often proved inadequate when administered individually or even in sequence. But during the 1960s doctors discovered that some cancers, such as leukaemia, could be cured when several drugs were used in combination. Unfortunately solid tumours such as breast cancer are only rarely curable with chemotherapy alone.[22]

Just as bacteria develop resistance to antibiotics, some tumours also quite quickly develop resistance to chemotherapy drugs. Indeed, some tumours can develop resistance to several drugs after only one drug has been administered. In my own case I was put on a course of treatment based on the drugs methotrexate, fluorouracil and cyclophosphamide. The first two work by 'pretending' to be other substances in the biochemical reactions of cells. For example, methotrexate is chemically similar to folic acid which is involved in replicating the strands of DNA that carry genetic information during cell division (mitosis). The substitution of methotrexate for folic acid incapacitates the ability of cells to replicate DNA. Cyclophosphamide (which is listed by the National Science Foundation of America as a carcinogen i.e. a cancer-producing substance) works by actually bonding chemically with particular DNA building blocks leading to breaks and inappropriate linkages between or within strands of DNA. As in the case of radiotherapy, chemotherapy depends on the ability of normal cells to recover while cancer cells are permanently destroyed because they have lost their DNA 'repair kits'.

My course of treatment was carried out each Thursday of two consecutive weeks and then I was given a break of about three weeks before being given the next treatment. This was to be repeated for six months making a total of twelve treatments. In general I was treated extremely well by Charing Cross Hospital and the staff did everything they could to minimise any discomfort or distress associated with the treatment. But it was still grim. In response to my request for an honest appraisal of my chances of survival so that I could plan for my children, try to prepare them for what was to happen and make arrangements for their future, I was told I probably had three months to live – six months if I was lucky!

Before beginning treatment I was taken through the procedures that would be followed on each day I attended. These began with being weighed and having urine tests and blood tests to ensure that my red and white cell count had not fallen so low that I could not tolerate further treatment. When the results were available I saw a doctor who then prescribed the chemotherapy drugs on the basis of the results of the tests obtained. I would then go to the hospital pharmacy myself in order to help the busy staff to get the drugs – something which, as you will see below, can be crucial. The drugs were administered in a large open ward full of others being given various chemo-therapeutic treatments for a range of different types of cancers. In my case the methotrexate was injected first and then the other bags of solution were attached to drips and administered through tubes into the veins in the backs of my hands.

There is no getting away from the unpleasantness of the treatment. I felt reasonably well until about four or five hours after leaving hospital when I would feel violently sick and would vomit even when there was nothing left to vomit. However, once my anti-sickness pills were changed to Andon-setron, which actually blocks the receptors in the brain which tell you to feel sick, I had much less of a problem and was able to return to work within a couple of days of each treatment.

There was one particularly unfortunate incident in which I was involved later, when I accompanied a friend for her chemotherapy at another hospital – it indicates how important it is to be fully involved if you are to stand the best chance of survival in a busy hospital, however good it is. The doctor took the results of the standard tests carried out before my friend's chemotherapy. He entered them into the computer to calculate her drug dosage based on her new weight (the dose is calculated on the basis of your height and weight). When we collected the drugs he had prescribed from the pharmacist, I read the labels (it was second nature for me to do this) and I became convinced that the solutions were about *double* the strength that they had been on previous occasions, whereas the concentration had been declining slightly as she had lost weight. When I gave the drugs to the sister in charge of chemotherapy treatment, I told her of my concern and urged her to check the drug doses carefully before giving them to my friend. After about an hour, I went with my friend to see what was happening and, after promising not to take legal action against the hospital, the nursing sister admitted that the doctor had indeed prescribed about double the strength of chemicals he should have done. Looking at the concentrations in the bags and thinking about the interview with the doctor, I actually worked out what had happened. The doctor had entered her new weight into the computer where her height should have been.

I did not and do not blame the young doctor concerned. Doctors at breast clinics in any hospital are working under incredible pressure. There should, however, have been a better quality control/quality assurance system in place. For example, the computer should have been programmed to flash a warning and refuse to carry out the calculation of dose (no one could have grown three and a half feet in three weeks!). I wrote to the hospital management describing what had happened to my friend. I also pointed out that my chemical laboratories at the British Geological Survey process tens of thousands of rock, soil and water samples every year, but we have a rigorous quality control/quality assurance system in place. What happened at one of the best hospitals in the National Health Service could not happen to a rock in the laboratory of the British Geological Survey! The NHS generally has extremely poor information technology with many doctors and nurses poorly trained (or not trained at all) in its use. Even now, less than two per cent of the budget of the NHS is spend on IT. In the organisation I work for, more than 25 per cent of our budget is spent on IT and the benefits in terms of efficiency, effectiveness, cost saving and the ability to collect data and compile information just keep on growing.

When I asked what would have happened to my friend if she had been given the wrong dosage of the anti-cancer drugs she was being treated with, I was told that it was likely that she would have died of liver or kidney failure. I have since heard of several people undergoing chemotherapy dying of liver or kidney failure, though not, I would stress, at Charing Cross hospital. I hope none of them have died because of inadequate quality systems or computer software in the hospitals where they were treated. By the time this happened to my friend, she was following my programme and her cancer had disappeared. It would have been ironic if she had been killed by the chemotherapy she no longer needed!

Despite the fact that my cancer disappeared early in my treatment (see Chapter Three), I was persuaded to complete the course, which I did. Apart from sickness, the only minor side effects I had were increased occurrences of cold sores (which I treated with raw garlic) and infections at the base of my nails (which responded to being bathed in warm salty water), reflecting damage to my immune system as a result of the treatment. I also had some abscesses in my teeth, which my dentist treated with special care (because I made sure he was fully aware of the type of treatment I was being given for my cancer). Also I had horrendous haemorrhoids or piles as a result of constipation caused by the anti-sickness pills I had been prescribed. I soon dealt with those by eating Linusit, which is organically-grown linseed (also called flax seed) and is widely available in health-food shops and has other benefits in combating cancer (*see* Chapter Five).

It was during this final, fifth round with cancer that things had really turned round for me. The cancer had gone, not to return. And, also important to me, I hadn't lost my hair. In fact, it became darker and thicker and I attribute this to the new diet and lifestyle I had adopted. Others on chemotherapy who have followed 'The Plant Programme' have not lost their hair either. My hairdresser's boss feared that my hair would end up on the floor of the salon, but my hairdresser, David, whom I have known a long time and trusted, believed me when I said I would accept the blame if this happened. He processed my hair as usual: it was permed straight and bleached; it even needed thinning to achieve the same smooth close-to-the-head hairstyle I like. In fact, David now actually hands out my diet to other clients who have cancer.

I am not sure exactly how my diet works to prevent hair loss, but I have some ideas. For example, the high content of folic acid it contains would exchange with the folic acid-like methotrexate molecule, speeding up its elimination from the body as soon as it had done its job.

My consultant radiologist (who it was agreed was also my oncologist – or cancer specialist – and remains on my case), while delighted that any sign of my cancer had disappeared by the end of my fifth treatment, was concerned that it would return once the chemotherapy treatment was over. It never has. Seven years later I remain cancer-free. Apparently the drugs I was given at the time were the cheapest standard preparations available and even reading medical textbooks now it is clear that it is highly unlikely that these would, on their own, have cured my cancer.

Two years after my recovery, I was offered a new, advanced form of chemotherapy by Charing Cross Hospital. The treatment I was offered this time is, I am told, extremely expensive but apparently the doctors were impressed by my positive approach and the fact that I had survived much longer than they had expected. They thought that they should help me as much as they could. I turned down their offer because I knew that the key to my cure lay elsewhere.

In the following chapters I will tell you why and how I recovered from cancer and, most importantly, how I remain cancer-free.

SUMMARY OF TIPS FOR COPING WITH ANTI-CANCER TREATMENT

General

1. Insist you are treated at a hospital with a specialist breast cancer team, which includes a breast surgeon – not just a general surgeon – a radiotherapist and a chemotherapist.
2. Try to take a partner or friend when you go for consultations with your doctors. Ensure they are equipped with a notebook and pen to take notes to minimise confusion and additional stress.
3. If you know you are panicking or feeling emotional, ask your doctors for more time before making irrevocable choices such as mastectomy versus lumpectomy and radiotherapy. Ensure you are as calm as possible when you make important decisions or choices.

Diagnosis

4. Listen and read instructions carefully and follow them closely to minimise the need for repeat tests and hence to minimise your exposure to radioactivity and other impacts of diagnostic medicine.
5. After having a bone scan, drink cola containing phosphoric acid to try to flush the radioactive agent used for testing from your body as soon as possible. (This agent is usually attached to a phosphate compound so it will attach to your bones during testing.)

Surgery

6. Before surgery, while you are awake and fully conscious, ensure the breast or lump to be removed is clearly marked with a felt-tip pen by the surgeon who will be operating on you.

Radiotherapy

7. Wash affected area with water only – using a low-power shower. Do not use soap. Use olive oil on the skin but no creams – even herbal ones – that could contain irritating preservatives.

8. Eat seaweed, an organic egg a day and lots of garlic to give your body cysteine-like chemicals used, for instance, by astronauts to repair DNA (*see* Chapter Five).

Chemotherapy

9. Buy a wig with guidance from your normal hairdresser and have him/her style it to your usual hairdo. Drink juices high in folic acid to minimise or prevent hair loss (*see* Chapter Five).

10. Drink only filtered water that has been boiled to kill organisms that can cause sickness and diarrhoea in immunosuppressed patients (*see* Chapter Five).

The update to this chapter can be found on page 246.

2 Cells Behaving Badly

In this chapter I explain what cancer is in a way I wish it had been told to me when I was first diagnosed with breast cancer. The material is drawn from recently published scientific papers but it is explained in unscary, everyday language.

When I first told my mother of my illness, she said: 'But we've never had anything like *that* in our family!'

At first, I was startled by her reaction. Then I remembered that older people – and younger ones too, sometimes – used to look upon cancer as something shameful: a family secret to be concealed at all costs, like sexually transmitted diseases or as mental illness once was. Instead of saying someone had died of cancer, obituaries often euphemistically said the person had died 'after a long illness'. Perhaps the reason for this was superstition and fear.

I think a lot of this phobia stemmed from a basic lack of understanding of what cancer is. Even today, most of us still don't seem to understand what cancer is. On one level, cancer is very easy to understand: it is a certain way in which some cells in the body begin to behave badly. What is 'bad' or odd or unusual about the behaviour of cancerous cells? Well, normally, parts of your body do not start to grow out of control, do not attack or consume other parts of your body and do not take off and start up a new colony elsewhere in your body. But cancer cells *do* act in these ways.

In order to understand why cancer is so hard to treat and cure, we need to look at it in a bit more detail and to acquire some basic information. If you're tempted to skip this short chapter, let me beg you not to – this isn't *Mastermind* and you're not going to be tested on it afterwards! Knowledge is power: if you understand the basic science of cancer, you're in a powerful position to protect yourself, to get involved in your treatment if you ever become a patient, and to play an important role in the increasingly public debate about the number one threat to women's health. As a scientist confronted with the disease, I had to find out as much as possible about what I was dealing with. I found that getting to grips with the most up-to-date facts enabled me to clear my mind of unhelpful old wives' tales and having a modern understanding of cancer and its treatment helped me to feel less frightened.

WHEN BAD THINGS HAPPEN TO GOOD CELLS

As you probably know, your body is made up of millions and millions of cells living in complex interrelationships with each other. Normally, your cells do not grow out of control, they do not invade each other's territory, and cells from, say, the lining of your intestines or the ducts of your breasts do not take off and start growing in other organs such as your lungs or liver. But, as explained above, it is the property of cancer cells to do precisely these three things that makes them so dangerous.

Even when cancer cells are removed from the human body and grown in a laboratory culture, they behave very differently from normal cells. For example, normal cells are fussy about the nutrients they consume, but cancer cells are not. Also, normal cells reproduce only until they just touch each other, and then they stop (a phenomenon known as contact inhibition). By contrast, cancer cells keep on propagating and will pile up in mounds because they produce a substance called telomerase which stops them from counting how many times they have reproduced themselves.

So *why* do cancer cells start behaving badly? Why do they grow out of control and eventually, if unchecked, start migrating across the body establishing secondary tumours in a process called metastasis? To understand why, you need first be aware of the simple fact that your body must make new cells when necessary – and in some tissues 'necessary' is, in fact, almost constantly. As your body 'wears out', new cells are created to replace older, dead or damaged ones. This process is called cell division or, more technically, mitosis.

When cells reach a certain critical size and metabolic state, they divide and create new daughter cells. The daughter cell inherits an *exact* replica of the heredity information (an exact replica of the types of genes in an exact sequence) of the parent cell. Not all cells divide at the same rate. For example, liver cells in the adult do not normally divide, but they can be stimulated to do so if part of the liver is removed surgically. On the other hand, the stem cells in human bone marrow are a good example of cells that divide rapidly and almost constantly. The average red blood cell lives only about 120 days. There are about 2.5 trillion of them in an adult body. To maintain this number, about 2.5 million new red blood cells must be produced every second. In total, about 2 trillion cell divisions occur in an adult human every 24 hours; that's about 25 million a second!

Normally, the cells in your body reproduce only when instructed or allowed to do so by the cells around them, according to a complex and highly evolved system, which maintains the size and shape of your body throughout your life. Hence your ears and eyes, feet and legs stay in proportion to the rest of your body.

Now you can begin to imagine what would happen if this process goes wrong. If something happens to increase the rate at which one group of cells reproduce, the result will be an ever-increasing number of cells that have no beneficial function to the body, yet are absorbing nutrition at an increasing rate. And that's what a tumour is. If the cells remain in their place of origin and do not directly invade surrounding tissues, the tumour is said to be benign. If the cells invade neighbouring tissue and cause distant secondary growths (metastases), the tumour is known as malignant. Because of this ability to invade other parts of the body, the Greek doctor Hippocrates called this abnormal cell process 'karkinos', literally meaning 'crab', from which the modern word 'cancer' is derived.

THE WRONG KNITTING PATTERN

How can this process go wrong? Well, it's all a matter of control. Cell division, mitosis, happens according to a well-established cycle. First, the cells increase in size and make new proteins before a resting phase; then they make two exact copies of the cell chromosomes. (Chromosomes are the strings of DNA that contain our gene sequence and they carry all the instructions about how to make us: blue eyes, freckles, and so on.) Next, the chromosomes line up and finally they divide into two. The whole process is designed to make new cells that are exact copies of the ones they are replacing. This sequence of events is controlled by the cell's genes.

Each cell in the human body contains tens of thousands of genes which provide detailed instructions that determine not only the colour of our eyes or hair, but also instructions about cell division, growth and death. Genes can be thought of as knitting patterns or computer programs which, in the case of cancer cells, have somehow had a few mistakes introduced. Just think how a sweater would turn out of it was made from a pattern with a mistake in it. It's the same idea.

Most cells, no matter what their shape or function, have an outer wall – the cell membrane – inside which is a thick fluid called cytoplasm. Then, with the exception of red blood cells, all cells have a 'control centre', called a cell nucleus. In the cell nucleus are the chromosomes, made of strands of a special substance called DNA that contains our genes. The genes specify how to make particular proteins that carry out their work. When a gene is activated it causes such proteins to be made. Mutations (mistakes in genes) can cause the wrong amounts or types of the protein to be produced thus sending the wrong message. Then, when the cell begins its cycle of mitosis, there are errors – just like the misshapen sweater made from the misprinted knitting pattern.

Many types of cells, including breast and prostate cells, have receptors. Receptors are special parts of the cell designed to allow particular hormones or growth factors, for instance, to 'dock' and deliver their messages. One end of each receptor protrudes into the fluid between the cells, the other end projects into the cell's cytoplasm and in this way creates a conduit along which the message starts to be transmitted. So, for example, when a growth factor 'docks' on to an appropriate receptor its message is passed directly into the cytoplasm. There it begins the relay of a message that is carried from one protein to the next until it reaches the cell nucleus. This relay occurs along what is sometimes called a pathway. Once in the cell nucleus, the message activates genes to initiate their instructions – in this case, for the cell to begin its growth cycle. But cells can receive other messages as well.

There are basically three types of genes in normal cells that can go wrong to produce cancer: those that say 'grow', called proto-oncogenes by doctors and researchers; those that say 'don't grow', called tumour suppressor genes; and those that say 'fix it', instructing the cell to either repair damage or, in extreme situations, self-destruct.[1]

Currently, most doctors think that the cells in a cancer are descended from a common ancestral cell that at some point in time – probably years before any tumour is detected – initiated a programme of inappropriate reproduction. Somehow one or more of the 'knitting patterns' for the 'grow', 'don't grow' and 'fix it' genes crucial to cell mitosis accumulated a series of mistakes resulting in the ancestral cancer cell. Normally, the body has a complex 'quality control' system to ensure that such errors are detected and eliminated – to the extent of causing damaged cells to self-destruct (the cell's ability to commit suicide, 'apoptosis'). But somehow, the ancestral cancer cell avoided the body's quality control safeguards and began to grow out of control. Normal DNA repair mechanisms didn't work and for some reason, the body's immune system didn't recognise the cancer cells as abnormal, and so failed to kill them off. Even the 'final solution' of apoptosis failed to work. You can see from this sequence of events that cancer is actually the result of a series of failures, starting from mistakes in the cell's genes – the knitting patterns.

These mistakes in the genes are called mutations, and most cancers possess mutations in one or more of the three main gene categories.

The first genes that can go wrong are the proto-oncogenes, the genes which in normal cells produce a series of proteins that relay 'grow' messages from receptors outside the cell into the cell nucleus, telling it to grow, develop and divide. When the genes that make these proteins are damaged, they can cause too much or the wrong types of protein to be produced, thereby instructing the cell to grow inappropriately.

The relay of information between a receptor and a cell nucleus is sometimes called a pathway. When growth factors – present in the fluid between cells – attach to cell receptors, a pathway is activated or 'fired'. That is, the relay of the 'grow' message is begun. In cancerous cells, the relaying proteins maintain their activity when they should have stopped, or 'switched off'. In the case of many types of breast cancers, the proto-oncogenes with the mistakes – those that keep telling the cell to 'fire' when it should have 'switched off' – are thought to be those that control how the receptors for growth factors behave.

Pharmaceutical companies are currently working on drugs intended to 'shut down' growth factor receptors that have gone wrong and produced breast cancer. Shut-down methods have been shown to work in cultures of cancer cells, but they have not yet been shown to work in the human body. For example, a research team led by Dr Michael Pollak at the Jewish General Hospital in Montreal, Canada, has shown that IGF-binding protein 3 can stop breast cancer cells in culture by regulating the activity of an insulin-like substance, insulin-like growth factor IGF-1, which has been implicated in breast cancer.[2] Research is in progress to formulate a substance that will increase the activity of IGF-binding protein 3 in breast cancer patients, either directly or by stimulating its production in the body. There is more about IGF-1, its role in breast and prostate cancer and its presence in our diet in Chapter Four.

The second class of genes which can go wrong to produce cancer are called tumour suppressor genes. In normal cells these genes encode for a sequence of proteins to restrict cell growth, including by cell to cell signalling via the fluid between cells – the intercellular fluid. So if a cell is growing out of control, these genes can make a set of proteins to send a different relay of signals to the nucleus. This time it is to say 'don't grow'. It is the inheritance of mutated forms of the BRCA-1 gene and the BRCA-2 gene (both of which are tumour suppressor genes) that is associated with inherited or familial breast cancer, thought to cause an estimated 5–10 per cent of all breast cancer cases. Within affected families, the gene can be passed directly from generation to generation, through either the male or the female line. However, not everyone who carries one of the known breast cancer genes goes on to develop cancer. Furthermore, just because a close relative has had breast cancer it does not mean that there is genetic breast cancer in your family.

Some researchers have suggested that faults in the BRCA-1 gene are involved in types of breast cancer other than familial. So presumably the genes can be damaged during an individual's lifetime. Unlike some other cancer genes, which produce proteins that are more unreachable because they are located deep within the cell near the cell nucleus, the proteins that the BRCA-1 genes encode for are secreted into the fluid between cells. In healthy cells, these proteins are thought to be the method by which the breast protects itself against unruly cell division and hence, cancer. Further, there is evidence that the same genes responsible for inherited breast cancer may be involved in inherited prostate cancer. According to a Reuters news agency report of 4 August 1999, work by a team led by Dr D Easton of the Cancer Research Campaign's Genetic Epidemiology Unit, Cambridge, UK, has shown that men who carry the mutated BRCA-2 gene are four to five times more likely to get prostate cancer.

It may be important for people to know if they have inherited the mutated forms of the tumour suppressor genes involved in predisposing them to breast (or prostate) cancer.

If you wish to find out whether or not you have inherited faulty genes, you will need to consult an appropriate medical specialist. However, I believe that since the inherited mutated genes implicated in breast cancer are tumour suppressor genes, they are simply failing to 'close the door after the horse has bolted'. I believe that changing certain aspects of your diet and lifestyle could help to reduce your individual risk by reducing your exposure to growth factors, as discussed under proto-oncogenes, above, and hormone and hormone-mimicking substances.

The third group of genes involved in cancer are those controlling the replication and repair of DNA – the 'fix it' genes. An example of this type of gene, which is defective in many human cancers, is the p53 gene. The protein that this encodes for has been called the 'guardian of the genome';[3] it instructs cells to repair damage and prevents replication of damaged DNA in normal cells. In extreme situations it promotes suicide, or apoptosis, of cells with abnormal DNA. However, when the p53 gene is damaged, it allows cells carrying damaged DNA to survive and even replicate so the abnormal cells can pass on and even accumulate their mistakes.

In several types of cancer the genes that have gone wrong encode for proteins deep within the cell. In the case of breast cancer, recent research is hopeful and suggests that the problems are related to proteins responsible for transmitting messages to stimulate or slow down growth, between the cells and intercellular fluid, rather than deep in the cell as in the case of some other cancers. This suggests that, in the case of breast cancer, changes in body chemistry such as those achieved through changes in diet or lifestyle, can help relatively easily and quickly. This is discussed further in Chapters Five and Six.

ALL IN THE GENES?

Because there is a clear, obvious and unambiguous genetic component in the causation of cancer, many scientists and lay people seem to take for granted that cancer is, by definition, a genetic disease. Let me explain the way this reasoning runs:

1. Cancer results from genetic errors
2. Cancer is therefore a genetic disease
3. There's nothing you can do about your genes, so there's nothing you can do about your risk of getting cancer
4. The cure for cancer will therefore be a genetic one: spend a few more billion on researching 'gene therapy' and we'll one day find the answer.

This is faulty logic and it is unscientific. Unfortunately, many people who ought to know better seem to believe this mistaken line of reasoning. I do not.

Even the term 'proto-oncogenes' which literally means 'first cancer genes' (it is quite a mouthful!) implies that we have genes in our body whose only purpose is to lurk in hiding just waiting for their opportunity to malfunction and cause cancer. In fact, these genes are *essential* for the growth cycle of normal cells. Only *mutated* or *damaged* forms of these genes lead to cancer. But you wouldn't think so from the name. I do not believe that most of those suffering from tobacco- or asbestos-induced lung cancer would be affected if they had not been exposed to cancer-causing agents. And neither do I believe that most of us have genes that will lead us to suffer breast cancer without us first exposing ourselves to something that causes it.

Genetic treatments for cancer are particularly hyped at the moment. These treatments attempt to deliver into the body new healthy genes or proteins in order to correct faulty genes. But there is concern that gene therapy may be causing deaths. According to Neil Boyce, writing in the *New Scientist* of 13 November 1999, 'Members of the advisory panel that oversees gene therapy in the USA fear that they have not been fully informed following revelations that deaths were not made public. Gene therapists in the USA are supposed to submit reports of deaths and side effects to the National Institute of Health's Office of Recombinant DNA Activities near Washington DC, so that they can be discussed by the Recombinant DNA

Advisory Committee (RAC). But some companies have demanded that these reports be kept confidential, while other researchers believed that they did not have to submit reports at all, unless they had evidence that gene therapy caused the death. The Food and Drug Administration will halt a study if it has evidence of harm to patients, and [in 1999] it said that no new patients should be enrolled into a liver cancer gene therapy study run by Schering-Plough of Madison, New Jersey.' According to the article, 'The company had reported information about side effects to the RAC, but asked for it not to be made public. However, it has now dropped this request.'

So why does all the research not lead to cures? Probably because all the 'new' methods face the same problems and must overcome many of the same obstacles faced by standard chemotherapy. Hence, for any method to be effective, it must find, penetrate and then change or destroy cancer cells without irreparably damaging normal, healthy cells.

One of the main results of all the recent scientific research activity has been to show that there are only minimal differences between cancer and normal cells.[4] Only a minute fraction of the tens of thousands of genes in individual cancer cells are damaged and altered. Hence it is extremely difficult to devise treatments against cancer that will not damage normal tissue as much as cancerous tissue.

Cancer treatments may work well in cultures of cancer cells or sometimes in laboratory animals. In the human body however, not only must the anti-cancer agent, whether chemical or biological, find the cancer, but it must also find a way to penetrate tumours sufficiently to be effective *without* causing such serious side effects that it cannot be used on human patients. For instance, solid tumours have many barriers to drug delivery; not much blood flows within them, and some agents do not easily diffuse out of the blood vessels into the cancer itself.[5] Also, there are the problems of toxicity, side effects and the emergence of drug resistance in the tumour cells and immune resistance to foreign proteins in the body generally. Moreover, cancer cells are genetically unstable and can mutate or change so rapidly that they can readily evade recognition by immunology-based treatments and/or rapidly become resistant to many different methods of treatment, including those based on chemicals or gene therapy. Finally, as discussed in Chapter

One, the cost of researching the 'new' methods of treatment is extremely high and any drugs developed are likely to be so expensive (according to an article in the *Canadian Press and Ottawa Citizen*, 28 July 1999, one new breast cancer drug costs $8,000 for one month's supply) that they are unlikely to be widely available to breast cancer patients – even if they could be made to work in human beings with active breast cancer.

Many new methods of cancer treatment are being developed. They include methods based on gene therapy to correct defective genes (though current procedures fail to deliver genes to a high-enough proportion of cells in cancers); molecular medicine aimed at correcting the proteins produced by faulty genes; methods to make cancer cells commit suicide (apoptosis); methods of blocking the formation of small blood vessels to choke off the blood supply that cancers need to grow (angiogenesis inhibitors); methods to prevent cancer cells migrating and reattaching to cells in different organs (metastasis). New immunological methods designed to stimulate the body's own immune system into recognising and destroying cancer cells are also under development. A new drug which has been strongly marketed recently is based on using monoclonal antibodies (these are antibodies produced by fusing antibody-producing cells with special cancer cells to make cells that are able to survive indefinitely) to bind to proteins, called antigens, which are present on all cells. The monoclonal antibodies are created to target a particular antigen or antigens carried on specific cancer cells. One such new drug increases the time to disease progression, for women with advanced breast cancer on chemotherapy, from 4.6 to 7.6 months. Hardly a triumph compared to my survival of seven years due to a simple, low-tech, low-cost approach based on science and common sense!

The update to this chapter can be found on page 279.

3 The Third Strawberry

In this chapter I explain how I used my science, my knowledge and my experience of working in China and Korea, and with scientific colleagues from these countries and Thailand and Japan – as well as a large dollop of good luck – to identify what I believe to be the main factor that promotes breast (and probably prostate) cancer.

Once the panic and fear had subsided after the breast cancer returned for the fifth time, I felt as certain as I ever had been that the only person who could save me was the scientist within.

It was all too clear from what my doctors said, and from reading medical, pharmacological and chemical textbooks that chemotherapy treatment alone was unlikely to cure me. For five years, I had done everything my doctors had advised and undergone all the treatments that they had prescribed. Also, I had followed to the letter the anti-cancer diet and lifestyle recommended in the famous Bristol diet. Nevertheless, I now had a hard, cancerous lump in my neck that looked like half a small boiled egg sticking out above my collar bone, and this had grown in only ten days. Clearly, my lymph system was badly affected by breast cancer cells. (Even when cancer cells spread and invade other organs, they retain the characteristics of the organ in which they first developed. So, for example, despite the fact that they may have spread to the lungs, brain, bones or liver, breast cancer cells and prostate cancer cells remain breast or prostate cancer cells. As you will see later, this knowledge was important in my eventual understanding of how to overcome my illness.)

Years before, I had worked with an American doctor who specialised in multiple sclerosis (MS). At that time, he had described the disease to me as a 'slot machine disease'. It was a strange expression, and the first time I heard it, I asked him what he meant.

'Think Las Vegas,' he replied. 'You're playing the slot machines. You get one strawberry – no big deal. You get two strawberries in a row – still nothing special. But if you get three strawberries, then you've hit the jackpot big-time.'

What he was saying is this: if a person had two out of the three factors that he thought were implicated in multiple sclerosis (or as he put it more graphically, two strawberries and a lemon) they would not develop any symptoms. But in the comparatively rare event of three strawberries coming up, then you would have problems – you would develop the disease. In the case of MS my colleague had suggested that the three factors were a genetic predisposition, an infection – and at the time slow viruses were the fashionable scientific interpretation – and an environmental or lifestyle factor. (My involvement in his work had been an attempt to identify potential environmental factors, particularly in the Orkney Islands and other parts of northern Scotland where the incidence of MS is unusually high.)

Cancer, like MS, can be seen as a multi-factorial, multi-stage disease. This thought gave me my first real glimmer of hope: although there was nothing I could do about whatever might originally have *initiated* my own cancer (probably many years previously), there might be a lot I could do to eliminate whatever might be *promoting* it right now.

Since breast cancer develops at different rates over different periods of time in different people, it seemed likely that something in the body maintains an environment that promotes the cancer cells, enabling them to multiply out of control and eventually allowing them to invade other organs in the body. Such a model could also explain why, in some individuals, cancer goes into remission for long periods of time, or even fails to recur. On that basis, I had to identify and eliminate that something, that one 'strawberry', in order to overcome my disease.

So here I was – a scientist about to embark upon the most vital piece of research I had ever faced in my entire life. Like a plot straight out of a nightmare, the deal was starkly, exquisitely terrible: if I got it right, I could have my life back; if not, then it would be the last piece of research I would ever do.

THE SCIENTIST WITHIN

Now, I want to tell you something about myself which greatly benefited me at the time. As an earth and environmental scientist I am trained to observe natural phenomena such as rocks, fossils, volcanoes and earthquakes and to piece together observations to develop theories to try to understand how the Earth and its systems have developed.

Natural scientists like me work in a rather different way to biological and medical scientists. If you think about it, we have to: the time scales of earth processes are so vast (up to thousands of millions of years) that it is impossible to carry out experiments in test tubes or under controlled laboratory conditions as biological scientists do.

Instead, natural scientists work by piecing together fragments of, often very sparse, information; producing, synthesising and refining their theories from observations, observations and yet more observations. If you remember the 'tree of knowledge' I described in Chapter One, natural scientists have traditionally worked further up the root system and trunk of the tree than many other disciplines.

This approach has been astonishingly successful. In less than a century and a half, such methods have allowed the amazing story of the Earth and the evolution of its life forms to be pieced together. We now know, for example, that the Earth was formed about 4,500 million years ago. It has been transformed by a complex interplay of physico-chemical and biological processes from a hot ball of dust spinning through space into a planet with a cool and varied surface environment where abundant water and an oxygenated atmosphere are capable of supporting complex and diverse life forms. We also know that the outer layer of the Earth is divided into huge plates. These move on million-year time scales in a complex interrelationship with convection currents deep in the Earth; with volcanoes and earthquakes concentrated along the plate margins. Life began more than 3,500 million years ago, since when various diverse life forms have evolved and become extinct, or survived, in response to changes in environmental conditions.

The findings of natural scientists have often been opposed by the scientific orthodoxy. For example, in the second half of the nineteenth century, the famous natural scientist Charles Darwin suggested, on the basis of careful and extensive observations of rocks and fossils in relation to the modern world, that the Earth and its life forms had required more than 3,000 million years to evolve. At the time Darwin's views were vehemently opposed by many other scientists. Lord Kelvin, in dismissing Darwin's findings, used physical calculations to show that the Earth was only 20 million years old. Kelvin was wrong by a factor of approximately one hundred and fifty in his calculation – an enormous error for a physicist to make! He made this mistake because he had failed to take account of the heat generated within the Earth by its own natural radioactivity. Darwin, the careful observer, was eventually proved right and the orthodox physical scientist was proved wrong.

Later, the earth scientist Alfred Wegener proposed the then heretical theory that the continents had once formed one large land mass that had split apart to form the present-day oceans and continents. Despite being founded upon careful observation, Wegener's theory was vehemently rubbished by orthodox scientists, who said there could be no mechanism for such a process. Again, as evidence mounted and Wegener's ideas became irrefutable, the theory of plate tectonics finally became widely accepted by the entire scientific community.

More recently, the suggestion of American scientist Walter Alvarez that there have been mass extinctions of life forms during the history of the Earth (such as the death of the dinosaurs because of the impact of a large meteorite) was ridiculed. Again, this suggestion is now widely accepted by the scientific establishment.

So, having no alternative but to die or find a way out myself, I decided to find a way out. I determined to take control of my situation using my training as a natural scientist. I would work in the way that had taken me to the top of my career.

I reminded myself that, despite the billions of dollars spent on cancer research worldwide, little had been achieved in combating the global upward trend in the cancer death rate. Despite the dedication of doctors working to treat patients with cancer, the tools that they had at their disposal were essentially the same as those of twenty years ago. If any other area of scientific research had produced so little benefit for such a high cost, it would have been closed down long ago. I would reject the orthodoxy that predicted – on the basis of a classification of the type of cancer I had and the stage that it had reached – that I would die in, at most, three to six months. I decided that, instead, I would look at breast cancer in a detached way as a natural scientist, and try to understand the disease as a type of natural phenomenon. I would try to look at it in a holistic way in the tradition of Darwin. This, therefore, was to be my initial approach: look at the facts, the figures, the statistics, the data and observe, observe, observe.

THE RIGHT HAYSTACK

When you're looking for a needle in a haystack, you must first find your haystack. Sometimes finding the right haystack can be as hard as finding the needle.

That's pretty much how I felt. I knew how I was going to tackle my crisis – by using the techniques of observation that I had been educated in – but where, precisely, should I start looking?

That was the problem. Current thinking at the time was that the factors involved in breast cancer were a genetic predisposition, total lifetime exposure to the female hormone oestrogen, total animal fat consumption, personality type and stress. I therefore had five major factors to investigate and, if possible, correctly evaluate. And, of course, not much time in which to do it. Quickly, I made preliminary assessments of each factor, as it seemed to apply to me. This is how my initial thinking proceeded:

Genetic Predisposition The first thing I did was to remind myself that neither my mother nor any of her sisters had had breast cancer (my mother is now 91 and her sister, 94); nor had my maternal grandmother or any of her sisters had cancer. They all lived to a ripe old age. Investigating women in my father's family, a similar story emerged. There was no evidence of any type of cancer in my family. There was therefore no evidence that I was genetically predisposed. Recently it has been shown that inherited mutations of two genes called BRCA-1 (also implicated in ovarian cancer) and BRCA-2 are significant genetic factors in the development of breast cancer.[1] However, only five to ten per cent of breast cancers develop because of inherited genetic defects.[2] Inheritance of one mutated copy of a 'Breast Cancer Gene' certainly does not guarantee that breast cancer will develop – although every breast cell contains the mutation. Within affected families, the genes can be passed down through the generations through the female or male line. But, as already mentioned, not everyone who carries the gene develops breast cancer. Moreover, the fact that the inherited mutated genes are tumour suppressor genes suggests that, if the factors that promote breast cancer could be removed, then breast cancer risk might be reduced even in those with damaged inherited genes (*see* also p. 61). I decided that, for me, this didn't present a promising line of investigation.

Oestrogen   The female hormone oestrogen has been implicated in breast cancer since the nineteenth century when a Scottish surgeon, George Beatson, observed that breast tumours regressed in women whose ovaries were removed. Factors thought to increase women's cumulative lifetime exposure to oestrogen include early menstruation, delaying childbearing until later life and late menopause. Some scientists have suggested that increased body weight and the use of birth control and hormone replacement therapy (HRT) pills contribute significantly to oestrogen exposure.

It seemed most unlikely to me that a woman's natural oestrogen could, on its own, be the main factor in her developing breast cancer. Otherwise why did all pregnant women not develop breast cancer, and why did women, even before HRT was discovered, develop breast cancer long after their menopause, when oestrogen levels were greatly reduced? Indeed, the older the woman (and hence the lower the oestrogen levels), the higher the risk. It seemed to me, as a natural scientist, more likely that oestrogen promotes breast cancer only when another more fundamental factor, or factors, has caused the body's chemistry to malfunction. I decided to look into this in greater detail and have discussed it further in the next chapter.

Fat   Many scientists continue to link increased risk of breast cancer to the Western diet and suggest that the factor is total fat consumption, especially the amount of animal fat in the diet, although investigations following up large numbers of women for a dozen years or more have failed to show any clear link.[3] It is now known that the types of fat in different diets vary greatly. For example, Eskimos, who consume large amounts of fat, mainly from whales, fish and other marine animals, are not subject to increased rates of breast cancer. In my own case, I'd eaten well within official guidelines for fat intake for years, consuming only lean, grilled meat or mince dishes and low-fat cheeses, skimmed milk and yoghurt. My fat intake, I felt sure, wasn't the factor I was looking for.

Personality Type and Stress American psychotherapist Lawrence LeShan has suggested that the type of person who internalises stress is more likely to suffer from cancer. Indeed, he has gone so far as to suggest that there might be a cancer 'personality type'. (In contrast, aggressive go-getting individuals – the stereotypical personality type-A people, are more likely to die of heart attacks or strokes.) On the question of stress, I, and many other women who have suffered from breast cancer, were under stress in our daily lives or had suffered tragic events. However, so have most people – and not everyone develops cancer. Recently, large well-controlled studies have suggested that there is little evidence to support the widespread belief that emotional factors, whether caused by incidents associated with grief or because of an anxious or depressive personality, cause cancer.[4] Nevertheless, at the time it seemed to me to be a good idea to develop coping strategies for stress, and this is discussed further in Chapter Six.

Having completed my assessments, I felt that none of the factors, with the exception of stress, seemed to fit my situation. For example my periods had started late, I had never taken contraceptive or hormone replacement pills, I had given birth to three children and breast-fed each of them although for different lengths of time. I had consumed very little animal fat and none of my female ancestors or female relatives had died before the age of 85 and then not of cancer (remember my mother's reaction: 'We've never had anything like *that* in our family!')

I felt that, somewhere, there had to be another factor. And I had to find it.

THE GAME'S AFOOT

'Come, Watson, come!' Sherlock Holmes used to cry when he was on the trail of a particularly exciting case. 'The game is afoot. Not a word! Into your clothes and come!'

There's a certain kick you get when you're doing scientific detective work, even when it's a rather grim race against time. Even though I was, at that time, undergoing chemotherapy and so from time to time feeling desperately sick, I still felt the thrill of the chase as I started to use my brain for my own survival. But I still wasn't sure where to start looking.

Scientists are supposed to be logical, dispassionate types who labour long and hard for their results, but you'd be surprised how many scientific breakthroughs would never have happened without a healthy dollop of good, old-fashioned luck. And that's what happened to me.

The first clue to understanding what was promoting my breast cancer came when my husband arrived back from working in China while I was being 'plugged in' for a chemo-therapy session. He had brought with him cards and letters as well as some amazing herbal suppositories sent by my friends and colleagues in China. The suppositories had been sent to me as a cure for breast cancer. To this day I do not know what they contained but they looked like firework rockets. I gave them to Charing Cross Hospital for their research, but I was never able to obtain the results. Despite the awfulness of the situation, we both had a good belly-laugh and I remember saying that if this was the treatment for breast cancer in China, then it was little wonder that Chinese women do not get the disease!

Those words echoed in my mind. *Why* didn't Chinese women get breast cancer? My mind flashed up the image of an atlas called *The Atlas of Cancer Mortality in the People's Republic of China*, which I had been given by Chinese colleagues when I had been working with them a few years earlier. I had been helping to develop a collaborative project between Britain and China, aimed at examining the links between soil chemistry and disease. Specifically, we were examining how low levels of the chemical element selenium might be related to the occurrence of a type of heart disorder called Keshan disease, and also a crippling condition characterised by enlargement and deformity as a result of the degeneration of cartilage called Kashin-Beck disease. Keshan disease is now accepted to be a selenium-responsive endemic condition that mainly affects children and women of child-bearing age and which, untreated, results in heart failure and death. Subsequent field trials of selenium supplementation involving thousands of children proved that selenium could effectively prevent Keshan disease.[5]

Initially, Western doctors and scientists had been highly sceptical of the findings of the Chinese scientists. It was not until organisations such as the famous Rowett Research Institute of Animal Health in Aberdeen, Scotland, replicated Keshan disease in laboratory animals by feeding them selenium-deficient diets, that the findings of the Chinese scientists were accepted. The scientific community, just like the wider community, can often be awfully chauvinistic when it comes to accepting the results of 'foreign' scientists. I call this the Raffy Syndrome: Refuse to Accept Foreign Facts Yet.

More recently, my own organisation, the British Geological Survey (BGS), has worked with Chinese colleagues to develop methods to identify and mitigate the problem of selenium deficiency caused by crops grown on certain soils and the incidence and death rates of Keshan in China are now greatly reduced. There is also a greater understanding of the risk factors for Kashin-Beck disease, which include selenium and iodine deficiency in crops. It is perhaps worth emphasising again that without an understanding of the fundamental *cause* of the problems – which lay in the environment – there would have been little or nothing that conventional Western medicine could have done.

THE NEWS FROM CHINA

The Atlas of Cancer Mortality in the People's Republic of China had always intrigued me. It shows the markedly different distributions of the various types of cancer over the country. The distribution of lung cancer, for example, shows the disease to be concentrated mainly in urban areas (consistent with research in the West, which indicates lung cancer rates in polluted cities exceed those in rural areas, especially among smokers); and locally in areas of tin or uranium mining where inhalation of radioactive aerosols is likely to be a factor. Overall, the mortality rate for stomach cancer in China is high; but the atlas shows that it occurs almost entirely in the cooler, wetter and mountainous areas of the north while levels are extremely low in the southern tropical areas of the country. This is consistent with the idea that this type of cancer is caused by microorganisms that grow in food stored for winter in poor and unhygienic conditions. In contrast, cancer of the nose and mouth is concentrated in south China in a well-defined region behind Hong Kong and Hainan island. The data in the atlas underlines the view that cancer is not one disease but many different diseases with different distributions and causes.

What struck me the first time I looked through the atlas was the amazingly low rate of breast cancer shown *throughout* China. The background rate on the map is 1 cancer death in 100,000 women, which is very much lower than rates in the

West which, as already mentioned, approaches 1 in 10 women in many Western countries. I knew, however, that data from different countries could not be compared this simply. They must first be converted to fit a model age distribution for the population using a method developed by Professor Sir Richard Doll of Oxford University (the man who first demonstrated the link between smoking and lung cancer). Otherwise, false assumptions might be made. For example, if a type of cancer affects mainly middle-aged and elderly people, as breast and prostate cancer does, and population A has many more young people than population B, then the overall cancer rate would appear to be much lower in population A than in population B – an erroneous impression. Therefore, statisticians have developed a simple method for adjusting data that takes these age differences into account. Data adjusted this way are termed 'age-standardised'.

Nevertheless, even using the age-standardised rates of incidence for breast and prostate cancer for China and Japan, compiled by the International Agency for Research on Cancer (part of the World Health Organisation) the breast cancer rates are *extremely* low compared to Western countries (see Table 1, p. 75).[6]

The age-standardised data shows that the lowest breast-cancer rates occur in rural China (Qidong county), where only 11 out of every 100,000 women contract it (prostate cancer is even lower – 0.5 men in every 100,000!). The rate doubles in Chinese cities (Shanghai and Tianjin) and at the time I thought this was probably because of the serious urban pollution problem the severity of which is rapidly overtaking anything the West can produce.

In highly urbanised Hong Kong, the rate trebles to 34 women in every 100,000. The Japanese cities of Hiroshima and Nagasaki have similar rates of breast cancer: and remember, both cities were attacked with nuclear weapons so, in addition to the usual pollution-related cancers, one would also expect to find some radiation-related cases of cancer.

The conclusion we can draw from this data strikes you with some force. If you, as a Western woman, were living a Japanese lifestyle in industrialised, irradiated Hiroshima, *you would slash your risk of contracting breast cancer by half*.

The conclusion is inescapable. Clearly, some lifestyle factor not related to pollution, urbanisation or the environment is

PLACE	Breast Cancer in Females	Prostate Cancer in Males
China, Qidong county (rural)	11.2	0.5
China, Shanghai (urban)	26.5	2.3
China, Tianjin (urban)	24.6	1.9
Hong Kong	34.0	7.9
Japan, Hiroshima	33.4	10.9
Japan, Miyagi	31.1	9.0
Japan, Nagasaki	27.1	9.1
Japan, Osaka	24.3	6.8
Japan, Saga	19.1	6.7
Japan, Yamagata	22.7	7.9
England and Wales	68.8	28.0
Scotland	72.7	31.2
USA (whites)	90.7	100.8
USA (blacks)	79.3	137.0

Table 1: Age-standardised rates (ASR) of incidence (per 100,000)[7]

seriously increasing the Western woman's chance of contracting breast cancer.

If we expand our view to include other countries, we can see a remarkable picture emerging. The graph on page 76 shows mortality (deaths) from breast cancer for ten countries. The second graph on that page shows the same comparison between countries for prostate cancer.

DECODING THE DATA

Let me just remind you that the statistics we are examining aren't simply the abstract results of some obscure laboratory experiment. They are real-world, real-life body counts. The knowledge that these studies give us has been obtained at an extraordinarily high price: the neat little graphs overleaf reflect the loss of hundreds of thousands of individual lives. The least we can do, as scientists, is to study these figures with all our attention and to learn everything we can.

Figure 1

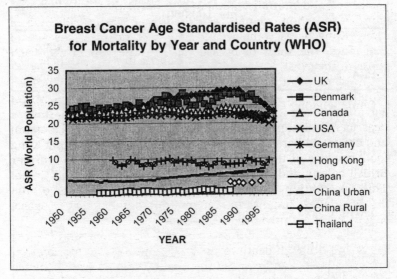

Breast Cancer Age Standardised Rates (ASR) for Mortality by Year and Country (WHO)

Figure 2

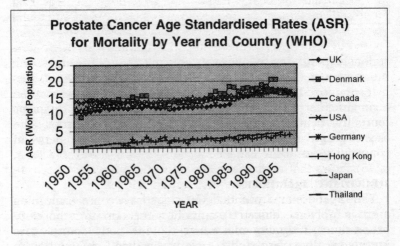

Prostate Cancer Age Standardised Rates (ASR) for Mortality by Year and Country (WHO)

Well, we know first of all that whatever causes the huge difference in breast and prostate cancer rates between oriental and Western countries, it isn't genetic. Migration studies show that when Chinese or Japanese people move to the West, within one or two generations their rates of breast and prostate cancer incidence and mortality approach those of their host community.[8] Also, when oriental people adopt a Western lifestyle in Hong Kong or as some wealthy Chinese do in Malaysia and Singapore, the rates of breast and prostate cancer approach those of the West.

The slang name for breast cancer in China translates as 'Rich Woman's Disease'. This is because, in China, only the better-off can afford to eat what is termed 'Hong Kong food'. The Chinese describe all Western food, including everything from ice cream and chocolate bars to spaghetti and feta cheese, as 'Hong Kong food' because of the availability of Western food in the former British colony and its scarcity, in the past, in mainland China. This observation suggests that genetic determinants of the disease are less important than environmental factors – suggesting in turn that prevention is possible.

The fact that rates of breast and prostate cancers are so low in Japan (although death rates have risen over the last decade) is particularly significant. Many parts of Japan are as industrialised as Britain and other Western countries. Indeed, serious illness caused by heavy metal industrial pollution was first identified in Japan in the 1950s. For example, Minamata disease, a serious neurological disease, had been shown to be caused by eating fish and shellfish contaminated by the industrial release of methyl mercury while Itai-itai or Ouch-Ouch disease, a painful bone condition, had been shown to be caused by eating food contaminated with cadmium. In 1945, Japan had been the first country to be attacked with nuclear weapons. Since that time, scientists have studied the cancer rates in Nagasaki and Hiroshima in detail to identify the types of cancers linked to the use of nuclear weapons, but Table 1 (on p. 75) shows that rates of neither breast nor prostate cancer are significantly higher than in other urban centres.

The Japanese environment is in many ways comparable to an average Western, industrialised nation. Yet, the differences in breast cancer mortality rates between the UK and Japan (Figure 1, opposite) based on reliable statistical data from the World Health Organisation suggest that, despite similar industrial cultures, there is a factor causing a fundamentally different level of risk of breast cancer between the two countries. This observation is also consistent with strikingly similar data from Thailand, China and other oriental countries. It therefore seemed a fair bet that the environmental lifestyle factor – the 'third strawberry' – that I was looking for was probably related to a long-standing cultural difference between oriental and Western countries.

I remember saying to my husband: 'Come on Peter, you have just come back from China. What is it about the Chinese way of life that is so different. Why don't they get breast cancer?'

Over the next couple of weeks Peter and I examined the results of the China–Cornell–Oxford project on nutrition, environment and health based on national surveys carried out between 1983–1984 in the People's Republic of China.[9] The study was led by T Colin Campbell at Cornell University in the USA, Chen Junshi at the Chinese Academy of Preventive Medicine (CAPM), Beijing, Li Junyao at the Chinese Academy of Medical Sciences (CAMS) in Beijing, and Richard Peto at Oxford University in the UK. Eventually the project involved about twenty collaborators around the world analysing blood and urine samples. The work was carried out in China because it represented a vast laboratory for health investigations with its huge population living in a wide variety of environments with varied mortality rates from various diseases, different dietary practice patterns and socio-economic conditions.

The China–Cornell–Oxford study established that the Chinese had a higher calorie intake than Americans, but there was much *less* obesity in China: attributed in part to higher levels of physical activity amongst the Chinese, and in part to what foods they ate. At the time of the survey, only 14 per cent of calories in the average Chinese diet was from fat, compared to almost 36 per cent in the West.

So the Chinese ate a low-fat diet: but so did I. The diet I had been living on for years before I contracted breast cancer was very low in fat and high in fibre. In any case, evidence for a simple link between dietary fat intake and breast cancer is at best ambiguous.[10] High total (typically animal) fat intake in adults has not been shown to increase risk for breast cancer in most investigations that have followed large groups of women for up to a dozen years.[11]

Peter and I persevered and discussed the suggestions made by some scientists that it was the high levels of soya consumption in oriental countries such as Japan and China that gave the female population protection against breast cancer. The soya bean is one of the most nutritious legumes known. It has provided the main source of protein in oriental countries for over four thousand years. It is used to make soya milk, soya sauce (made by fermenting soya beans), tofu or beancurd (made by coagulating soya with a setting agent such as calcium or magnesium salts) and other products, as well as being eaten raw as beanshoots.

There is good evidence that the soya bean contains substances which are cancer-protective. In particular, it is the high content of chemicals called phyto-oestrogens (chemicals derived from plants, which are closely similar to the female hormone oestrogen) in soya that is thought to be protective against cancer. These substances are thought to block the effect of oestrogen on receptors in breast or breast cancer cells – an effect implicated in the growth of certain types of breast cancers – in a manner similar to that of the anti-oestrogen drug Tamoxifen. Most legumes (plants such as peas and beans which fix nitrogen from the atmosphere to make proteins) also contain powerful anti-oxidants which may also explain their protective effect against cancer. One of the soya isoflavones – genistein – seems to prevent cancer through several means, including preventing the growth of new blood supply systems (angiogenesis) that cancer needs in order to grow, and by inhibiting several key enzymes thought to be involved in carcinogenesis. Soya added to the diet of rodents has been shown to decrease the incidence of mammary tumours. Chick peas – the basis of houmous eaten throughout the Middle East – as well as lentils and red clover contain a complete range of the isoflavones while beans, which are the staple foods in some Central and South American countries such as Mexico, also contain isoflavones. Although these populations have breast cancer rates lower than those of the industrialised West, they do not have the exceptionally low rates of China or Japan.

Soya, provided it is organically grown and not genetically modified, is an excellent source of protein that I include in my diet, and it has many other benefits, especially for menopausal women. However, at that time I had been consuming so much soya in various forms, including as traditional Chinese bean curd or tofu as it is called by the Japanese, that I did not believe that this could be the factor that I was looking for.

A BELL RINGS
Then one day a couple of weeks later something rather special happened.

Peter and I have worked together so closely over the years that I am not sure which one of us first said:

'The Chinese don't eat dairy produce!'

It is hard to explain to a non-scientist the sudden emotional and mental 'buzz' you get when you know you have had an important insight. It's as if you have had a lot of pieces of a jigsaw in your mind and suddenly, in a few seconds, they all fall into place and the whole picture is clear. Whenever that has happened to me in the past, I have always been proved right – even if, initially, my suggestions were regarded as controversial and unlikely.

This is precisely the feeling I experienced. I felt the same 'buzz' or to use the German-derived word which sums up the feeling so well: *gestalt*. Suddenly, I recalled how many Chinese people were lactose-intolerant, how the Chinese people I had worked with had always said that milk was only for babies, and how one of my close friends, who is of Chinese origin, always politely turned down the cheese course at dinner parties. I know of no Chinese people who live a traditional Chinese life who ever used cow or other dairy food to feed their babies. The tradition was to use a wet nurse but never, ever dairy products.

Culturally, the Chinese find our Western preoccupation with milk and milk products very strange. I remember entertaining a large delegation of Chinese scientists shortly after the ending of the Cultural Revolution in the 1980s. On advice from the Foreign Office, we had asked the caterer to provide a pudding that contained a lot of ice cream. After enquiring what the pudding consisted of, all of the Chinese including their interpreter, politely but firmly refused to eat it and they could not be persuaded to change their minds. At the time we were all delighted and ate extra large portions!

More recently, I attended an international conference in Beijing and was having lunch with two senior Chinese women scientists. A man smelling strongly of spices and garlic walked past, and I suppose my reaction showed. One of my companions giggled, and shyly asked me 'What do Chinese people smell of to you?'

I thought about it carefully and replied honestly, 'Nothing in particular.' Then, deciding that I could legitimately ask the question in reverse, I said:

'And what do we Westerners smell of to you?'

There was considerable laughter – usually reflecting embarrassment in Chinese people – but after encouragement on my part, they finally said:

'Westerners smell to us of sour milk!'

Recently I checked several Oriental (Chinese, Japanese, Korean and Thai) cookbooks. None mentioned dairy produce.

THE FINGER POINTS

In my years of exploring alternative health systems – since I first had breast cancer – I have learned that many naturopaths believe that the part of the body that is diseased provides a clue as to the cause of the illness. This seems to be particularly the case for cancers for which we know the cause. For example, lung cancers reflect inhalation of cancer-causing cigarette smoke, radioactive aerosols such as the naturally occurring radioactive gas radon, or asbestos dust. Skin cancers frequently reflect excessive exposure to sunlight whilst cervical cancer is associated with infection by sexually transmitted human wart (or papilloma) viruses. It seemed highly likely that consuming a powerful biochemical solution from the mammary gland of one species of animal (milk) could be sending the wrong signals to my own mammary glands – my breasts.

And I'd certainly been a big milk drinker. Before I had breast cancer the first time, I had consumed a lot of dairy produce as skimmed milk and particularly as low-fat cheeses and yoghurt, which I had used as my main source of protein. I also ate cheap but lean minced beef (which I have since realised was probably often ground up dairy cow) as hamburgers with my children, especially when we went out for treats, or made it into spaghetti bolognese or other low-cost meat dishes.

At the time of my last recurrence of cancer in the lymph nodes in my neck, I had been eating yoghurt and some skimmed organic milk which I boiled before drinking, as allowed in the Gerson and Bristol diets. The Bristol diet recommended Indian-style ghee (clarified butter) for cooking and one of the salad dressings for which a recipe is given is based entirely on yoghurt. A detailed case history describing a breast cancer cure in the Bristol diet book also refers to the extensive use of yoghurt. I had been careful to choose only those brands of yoghurt labelled as 'live' and 'organic' or I had often made my own yoghurt using milk labelled as 'organic'. In order to cope with the chemotherapy, I had initially been eating organic yoghurts as a way of helping my digestive tract to recover and repopulate my gut with 'good' bacteria.

However, following Peter's and my insight into the Chinese diet, I decided to give up all dairy produce immediately. Cheese, butter, milk and yoghurt and anything else that contained dairy produce – it all went down the sink or into the rubbish bin. It is surprising how many products, including commercial soups, biscuits and cakes, contain some form of dairy produce. Even many proprietary brands of margarine marketed as soya, sunflower or olive oil spreads can contain dairy produce. I therefore became an avid reader of the small print on food labels. Many prescription drugs are in a lactose base.

Recently, I discovered that way back in 1989 yoghurt had been implicated in ovarian cancer.[12] Dr Daniel Cramer of Harvard University studied hundreds of women with ovarian cancer, and had them record in detail what they normally ate. He compared them to a group of women who were similar in age and other demographic variables, but who did not develop cancer. There was one thing that the women with cancer had eaten much more frequently than women without cancer: dairy products, especially the supposedly 'healthy' products, such as yoghurt.

Dr Cramer suggested that the culprit might be a normal breakdown product of the milk sugar, lactose. Lactose is broken down in the body to another sugar called galactose. In turn, galactose is broken down further by enzymes in the body. According to Dr Cramer, when dairy product consumption exceeds the enzymes' capacity to break down galactose, there is a build-up of galactose in the blood, which may damage a woman's ovaries. Some women have particularly low levels of the enzymes needed to break down galactose, and when they consume dairy products on a regular basis, their risk of ovarian cancer could be triple that of other women. Dr Cramer observed that the problem was the milk sugar, not the milk fat, so it is *not* solved by using low-fat dairy products. In fact, yoghurt and cottage cheese seem to be of most concern because the bacteria used in their production increase the production of galactose from lactose. Although I am not sure that this mechanism explains breast cancer, the link certainly explained my situation and my observations and hypothesis. How I wish Dr Cramer's information had been more widely publicised at the time.

I BECOME A HUMAN GUINEA-PIG

Up to this point, I had been steadfastly measuring the progress of my latest and greatest lump with callipers and plotting the results. Despite all the encouraging comments and positive feedback from my doctors and nurses, my own precise observations told me the bitter truth: the first chemotherapy sessions had produced no effect – the lump was still the same size.

Then I eliminated dairy products.

Within days, the lump started to shrink. About two weeks after my second chemotherapy session and one week after I gave up dairy produce the lump in my neck started to itch, and then it began to soften and to reduce in size. The line on the graph, which had shown no change was now pointing downwards as the tumour got smaller and smaller. And, very significantly, I noted that instead of declining exponentially (a graceful curve) as cancer is meant to do, the tumour's decrease in size plotted on a straight line heading off the bottom of the graph, *indicating a cure*: not suppression or remission of the tumour.

One Saturday afternoon after about six weeks of excluding all dairy produce from my diet, I practised an hour of meditation (more of that later) then felt for what was left of the lump. I could not find it. I went downstairs and asked my husband to feel my neck. He could not find any trace of the lump either. On the following Thursday I was due to be seen by my cancer specialist at Charing Cross Hospital. He examined me thoroughly, especially my neck where the tumour had been. He was initially bemused and then delighted as he said, 'but I cannot find it'. He was as overjoyed as I was. When I saw the same specialist for my most recent annual check-up (1999), he told me that my chemotherapy treatment had been only the same basic type that has been used for breast cancer for the past twenty years. None of my doctors, it appeared, had expected someone with my type and stage of cancer (which had clearly spread to the lymph system) to have survived, let alone be so hale and hearty.

When I first discussed my ideas with my cancer specialist he was understandably sceptical. But I understand that he now uses maps from *The Atlas of Cancer Mortality in the People's Republic of China* in his lectures and recommends a non-dairy diet to his breast cancer patients.

I now believe that the link between dairy produce and breast cancer (and probably prostate cancer) is similar to that between smoking and lung cancer. In fact, epidemiological studies have indicated a positive correlation between dairy product consumption and breast cancer risk in publications going back two decades and more. For example, a study in 1970 found low death rates for breast cancer where dairy product consumption was low and intake of other fats was high.[13] Other studies have found a dose-dependent increase in breast cancer risk among women who consumed milk (especially whole milk) and/or cheese. For example, in 1977 scientists examined the incidence of breast cancer in Japan and found a significant increase in both the consumption of dairy products and the occurrence of breast cancer in urban areas where the average intake of other fatty foods was at or below average.[14]

I believe that identifying the link between breast cancer and dairy produce, and then developing a diet specifically targeted at maintaining the health of my breast and hormone system, cured me. Initially, it was difficult for me, as it may be difficult for you, to accept that a substance as 'natural' as milk might have such ominous health implications. In the next chapter, I want to show you some of the factors in dairy products that may be to blame.

The update to this chapter can be found on page 293.

4 Rich Woman's Disease

*In this chapter I explain much of the hard scientific evidence that I
have collected over the years linking the consumption of dairy
produce to breast and prostate cancer. It also explains why giving
up dairy is unlikely to cause health problems, but is likely to cut
your risk of suffering from many other diseases as well as breast or
prostate cancer.*

Just as many Chinese people giggle in astonishment when they
see Westerners consuming so much milk and dairy products, so
we find it difficult to understand how anyone could possibly live
healthily without it.

It all boils down to a matter of cultural perceptions. To mix
metaphors a bit, one person's milk is another person's 'yuk!'.

In most of Western society, milk is seen as a healthy, natural
food: vital for babies, essential for women at risk of osteoporosis, full of protein for hard-working men, a slimming drink for
svelte catwalk models. In short, it's all things to all people.

But this carefully crafted image is just that: an image. We
have no scientific requirement to consume milk after weaning
– in fact, we're the only species that intentionally does so. Even
stranger is our obsession with the milk of another species: the
cow. It would be just as logical (or indeed, illogical) to drink
dogs' milk, pigs' milk, or rats' milk. Those thoughts fill us with
disgust – maybe that's how we ought to feel about cows' milk,
too.

Cows' milk isn't intended by nature for consumption by any
species other than baby cows. If you compare its nutritional
profile to human breast milk, you'll see some major differences.[1] The vertical line on Table 2 on page 87 represents the
nutritional profile of human mother's milk; the horizontal bars
show how cows' milk compares, gram for gram. You can see
that cows' milk contains about three times as much protein as
human milk, and far more calcium – both of which may place
an excessive burden on young human kidneys. Basically, cows'
milk is a perfect food for a rapidly growing baby calf (about a

kilogram or so gained every day). But that doesn't mean it's good for human babies – or adults!

Many scientists believe that the amount of dairy produce in our diet is now far too high. According to the Statistical Abstract of the US, Americans in 1992 each consumed an average of 564.6 pounds of cows' milk products, or about 1.54 pounds per person per day; this included milk, cream, ice cream, ice milk, buttermilk, cheese, cottage cheese, various 'dips' and yoghurt.[2] The United States Department of Agriculture recently estimated that the average American's diet comprises more than 40 per cent dairy produce, more than double most official guidelines. According to Willet and others, the prevalence of obesity in the US rose by 33 per cent between 1980 and 1991.[3]

In Bill Bryson's book *The Lost Continent* he repeatedly refers to the obesity of the American population:

> Iowa women are almost always sensationally overweight – you see them at Merle Hay Mall in Des Moines on Saturdays, clammy and meaty in their shorts and halter tops, looking a little like elephants dressed in children's clothes, yelling at their kids, calling out names like Dwayne and Shauna.

HOW HORMONES INFLUENCE OUR BREASTS – AND VICE VERSA

The breast is a special gland that develops early in foetal life out of the same type of tissue as the skin.[4] It has a structure that has been likened to a tree, with the tiny sacs in which milk is produced equivalent to leaves, the milk ducts leading from the sacs forming the branches, and then the trunk of the tree behind the nipple from where milk is expelled.

As every woman knows, breasts change with age – especially during puberty and the menopause and with stages in the menstrual cycle, pregnancy and sexual arousal. This is because breasts are involved both in bonding with our sexual partners and in feeding and bonding with our babies. Breasts can be a source of great pleasure for example during sexual activity or breast feeding children. But at other times they can feel like large, aching, lumpy boils, especially for example, in women affected by pre-menstrual tension. They can also become a centre of disease, the most lethal of which is breast cancer.

Table 2: Comparison of the composition of typical cows' and human milk.

(The vertical line represents the composition of typical human milk.)

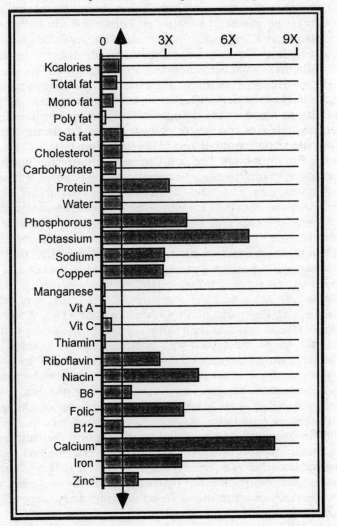

Changes in the size, weight, sensitivity and health of the breasts generally reflect changes in the type and concentration of different chemicals circulating through our bodies. The changes in concentrations of the chemicals can be minute, and it is only in the past ten to twenty years that it has been possible to measure them accurately as a result of advances in analytical methods. The most important chemicals affecting breast function and physiology are chemical messengers, or hormones, which are released in minute quantities, for example, from special parts of the brain or ovaries, in response to biological or physiological factors or outside stimuli. At puberty, growth hormones such as insulin-like growth factor-1 (abbreviated as IGF-1) stimulate breast tissue to develop into breasts. During pregnancy, hormones are also released from the placenta, helping to prepare the breast to feed a new baby when it is born. Breast tissue increases, and the milk ducts in the breast sprout extensively under the influence of increasing amounts of oestrogen circulating in the blood.[5] As early as five to eight weeks into pregnancy, the quantity and volume of the milk sacs and ducts in the breast have increased so rapidly that the breasts are heavy and enlarged, the nipples are darker and the superficial veins in the breast become dilated.

Hormones are chemical messengers used to carry information from one part of our body to another. Mammalian hormones have many features in common. They are usually relatively small molecules and many, such as insulin, are proteins (although testosterone and oestrogen are steroids). They are made in endocrine (meaning secreting to the inside) glands, so called because they secrete hormones into blood capillaries within glands for distribution throughout the body via the blood circulation system. The concentrations of hormones in human blood are very small. For any one hormone, the concentration is rarely more than a few micrograms per ml of blood and the rate of secretion is also very low. This is because hormones are so POWERFUL and even the tiny quantities of hormones in our blood can have very large effects on the body.

Each hormone has a particular group of target cells that it affects because they have receptors specific for the hormone. Receptors for protein hormones are on cell surface membranes and their attachment to the membrane sets off a chain of reactions inside the cell whereas steroid hormones, which are lipid soluble, pass into the cell where their receptors are located.

The interaction of the hormones involved in milk production is particularly complex. Following the birth of the baby, milk production begins. The breasts first fill with colostrum, a thick, yellowish fluid, before changing to milk as the amount of lactose (milk sugar) increases (lactose is one of the major carbohydrates in milk, and is a sugar found only in milk). A number of hormones, including prolactin and oxytocin, cortisol, insulin, thyroid and parathyroid hormones, and growth hormones enable this process to commence. Prolactin, in particular, is a key milk-supporting hormone.[6] The normal levels of this hormone in the blood of non-pregnant, non-milk-producing women is about 10ng/ml, but in breast-feeding women it is two or three times higher. (A ng, or nanogram, is one thousand millionth of a gram.)

Just as hormones profoundly affect every aspect of the breasts' growth and function, so breast milk itself contains a powerful cocktail of hormones and hormone-like substances. If you have always been used to thinking of milk as a pure, white, inert substance, full of vitamins, minerals and other good things for our bodies to absorb, then you may perhaps be surprised to think about it in this new way: as a concentrated source of chemical messengers, each one with a particular mission to accomplish in influencing the growth and development of the newly-born. For example, research indicates that certain components in milk can exert control over aspects of metabolism, including cell division, in the newborn. Since ancient times, milk has been referred to as 'white blood'.[7]

Some of the hormones naturally present in milk include oxytocin, prolactin, adrenal and ovarian steroids, Gn-RH (gonadotropin-releasing hormone), GRF (growth hormone-releasing factor), insulin, somatostatin, relaxin, calcitonin and neurotensin, and prostaglandins (hormone-like substances made in many parts of the body rather than coming from one organ as do most hormones), all at levels greater than those in the breast-feeding mother's blood; and TRH (thyrotropin-releasing hormone), TSH (thyroid-stimulating hormone), thyroxine, triiodothyronine, erythropoietin and bombesin although these substances are at lower levels in milk than in maternal blood. Milk also contains numerous growth factors including epidermal growth factor (EGF), insulin-like growth factor (IGF-1) and nerve growth factor (NGF). It also contains over 40 enzymes, which have many functions including the development of the infant's immunological function and in some cases the maturation of certain cells.[8]

In fact, all mature breast milk, whether from humans or other mammals, is a medium for transporting hundreds of different chemical components. And it varies in composition between species, between mothers, between breasts, between feeds and during the course of lactation.[9] Different breast teats have even been shown to produce milk of different composition to suckle different young animals with different nutritional needs.

The point is this: *all* mammalian milk, whether from humans, cows or other species, is a powerful biochemical solution of great complexity, uniquely designed to provide for the individual needs of young mammals of the same species. It's not that cows' milk isn't a good food: it's a *great* food – for baby cows.

And therein lies the source of the problem.

SOME PROBLEMS WITH MILK

Scientists have linked cows' milk consumption to a wide range of human health problems. Here are some of them:

- Babies who are fed whole cows' milk in the first year of life are at risk of developing iron deficiency. Indeed, many authorities, including the American Academy of Pediatrics Committee on Nutrition recommend that whole cows' milk should be *excluded* from the diet in the first year of life.[10] The iron in cows' milk isn't easy for babies to absorb and, in addition, cows' milk appears to interfere with the body's absorption of iron from other foods. Even worse, cows' milk has been shown to cause iron loss by producing gastro-intestinal bleeding.[11] Paediatricians learned long ago that cows' milk was often a cause of colic in young infants. We now know that breast-feeding mothers can have colicky babies if the mothers are consuming cow's milk, since the cows' antibodies can pass through the mother's blood stream into her breast milk and to the baby.[12] This is how one British consultant paediatrician describes allergy to cows' milk in infants: 'An infant receiving cows' milk protein (CMP) may be persistently restless and unhappy, screaming at intervals and appearing in pain. His appetite may be excessively greedy, he may regurgitate freely and he may have loose, mucousy stools in which blood and sometimes sugars are detected. There may be impaired weight gain and anaemia is common. Infants, especially if their parents or siblings suffer from eczema/hay fever/ asthma, may develop facial or generalised eczema, persistent nasal congestion and noisy wheezing when CMP is introduced, or these symptoms may be accentuated at that time, with or without gastrointestinal disturbance.'[13]

- Insulin-dependent diabetes (Type I or childhood-onset) is linked to dairy products. Epidemiological studies of various countries show a strong correlation between the use of dairy products and the incidence of insulin-dependent diabetes.[14] This disease, which tends to strike in early teenage years and accounts for many deaths a year in the UK alone, starts with the immune system destroying the beta cells in the pancreas that produce insulin. There is probably a genetic predisposition but mounting evidence suggests that the disease is linked to an allergy to bovine (cows') serum protein.

- Milk is one of the most common causes of food allergies, and it is the *single most common* cause of allergy in infants.[15] Milk proteins, which some people's bodies recognise as foreign proteins, have frequently been implicated in cases of eczema, asthma and migraine. A meeting of the American Society of Microbiologists suggested that some of the thousands of cases of cot death occurring in the USA every year might be attributed to cows' milk allergy, as babies who are breast fed are less likely to succumb to cot death.[16] Respiratory problems, canker sores, skin conditions, and other subtle and not-so-subtle allergies can all be caused by dairy products. Over 70 per cent of the world's adult population are unable to digest the milk sugar, lactose, which has led nutritionists to believe that this is the normal condition for adults, not some sort of deficiency.[17] The symptoms, which include abdominal pain, flatulence and diarrhoea, are relieved by taking the enzyme that breaks down lactose, called lactase. Lactose intolerance may be nature's early warning system: perhaps nature is trying to tell us that we're eating the wrong food!

- Milk is an excellent culture medium for the growth and transmission of many unpleasant bacteria and micro-organisms. Pasteurisation was originally developed to destroy Coxiella burnetii (the organism responsible for Q-fever) and Mycobacterium tuberculosis (the organism re-sponsible for tuberculosis), which were thought to be the most heat-resistant pathogens likely to be present in raw milk. However, results of two studies suggest that a microbe called Mycobacterium paratuberculosis may survive heat treatment at 63°C for 30 minutes (equivalent to one type of pasteurisation) and 71.7°C for 15 seconds (another type of pasteurisation) before it is rapidly cooled to 10°C (equivalent to high-temperature, short-time pasteurisation) if it is present in high numbers prior to heat treatment.[18] Mycobacterium paratuberculosis causes chronic enteritis in cows, known as Johne's disease, which is an incurable, chronic, infectious disease characterised by diarrhoea, weight loss and debilitation. It is one of the most widespread bacterial diseases of domestic animals throughout the world, and is believed to be associated with irritable bowel syndrome in humans[19] (which affects 20 per cent of the population in the USA.[20])

- Listeria monocytogenes is a bacterium which can occur in soft cheeses to such an extent that it causes very serious illness, including meningitis and septicaemia; the mortality rate from Listeriosis can be as high as 30 per cent of those affected.[21] The most vulnerable people are pregnant women and their infants, the elderly and people who are immunosuppressed, which of course includes those on chemotherapy. These vulnerable groups form a considerable proportion of the population. The incubation period before the development of the disease can be as long as ten weeks, and this causes considerable difficulty in determining the food implicated in the infection.

- As if this were not bad enough, a wide range of chemicals can be administered legally to dairy animals.[22] These chemicals include antibiotics to treat infection and as growth promoters, and anti-parasitic drugs including those active against worms. In the USA and some other countries, prostaglandins and pituitary hormones, including oxytocin, luteinizing hormones and follicle stimulating hormones are used as veterinary prescription drugs. It is claimed that their use in cows does not pose human food safety concerns, provided that they are used according to label directions. They can, however, be misused – for example oxytocin can be used to increase milk production – and highly effective policing is needed to ensure milk does not contain excess residues of hormones administered by dairy farmers.[23]

- The trend towards intensive farming means that fewer and fewer cows are being unnaturally forced to produce more and more milk (if you thought that there was a milk surplus, you're right: but that doesn't have anything to do with the economics of the dairy industry). In the USA for example, there has been an almost constant annual increase in milk yield per cow of 1.5–2 per cent. Cows now become pregnant much earlier in their lives with the shortest possible time between calving. Their young are removed from them, after which they are milked more intensively and for longer periods of time than ever before. Then they are slaughtered. One of the consequences of this highly artificial, high-pressure environment is an increase in mastitis and other infections of cows' udders, which can cause pus to be present in milk. Do you realise that even in the European Union, milk for human consumption can be sold legally even when it contains up to 400,000 somatic pus cells/ml? (EU directive 92/46/EEC). So one teaspoon of milk can contain 2 million pus cells. Because increased pus diminishes the value of milk, dairy farmers use antibiotics on their animals. In 1990, a US Food and Drug Administration survey found antibiotics and other drugs in 51 per cent of 70 milk samples taken in 14 cities.[24] There is growing concern that residues such as these may increase the human allergic response to drinking milk, as well as increasing the immunity of bacteria to antibiotics, making human diseases more difficult to treat. It is estimated by the European Union that 3–10 per cent of the human population is allergic to penicillin and the other antibiotics most commonly used to treat mastitis in cows. Their report also states that increased use of anti-microbial substances in treating mastitis (related to the use of rBGH – see over) might lead to the selection of resistant bacteria.[25]

- Milk is designed to be a concentrated source of chemicals which ensure the growth and well-being of newly-born and young mammals. Unfortunately, many man-made chemicals which the body cannot distinguish from natural substances *also* become concentrated in milk by the same process. It has been hypothesised that contaminants in milk were implicated in doubling the Israeli breast cancer mortality rate before 1976 (compared to other countries with the same average consumption of dietary fat).[26] Three carcinogens found in Israeli milk, one of which was DDT, possess characteristics similar to oestrogen. Public disapproval of these contaminants resulted in Government action in 1978 which drastically reduced their levels in milk. Subsequently, there was a decline in Israeli breast cancer deaths between 1978 and 1986. Pollutants such as the fat-soluble PCBs and dioxins, some of which can cause cancer and which are powerful endocrine disrupters, can be particularly concentrated in milk from pasture or feed (*see* Chapter Six), together with some radioactive isotopes released as a result of nuclear accidents in the past. Recent studies have shown that even breast milk from 'clean human beings' has up to 350 artificial chemicals or pollutants in it.[27]

HARD EVIDENCE

We've now seen how cows' milk, although an ideal food for young bovines, is far from ideal for adult humans. But how could dairy products be linked to breast and prostate cancer?

I believe that the evidence suggests that consuming dairy products (milk and meat), including low fat products such as yoghurt, does indeed increase the risk of breast and prostate cancer in exposed populations. When I eliminated *all* dairy products from my diet, a large 'secondary' tumour comprising cancer cells in the lymph nodes in my neck, which was thought to be incurable, disappeared in weeks. For me, this is pretty compelling evidence.

But that's not all. Since many of the powerful chemicals contained in milk are known to have an important role in the development of young mammals, including cell division, and milk is designed for this purpose, it is worth asking the question: what happens if the chemicals designed to stimulate cell growth in newly-born animals send similar signals to adult tissue?

Let's look at some of the suspect chemicals, starting with the previously mentioned growth factor, IGF-1. Both insulin and insulin-like growth factors cause cells to increase in size. Insulin has a simple short-term action of cleaning excess nutrients from the circulation and storing them in cells. In contrast, insulin-like growth factors (IGFs) are involved in cell proliferation and differentiation, and a complex set of factors have evolved to ensure that IGF activity occurs only when conditions are optimal for growth. Zinc levels are particularly important in this respect.[28]

In 1994, a genetically engineered copy of natural bovine growth hormone, BGH,* called recombinant bovine growth hormone – rBGH (also known as bovine somatotropin or BST), was marketed in the USA following approval by the American Food and Drug Administration. The hormone is manufactured by taking the specific gene sequence that carries the instructions for making BGH from the DNA of cows and inserting it into E-coli bacteria which are then cultured to produce commercial quantities of rBGH.

The effect of rBGH on the mammary glands of lactating cows is to increase secretory activity, bloodflow, nutrient uptake and milk synthesis. That's what the hormone is supposed to do: when injected into cows it is capable of increasing milk production by an average of 12 per cent. There is a moratorium on its use in Europe and Canada but its use in the USA and several other countries is increasing. For example between 1995 and 1996 its use increased by 45 per cent in the USA alone. Unlike most other hormones used on agricultural animals in the States, a veterinary prescription is not required for rBGH. Under the General Agreement on Tariffs and Trade (GATT), the EU is unable to ban the imports of milk or milk products from rBGH-treated cows from the USA or other countries.[29]

What effect might bovine growth hormone have in humans? Since it is structurally different by approximately 35 per cent from its human equivalent, it is argued that it has no effect,

---

* Growth hormone or somatotropin is structurally different in different species, therefore it has to be specified as bovine (B)GH or porcine (pig) (P)GH or human (H)GH growth hormone for example.

because it would be unable to bind to appropriate receptors in human tissues (such as the breast). However, it has also been suggested by other scientists that the extra amino acids on the genetically modified substance make it exceptionally potent to cows and dangerous to humans.

What really is of concern, however, is what rBGH does to milk. Changes in the composition of milk from rBGH-treated cows were noted as early as 1985 by scientists who reported changes in the proportion of short- and medium-chain fatty acids, and of long-chain fatty acids, findings confirmed recently.[30]

One of the most important effects of rBGH, as far as breast and prostate cancer studies are concerned, is that it releases extra quantities of the insulin-like growth factor IGF-1. Insulin and the insulin-like growth factors (IGF-1 and IGF-II) are secreted by cells into the bloodstream and intercellular spaces in all mammals. IGF-1 stimulates cell division, especially in the first phase of the cell cycle when the cell enlarges and makes new proteins. It also has insulin-like effects, such as the stimulation of glucose storage in fat cells. The highest proportion of IGF-1 is made by the liver. The liver also makes two proteins which inactivate it – IGF-binding proteins 1 and 3.

Unlike bovine growth hormone, IGF-1 is exactly the same chemical whether it is in the milk of goats, sheep, cows, humans or other mammalian species. Levels of IGF-1 are naturally higher in cows' milk than human milk: but its average concentration in milk from cows treated with rBGH is *even higher* (estimates vary from 2 to 5 times higher concentration in treated milk) and there is about two times more IGF-1 in the meat of treated cows than in that of untreated cows.[31] Different breeds of cows have different levels of IGF-1. For example, the Brahman breed generally has higher blood levels of IGF-1 than the Angus breed of cattle.[32]

Over the years, the dairy industry has chosen to increase the average milk yield by selectively breeding from cattle which are better milk producers. This has resulted in the selection of cows which have higher levels of naturally occurring BGH, so that even before the era of rBGH, levels of IGF-1 in milk were increasing anyway. Also, the long-term treatment of cows with the hormone implant oestradiol as a growth promoter increases secretion of IGF-1. IGF-1 is not destroyed during pasteurisation of milk. In experiments, after being treated at 175°C for 45 seconds (longer than the US Department of Agriculture Pasteurisation Protocol), the concentration of IGF-1 was not reduced.[33]

Because IGF-1 is known to be biologically active in humans – causing cells to divide including breast tissue in girls during puberty – the increased levels in milk raise the question: *Will IGF-1 from milk or the meat of dairy animals cause inappropriate cell division and growth and hence cancer in humans?*

In 1998, an American and Canadian research team led by Dr Susan Hankinson showed that among premenopausal women, those with the highest IGF-1 concentration in their blood had almost *three times the risk* of developing breast cancer compared to those with the lowest amount of IGF-1.[34] Among women younger than 50, the risk was increased *seven times!* The authors of this study state that there is 'substantial indirect evidence of a relation between IGF-1 and the risk of breast cancer' and point to experiments showing that IGF-1 enhances the growth of cancerous breast cells in mice. This study and that of Chan and others, 1998,[35] into IGF-1 levels and prostate cancer, discussed below, are both prospective studies whereby symptomless groups of patients are followed for years and data for those developing disease compared to data for those who do not. Generally, prospective studies are the most convincing for indicating causal relationships, rather than retrospective studies carried out when the disease has already developed, in which case there is a chance the disease could be causing the high measured levels of IGF-1.

According to a team led by Dr MN Pollack, Professor of Oncology at McGill University in Montreal, further studies of the association are needed to provide more precise estimates of the effect of IGF-1 on breast cancer and to investigate the possibility of a relationship also between premenopausal levels of IGF-1 and breast cancer in postmenopausal women. The levels of IGF-1 in the blood are highest during the years of puberty which is, of course, a time of rapid growth. Indeed, at the onset of puberty, IGF-1 signals to breast cells to begin dividing so that the breasts will grow. According to Dr Pollack, the substance plays the same role in stimulating breast cancer cells. And significantly, one of the ways in which the drug Tamoxifen is thought to work is by reducing circulating IGF-1 levels.[36]

Researchers from McGill University and the Harvard School of Public Health in the United States have also found increased levels of IGF-1 circulating in the blood to be a strong predictor of prostate cancer.[37] Men with the highest levels of circulating IGF-1 had a 4.3-fold increased risk of developing prostate cancer compared with those with the lowest IGF-1 levels. In the article in the magazine *Science*, Professor Pollack writes that 'until now, researchers interested in prostate cancer have focussed on male hormones such as testosterone, but these (IGF-1) results open up a whole new direction of research. This is of the same order of magnitude as the relationship between cholesterol levels and the risk of heart disease'.

According to Professor Pollack's team, insulin-like growth factor 1 (IGF-1) is a mitogenic (stimulating cell division) and anti-apoptotic (preventing cell death or suicide) substance that influences the prolific behaviour of many cell types, including certain normal breast cells. Pollack's work is confirmed by another study which also suggests a connection between IGF-1 and prostate cancer risk, again finding that men with high levels of IGF-1 in their blood are four times more likely to suffer from prostate cancer compared to those with lower levels.[38] And yet another recent study from 1998 confirms that increased IGF-1 levels in blood are associated with large relative risks for common cancers.[39] None of these researchers has specifically linked IGF-1 levels in the human body to consumption of milk or dairy products, but in 1996, Dr Samuel S Epstein of the University of Illinois in Chicago published a paper arguing that IGF-1 from rBGH-treated cows could indeed promote cancer of the breast and of the colon in humans who drink such milk.[40] Other studies including that of Outwater and others,[41] which was based on a review of more than 130 peer-reviewed publications, have also suggested such a link.

All this is, in my view, starting to look like a strong *prima facie* case. In 1995 the European Union successfully opposed approval for the use of rBGH in the EU.[42] Recently a European Commission (EC) committee has confirmed the findings of excess levels of IGF-1 in the milk of cows injected with rBGH.[43] The report of the EU Scientific Committee concludes that the excess levels of IGF-1 pose a serious risk of breast and prostate cancer, stating that 'risk characterisation has pointed to an association between circulating IGF-1 levels and an increased relative risk of breast and prostate cancer'. The report cites experimental and epidemiological evidence for such an association. It also concludes that the various ways of measuring IGF-I concentrations and those of its much more potent, truncated forms need to be evaluated. It may be, for instance, that available analytical techniques underestimate the actual levels of IGF-1 in milk by neglecting the protein bound fraction.

While there is still much to be learned about the precise way in which IGF-1 may be implicated in breast and prostate cancer, we already know enough, in my view, to start to take defensive measures. It has been hypothesised that IGF-1 contributes to breast cancer cell proliferation through actions on IGF-1 receptors[44] and it has already been shown that:

- Breast cancer cell cultures respond to minute IGF-1 concentrations by multiplying as much as 4–5 fold.[45]
- Nearly all breast cancer cell lines (cultures) and breast cancer cells from fresh tumour biopsies have receptors for IGF-1, and binding of IGF-1 to breast tumours is increased compared to normal breast tissue.[46]
- Median IGF-1 concentrations in primary breast cancers have been found to be significantly higher than in normal breast tissue.[47]
- IGF-1 also causes changes in the cell cycle and cancer causing genes, 'oncogenes'. Tiny concentrations of IGF-1 alter the relative number of breast cancer cells in each phase of the breast cancer cell cycle.[48] Such alterations may cause the unregulated growth of cancer.
- Evidence suggests that over-expression of IGF-1 receptors is a key factor in transforming normal breast tissue to breast cancer. In fact, one criterion for the effectiveness of cancer treatments is their ability to successfully lower IGF-1 levels or block IGF-1 receptor binding. Additionally, other hormones and growth factors may interact with IGF-1 in encouraging tumour growth. The problem with IGF-1 may be due to its ability to make transformed cells more responsive to signals from other growth factors.[49]

The argument of the pro-rBGH lobby is that IGF-1 occurs in milk naturally, and that although administration of rBGH to dairy cows increases IGF-1 levels in milk, 'the levels are within the range of milk from untreated cows, especially those at the stage of early lactation'. They also point out that IGF-1 occurs naturally in the human body (but the extent to which the levels reflect the Western dairy-rich diet is not known). However, it would also be true to say that we manufacture our own cholesterol, but cholesterol-related disease (e.g. heart disease) is caused by consuming *extra* amounts of the substance from dairy and other animal products. Could a similar situation not apply in the case of IGF-1? Specifically that, yes, we manufacture our own IGF-1 but could not *disease* be caused by consuming extra quantities of IGF-1 from dairy produce and the meat of animals used for dairying? According to Macaulay, 1992, although IGF-1 is a normal body component, it may well be associated with malignant disease when present in excess.[50]

In humans, free, or circulating IGF-1 levels decline with age consistent with their role in growth. IGF-1 levels are higher in teenage girls than boys and the difference extends into adulthood. Levels are elevated in pregnant women. Although IGF-1 is essential for growth, its levels do not correlate closely with growth rates; suggesting amongst other possibilities that some IGF-1 may be of external origin. It has been suggested that IGF-1 levels may be affected by nutritional status.[51]

We also know that IGF-1 has growth promoting effects in response to concentrations as low as 1ng/ml. Milk contains approximately 30ng/ml so that two, 8oz glasses of milk a day would contain 200ng of IGF-1 per kilogram of body weight per day for a person weighing 70kg.[52] Also, milk secretions of mammals contain special forms of IGF-1 which is ten times more potent than normal IGF-1. In normal cows' milk 3 per cent of the IGF-1 is reported to be in this form.[53]

Champions of the dairy industry argue that the hormones and other powerful chemicals in milk do not enter the bloodstream because they are destroyed during the digestive process. For example, in the case of rBGH or natural BGH and IGF-1, both of which are proteins, it is argued that they are broken down by enzymes in the digestive tract into simple amino acids prior to absorption. (Hence the need to administer rBGH to cows by injection). Yet since the early 1990s there have been concerns about effects of increased IGF-1 levels in milk on the digestive tract. When the American National Institutes of Health (NIH) reviewed the safety of rBGH back in 1991 (concluding that it was safe), it was stated that 'further studies will be required to determine whether ingestion of bovine IGF-1 is safe for children, adolescents and adults'.[54] They acknowledged that 'Whether the additional amount of insulin-like growth factor in milk from [rBGH-treated cows] has a local effect on the oesophagus, stomach or intestines is unknown'. Three studies suggest a possible link:

- Some humans suffer from a condition called acromegaly, or gigantism, which is characterised by excessive growth of the head, face, hands and feet. It is caused by natural over-production of IGF-1. Importantly, a recent report indicates that people who suffer from acromegaly have an increased incidence of tumours of the colon (a portion of the intestines).[55]
- Two British researchers, Challacombe and Wheeler, experimented with IGF-1 on human small intestine cells. They reported that IGF-1 promoted cell division (and cancer is uncontrolled cell division).[56]
- A study published in 1995 in the journal *Cancer Research* indicates that IGF-1 promotes the growth of cancer tumours in laboratory animals and in humans by preventing programmed cell death (apoptosis).[57]

Even researchers who support the use of rBGH have admitted that 'many more potential effects of ingested IGF-1 on the gastrointestinal tract need to be explored'.[58] Certainly, the human gut is quite different from that of ruminant animals such as cows, sheep and goats, from which we obtain dairy produce. The digestive tracts of these animals are designed to digest large quantities of vegetable matter such as grass. Moreover, could certain people have digestive tracts that are poorly adapted to the digestion of dairy products and so allow the biologically active chemicals into the bloodstream? Could this 'leakiness' of the digestive tract to hormones increase under stress? Could it be differences in the ability to digest dairy produce which are partly responsible for differences in individual susceptibility to breast or prostate cancer?

One of the arguments of the dairy lobby is that human saliva contains IGF-1 which is known to be broken down during digestion. Independent studies show, however, that growth hormones contained in milk closely similar to IGF-1 are *not* destroyed by the digestive system because of the protective effect of casein (the principal protein in milk).[59] The 1999 report of the EU Scientific Committee (see reference 53) states 'there is clear evidence that orally ingested IGF-1 reaches the receptor sites in the gut in its biologically active form'.

Also, it has been suggested that homogenisation and other methods of processing milk could increase the risk of cancer-promoting hormones and other chemicals reaching the bloodstream and hence affecting the breast or prostate. Homogenisation distributes fat globules through milk so that there are no longer separate milk and cream components. The process involves passing milk through an extremely fine filter at very high pressure to reduce the fat globules (which would otherwise separate out as cream) to about a tenth of their size. By definition, homogenisation ensures that the fat molecules are evenly dispersed in the milk so that after 48 hours of storage at 45°F, there is no visible separation of cream. According to some scientists, homogenisation encapsulates in fat the biologically active proteins and hormones present in milk (rather like a gelatine time-release capsule protects cold remedies) until they have passed through the part of the digestive system capable of breaking them down. These hormones would therefore survive digestion and risk being absorbed into the bloodstream. Once in the bloodstream, such chemicals would be able to affect breast and prostate tissue, and could also promote cancer cells wherever they have reached – for example, where they occur as secondary tumours in the lungs or liver (remember, breast cancer cells are still breast cancer cells and prostate cancer cells are still prostate cancer cells!). Because of advances in food processing, milk can now be engineered to fit its minimum legal definition and excess fat, whey or lactose for example, can be removed and sold on and added to other food. Hence dairy products now turn up in products that one would never suspect to contain milk-derived components (*see* Chapter Five).

Breast and prostate cancers have existed in Western populations for a long time. A mid-seventeenth century painting (p. 103) by Rembrandt entitled *Bathsheeba at her Toilet* (1654), which hangs in the Louvre in Paris, clearly shows that the model Rembrandt painted had a large tumour in her right breast. Since the time Western man developed stable, farming communities they have consumed significant quantities of milk, and it is worth remembering that, even without the use of rBGH, milk contains quantities of IGF-1 that have been steadily increasing over the centuries because of the selection of higher yielding dairy cows. In fact, the recent debate about rBGH may have served mainly to draw the potential problem of IGF-1 in milk to public attention, which otherwise only a few specialist scientists would have known about.

And yet, IGF-1 is only *one* of the powerful chemicals in milk which may have a significant role to play in the development of breast and prostate cancer. What about all of the others?

IGF-II

According to Outwater and others,[60] IGF-II is also a potent mitogen (a substance that induces cell division) present in human and cows' milk. The US Food and Drug Administration

(FDA) reported that IGF-1 levels are approximately 30ng/ml. Those of IGF-II are approximately 350ng/ml – more than ten times greater. Most studies have concentrated on IGF-1 because of the effects of rBGH on its concentration and there is little about IGF-II in the literature. One experiment, however, which involved increasing IGF-II levels in transgenic mice 20–30 fold, indicated the development of a wide range of tumours after eighteen months.

PROLACTIN

The hormone prolactin is a growth factor required for the proliferation and differentiation of the human breast and is a key milk-supporting hormone. Prolactin is found in all milk, although there are differences between human prolactin and that of other species. Prolactin has been linked to breast and prostate cancer by several research groups. For example, Haraguchi and others[61] from the University of South Florida wrote in the *International Journal of Cancer* in 1992: 'Prolactin plays a key role in the regulation and growth of mammary cells and influences tumour promotion'. Their studies were based on cultures of human ductal carcinoma cells using human prolactin.

Clevenger and others[62] from the University of Pennsylvania writing in the *American Journal of Pathology* in 1995 concluded that their data suggested a role for prolactin in the pathogenesis of breast cancer. In 1989 Vonderhaar,[63] of the National Cancer Institute (USA) found that the same cell culture responded to the presence of sheep or human prolactin (in the absence of oestrogens) with a two- to three-fold increase in cancer cell numbers. The second generation of cells produced an even greater response. Vonderhaar concludes that 'the data indicates that prolactin alone is a mitogen (causes cell division) in human breast cancer cells in long-term culture'. Research at the University of Turku, Finland into prolactin receptors in the prostate has also concluded that prolactin may increase prostate cancer progression because it increases epithelial cell DNA synthesis.[64] Some of the experimental evidence on the ability of bovine (cow) prolactin to stimulate human breast cancer cell cultures is conflicting.[65] The ability of bovine prolactin to act as a mitogen in cultures of rodent breast cancer cells is undisputed, however. According to Vonderhaar, 80 per cent of human breast cancer cell lines respond to prolactin as a mitogen.[66] Struman and others in 1999[67] also showed that the human prolactin/growth hormone family are angiogenic – that is they promote the development of microvascular structures – remember from Chapter Two that cancers need to develop a blood supply system and scientists are trying to develop anti-angiogenic substances to effectively starve cancers. The same molecules however, can have anti-angiogenic properties. These properties are thought to be important in the development of the vascular connections between the mother and developing foetus (stress and some drugs, including some for treating psychotic disorders, increase the body's circulating prolactin). Prolactin has also been shown to be a significant driver in breast cancer metastasis by research at the University of Pennsylvania Medical Center.[68]

Most amazingly, in the lab prolactin is actually measured by adding milk to cultures of a type of cancer cell (rat lymphoma) and weighing the increase in the mass of the cancer to calculate the concentration of prolactin! This technique has been shown to be a sensitive bio-assay method (relies on biological rather than chemical reaction) for determining the levels of prolactin in milk, and it *depends upon* prolactin's ability to stimulate cancer cell growth. I actually first discovered this in a book entitled *Breast Feeding – A Guide to the Medical Profession*.[69] Genetically engineered prolactin is also marketed and sold for experiments on prolactin-dependent tumours.[70]

Prolactin in milk has been described as biologically potent and in new, suckling infant mammals it influences fluid, sodium, potassium and calcium transport. Again, we manufacture our own prolactin. Is it not likely that, as in the case of cholesterol, triglycerides and IGF-1, disease could be caused by consuming foods (especially in large quantities) in which *extra amounts* of this chemical is concentrated? Especially since this is a somewhat different version to that meant to be circulating in the human body.

Hence, at least one hormone – IGF-1 – contained in milk and the meat from slaughtered dairy cows has been shown to be a cancer promoter. There is evidence that prolactin and IGF-II are also cancer promoters. And these are only three of the many powerful biologically active chemicals in milk designed to influence development of the newborn of the same species.

Epidermal growth factor (EGF), which is also a mitogen (promoting cell division), also occurs in milk. It is well established that EGF stimulates the proliferation of epidermal and epithelial tissues.[71]

In 1998, some fascinating work was carried out at Yale University in the USA showing that breast tissues from patients with tumours contained closely associated deposits of calcium oxalate or of calcium phosphate.[72] It is these deposits which are detected by mammograms and indicate the presence of tumours. The deposits have different calcium to phosphorus ratios depending on where they occur in the breast. The mineral precipitates associated with tissues near the milk ducts in the breast have Ca:P ratios which are closely similar to those in human breast milk.

Does this suggest that breast tumour cells were trying to produce milk? Had they become malignant and cancerous because some chemicals were telling them to produce milk when other conditions were wrong so that the cells became confused, stressed and finally made mistakes in copying their own DNA (their own knitting pattern for cell function and behaviour)? Could not hormones and growth factors that are derived from food and are circulating in the blood, confuse the body's own hormone signalling system?

If breast tissue were frequently bathed in fluid with elevated levels of a growth factor used in nature to signal to females to develop breasts during puberty, and/or a hormone which is the main milk-supporting hormone in lactating animals, it is not surprising that cells make mistakes that can lead to cancer?

OESTROGEN

Officially, exposure to oestrogen continues to be considered one of the main risk factors for breast cancer, with testosterone similarly thought to affect prostate cancer. Oestrogen is involved in the changes that take place at puberty in girls, such as the growth and development of the vagina, uterus, and Fallopian tubes. It causes enlargement of the breasts through growth of ducts, stromal (supporting) tissue, and the accretion of fat. Oestrogen contributes to moulding of female body contours and maturation of the skeleton. It is responsible for the growth of axillary and pubic hair and pigmentation of the nipples and areolae.

The human menstrual cycle involves the monthly preparation of a specially thickened and blood-filled lining in preparation for possible pregnancy. The lining is shed as a vaginal flow of blood if pregnancy does not occur. This cycle of preparation and shedding occurs at approximately monthly intervals. This uterine cycle is under the control of ovarian-secreted hormones, oestrogen and progesterone.

Oestrogen (from 'oestrus' meaning heat or fertility) dominates the first week or so after menstruation, starting the build-up of the special lining of the womb as the ovarian follicles begin their development of a matured ovum. About twelve days after the beginning of the previous menstruation, the rising oestrogen (primarily oestradiol) level peaks and then tapers off just as the follicle with the egg matures and just before ovulation, when the egg is shed into the womb via the Fallopian tubes in preparation for fertilisation. Progesterone production, also by special bodies in the ovary, dominates the second half of the menstrual month. The rise of progesterone at the time of ovulation causes a rise of body temperature of about 1 degree Fahrenheit, a finding used to indicate ovulation. If pregnancy does not occur within ten to twelve days after ovulation, oestrogen and progesterone levels fall abruptly, triggering the shedding of the accumulated secretory lining of the womb and menstruation and the cycle begins again. If pregnancy occurs, progesterone production increases and shedding of endometrium is prevented, thus preserving the developing embryo. As pregnancy progresses, progesterone production is taken over by the placenta and its secretion increases gradually to much higher levels, especially during late pregnancy.

Thus, the monthly rise and fall of oestrogen and progesterone levels explains the events of menstruation and is in turn controlled by other hormones secreted by the master gland – the pituitary gland near the base of the brain.

The whole complex cycle is part of a bio-feedback information and control system, with multiple neural centres sharing and integrating many biochemical, hormonal, immunological and emotional conditions. The system functions as a giant analogue computer with the capacity to formulate and send chemical messages or hormones to the pituitary, as well as to control many other body functions, including our immune system and our emotional well-being. It is no wonder that menstruation (and a great number of other body functions) can be affected by diet, emotional states of mind, stress, other hormones, illness, or drugs of all sorts.

Progesterone and oestrogen are closely interrelated in many ways. Progesterone is a precursor of oestrogen. The three most important hormones of the oestrogen class are oestrone, oestradiol, and oestriol. In popular writing, however, each of the specific members of the class continues to be referred to as oestrogen. In the case of progesterone, only a single hormone is found. Thus, 'progesterone' is both the name of the class and of the single member of the class.

The word 'oestrogen' generally refers to the class of hormones produced by the body with somewhat similar oestrus-like actions. Phyto-oestrogens refer to plant compounds with oestrogen-like activity. The three main groups of dietary phyto-oestrogens are isoflavones (enriched in soya beans), coumestans (clover and alfalfa sprouts) and lignans (oil seeds such as flax seeds). Xeno-oestrogens (literally 'stranger oestrogens') refer to other man-made chemical compounds (usually derived from petrochemicals) with oestrogen-like activity. Some of the xeno-oestrogens are very potent oestrogenic compounds even at extremely small doses. They are discussed in the section on endocrine-disrupting chemicals in Chapter Six.

Because oestrone is generally synthesised first, it is referred to as E_1, oestradiol as E_2, and oestriol as E_3. (These hormones are given 'E' titles because, in America, oestrogen is spelt without the initial 'o'.) In non-pregnant women, E_1 and E_2 are produced by the ovary in relatively large quantities and E_3 is only a scant by-product of E_1 metabolism. Relative serum E_1 and E_2 levels are determined mainly by the activity of the liver, which can convert one into the other, resulting in higher levels of E_2.

During pregnancy, however, the placenta is the major source of oestrogens; E_3 is produced in higher quantities while E_1 and E_2 are produced in lesser amounts. The placenta also becomes the major source of progesterone, producing relatively large quantities, especially during late pregnancy. Oestriol (E_3) and progesterone are the major sex steroids (fat-based hormones) during pregnancy. Both oestriol and progesterone are essentially devoid of the ability to affect secondary sex characteristics and thus the sexual development of the foetus is determined solely by its own DNA and not the sex hormones of the mother.

Among the three oestrogens, oestradiol (E_2) is the most stimulating to the breast and oestriol (E_3) is the least; their relative ratio of activity being 1,000:1. Studies of two decades ago found oestradiol (and oestrone to a lesser extent) to increase one's risk of breast cancer, whereas oestriol is protective.[73]

Dairy milk does contain oestrogen (and testosterone) although it has been suggested that the levels are so low that cows' milk oestrogen is biologically insignificant.[74] Yet for some chemicals, even *very* low levels can cause severe biological damage (just remember what the tiny changes in our own hormones do to our breasts during the normal menstrual cycle, for example). One illustration of this was the problem caused by the effects of a chemical called tributyl tin on dog whelks on Britain's south coast. The chemical was developed for use in paint to coat the underside of ships to prevent 'fouling' or the growth of creatures such as barnacles that increase friction and thus slow down ships and boats. The levels of tributyl tin in water were only of the order of five parts in a millionth of a millionth of seawater and were barely detectable. Nevertheless, in the 1980s, over a wide area of Britain's south coast where minute traces of the chemical occurred female dog whelks died as a result of their egg tubes becoming blocked by their own eggs because they had developed male organs which had overgrown their female organs. It is difficult to comprehend that such an infinitesimal amount of a substance could, in the open sea, have such a profound effect: but it did. Unfortunately, the chemical is still licensed for use in larger ships including those used by the British Navy and the chemical is accumulating in some of our offshore sediments to levels well above those known to cause problems in vulnerable marine organisms.

According to Outwater and others, although oestrogens in milk may or may not exert a direct effect, they may stimulate expression of IGF-1 resulting in indirect long-term tumour growth.[75] Free oestrogens have been found in commercial pasteurised whole cows' milk and, although their levels are lower, they are still present in skimmed milk. These authors suggest that the correlation between oestrogen levels and milk fat may offer a partial explanation of why, in some epidemiological studies, breast cancer has been correlated with high fat diets containing dairy products. In a report published in June 2000 (Royal Society document 06/00), a list of factors that may have altered exposure to oestrogens in the latter half of the twentieth century includes increased consumption of dairy produce. The report also notes that dairy practices have changed over the same period, such that pregnant cows (which produce high levels of oestrogens) continue to be milked.

Let me finish by quoting from the final conclusions of the review paper by Outwater and others who studied the findings of about 130 peer-reviewed publications: 'The existing evidence indicates possible cancer risks associated with the consumption of dairy products. Bovine GH has not been considered to be of health concern because subsequent increase in bovine milk IGF-1 levels are within the 'normal range' based on untreated cows' and human breast milk. However, it is possible that the 'normal range' could be carcinogenic when milk is ingested regularly over a lifetime. Hormones and growth factors in milk, such as IGF-1, are consumed in nature by the fast-growing infant; it may be that regular milk ingestion after the age of weaning produces enough IGF-1 in mammary tissue to cause the cell cycle to supercede its boundaries of control, increasing the risk of cancer.'

This same point is also made by the EU Scientific Committee on Veterinary Measures Relating to Public Health.[76] They state 'The physiological actions of IGF-1 and IGF-II relate to growth and development of the embryo and fetus and to cellular differentiation, proliferation and cancer.' Is this not just a modern, high-technology way of saying what the Chinese have always known: that milk is just for babies?

IN SUMMARY

This chapter has presented you with a lot of scientific evidence drawn from peer-reviewed scientific papers published in reputable international scientific journals or from the findings of international panels of experts about the potential causes of breast (and prostate) cancer. Let me summarise what all this information means.

- A rational explanation of cause and effect has been found now for many types of cancer, following Professor Richard Doll's breakthrough in the 1950s, which showed the link between smoking tobacco and lung cancer. For many types of cancer, we know that the disease is caused or triggered by something we do or are exposed to, including industrial chemicals and viral or bacterial infections. Some members of the exposed population may be more likely to be affected because of their genetic make-up, but many cancers for which there is now a well-established rational cause, are related to lifestyle or environmental factors.

- The incidence of breast cancer in some Western countries, especially the eastern seaboard of the USA, which includes many ethnic groups and hence a mixed gene pool, is similar to that of the incidence of lung cancer among heavy smokers. *This strongly suggests that something is causing the disease and that the cause relates to something that the higher socio-economic groups in rich countries are doing.*

- Oriental communities have traditionally had exceptionally low rates of breast and prostate cancer (compared to Western countries). However, when oriental people move to live in the West their rates of breast and prostate cancer approach those of Western countries.

- The rates of breast and prostate cancer also increase when oriental people adopt a Western lifestyle in their own countries: in China the slang name for breast cancer translates as 'Rich Woman's Disease'. Typically oriental diets have included most of the things eaten in the West, including meat such as pork, chicken and duck (although in smaller quantities), but traditionally oriental diets have *not* included dairy products.

- The consumption of Western food including dairy products such as milk, ice cream and reprocessed dairy cow meat such as sausages and burgers, is increasing as countries such as Japan embrace 'development'. This process of Westernisation typically begins in urban centres. Breast and prostate cancer rates are increasing in these countries and as we have seen from the data in Chapter Three, breast and prostate cancer rates in oriental countries are significantly higher in urban areas than in rural ones.

- Modern genetic research and molecular protein studies indicate that in the case of breast cancer the damage to the cell, which causes the wrong chain of protein signals to be relayed causing the uncontrolled growth that is cancer, is at a superficial level in the cell (between the receptors and intercellular fluid) – not deep inside the cell as is the case in some other types of cancers.

- Only five to ten per cent of breast cancers are the result of inherited mutated (damaged) genes (BRCA-1 and BRCA-2), which are called tumour suppressor genes. These genes normally produce proteins to slow down cell growth. However, the disease does not always develop, even in those carrying the mutated gene. This observation and the fact that they are tumour suppressor genes suggests that even where people have inherited mutated genes their risk of cancer *can be reduced* if factors signalling to the cell to produce too much, or the wrong sorts of, growth factors are removed.

- Milk and the meat of dairy animals contain significant amounts of a growth factor called insulin-like growth factor-1, or IGF-1, and hormones such as prolactin.

- The levels of IGF-1 in milk have probably increased due to selective stock breeding and the adoption of high-yielding species for dairying.

- The use of the genetically engineered hormone rBGH, or BST, to increase milk yield is associated with IGF-1 levels in milk at the highest part of the normal range.

- IGF-1 and prolactin are known to promote the growth of breast and prostate cancer cells in laboratory cultures. This strongly suggests that they can do the same in humans, too, if they enter the bloodstream. Breast tissue has receptors for IGF-1, IGF-II and prolactin.

- Casein, the main milk protein, has been shown to protect growth hormones contained in milk from being broken down during digestion.

- Modern methods of processing milk (including, for instance, homogenisation) may further protect the cancer-promoting chemicals from breaking down in the gut, so that significant quantities are absorbed into the bloodstream. The direct effect of these chemicals on the digestive tract has been suggested by some scientists to cause colon cancer.

- Research on humans shows that premenopausal women with high levels of circulating IGF-1 have a higher risk of breast cancer, and men with high levels of this circulating growth factor are at greater risk of suffering from prostate cancer than those with lower levels.

I RECOMMEND

Overall, I find the evidence of a connection between dairy consumption and breast and prostate cancer compelling. It would, for example, explain the increase in breast and prostate cancer incidence with increasing age if, by consuming dairy produce on a daily basis, we are exposing breast and prostate tissue, which should be turning off or turned off, to growth factors and hormones designed to cause the tissue to grow and proliferate. In the first version of the book I wrote 'However, further research is needed to confirm the hypothesis. For example, studies are needed to show the extent to which those consuming dairy products and certain types of meat, especially if badly cooked, see page 201, have higher levels of free circulating IGF-1 in their blood than those consuming traditional Eastern diets. This should be carried out in experiments timed to follow consumption of suspect food types. Such research should be carried out by scientists working in independent organisations entirely free from commercial or political pressure.' Since then research published by the Cancer Epidemiology Unit at Oxford University[77] has shown that serum IGF-1 was 9 per cent lower in vegan men than in meat eaters (also thought to consume dairy produce) and milk-consuming vegetarians. Because Chan and co-workers[78] found that men who developed prostate cancer had 8 per cent higher serum IGF-1 concentrations than men who remained healthy, the new work from Oxford appears highly significant. I recommend that all women who wish to prevent or treat breast cancer and all men who wish to prevent or treat prostate cancer *totally eliminate all forms of dairy produce from cows, goats or any animal source from their diet*. The precautionary principle should be applied with the onus on the dairy industry to prove their product is safe. Also, I repeat that those with active cancer should try to base their diets on foods of vegetable rather than animal origin until they are better.

THE RISK WE RUN

I know that there will be many people who will read this book, or hear about its suggestions, and say that they have consumed dairy produce all their lives with no ill effect – just as there are people who point out that they or someone they know has smoked 40–60 cigarettes a day and lived to be 100. The problem is one of increasing risk to those in the population who, for genetic or other reasons, are more vulnerable. Risk is a difficult idea to explain. Many scientists who are specialists in risk (which is a concept based on probabilities) point out that no one would buy lottery tickets if they understood the subject, but human behaviour is based more on personal experience and emotions than mathematical concepts.

The best way of explaining cancer risk is perhaps the aeroplane analogy, which I use to try to persuade people to stop smoking. According to this example, you should think how you would feel if you were going to fly in an aeroplane and you knew with certainty that one out of every ten flights was going to crash. Would you fly? I don't think you would! Perhaps because they understand risk, very few scientists smoke.

I have never smoked and knowing that I am vulnerable to breast cancer I will no longer eat any dairy produce (including meat from animals used for dairying) in any form, at any time. I have lived without any dairy produce whatsoever in my diet for almost seven years. Since then, a large cancer in my neck that was thought to be incurable, shrivelled and disappeared and has not returned. My previously brittle nails are now long and strong, my skin is in excellent condition and I have no signs of osteoporosis. My hair is in excellent condition with very few grey hairs and most people think I am much younger than my 55 years. I feel fitter and healthier than ever before. This advice to give up dairy is similar to that given by Dr RM Kradjian, MD, the Chief of the Breast Surgery Division at the Seton Medical Center, Daly City, California, in his book, *Save Yourself from Breast Cancer*,[79] and in a letter entitled 'The Milk Letter: A Message to my Patients' (see http://www.afpafitness.com/milkdoc.htm).

I believe that I, and all those who have suffered from breast cancer but shared in my advice, have avoided death by dairy.

The update to this chapter can be found on page 321.

5 The Plant Programme – The Food Factors

In this chapter I explain the seven dietary factors to help you cut your risk of suffering from breast or prostate cancer.

First of all, let me say that The Plant Programme *isn't* a diet. Diets, as many of us know from personal experience, generally don't work. Diets aren't much fun to follow, and sooner or later, we slide back to our old ways.

Instead, The Plant Programme consists of seven Food Factors, and five Lifestyle Factors, which together I have used to overcome advanced breast cancer and which I continue to follow to keep myself cancer free against all the odds. The Plant Programme not only helps to prevent and overcome breast and prostate cancer, but is also protective against osteoporosis and other ills that are wrongly supposed to accompany a dairy-free diet. Together, these factors are quite easy to incorporate into your life: they should be seen as helping hands, not as severe dietary constraints.

The Plant Programme is not a general anti-cancer diet like those published previously, such as the Bristol and Gerson diets. As discussed earlier, cancers and their causes are different. The Programme that I describe here is targeted specifically at breast and prostate cancer and aims to eliminate or reduce chemicals in our food and from the environment that could disrupt our endocrine systems (the systems by which chemical messengers – especially hormones – regulate body function). The Programme is also designed to ensure that the body has available to it the chemicals such as iodine and zinc that it needs to maintain breast and prostate tissue in a healthy condition.

The main aims of the Programme are to:

- Reduce the intake of hormones, including growth factors, from food; and of man-made chemicals for which there is evidence or a suspicion of carcinogenicity, including endocrine-disrupting chemicals.

- Increase the proportion of food containing substances that are protective against cancer.
- Ensure that the body has adequate quantities of the key nutrients in a bioavailable form, so that at least a significant proportion can be absorbed by the body, especially nutrients such as zinc, iodine and folic acid which play a crucial role in cell division in the body (when the errors causing cancer are most likely to arise).
- Reduce the amount of free radicals in the body that are capable of damaging DNA.
- Give emphasis to food that is organically grown and as fresh as possible.
- Eliminate or reduce to a minimum food that has been refined, tinned, preserved or overcooked so that its content of fibre, vitamins, minerals, natural colours or other natural constituents have been removed or reduced. (For example, molasses contains fluoride which is protective against tooth decay, but in the refined white sugar prepared from molasses, fluoride and other nutrients have been removed so we have to add fluoride back into our toothpaste). The aim is to eat whole food that has not been tampered with by the food processing industry and which does not contain chemical preservatives. Chemical preservatives and other additives in lists of ingredients on food labels are usually denoted by E numbers or chemical names. For further details see *Secret Ingredients*, Peter Cox and Peggy Brusseau, Bantam 1998.
- Provide the nutrients to help your body withstand and recover from surgery, radiotherapy and chemotherapy. The tips to help with radiation therapy described here are based on treatment methods developed to help astronauts withstand irradiation while in space. Many drugs, including those used in chemotherapy, destroy vitamins; also stress means you need more vitamins and antibiotics can prevent them being absorbed.
- Provide maximum choice and variety so that healthy eating can be maintained.
- Provide a varied diet without undue reliance on any one component.

BASED ON GOOD SCIENCE

It is acknowledged by such authorities as the British Department of Health and the United States Food and Drug Administration, as well as cancer specialists at Harvard University in the USA and Oxford University in Britain, that diet accounts for at least 30 per cent of all cancers. According to the Mayo Foundation for Medication Education and Research in the USA, individuals who eat five servings of fruit and vegetables (including cruciferous vegetables, that is, plants whose four petal flowers resemble a cross – e.g. pak choi, broccoli, Brussels sprouts, cauliflower, cabbage, kale, kohlrabi and watercress) a day cut their risk of cancer by half when compared to those consuming one serving or less. In Britain, official Government advice now recommends that we eat at least five portions of fruit and vegetables a day and, following the pioneering work of Michael B Sporn, Professor of Pharmacology and Medicine, Dartmouth Medical College, USA, it is now widely acknowledged that plants contain many anti-cancer chemicals, the most important of which are described in the following pages.[1]

No intelligent doctor, therefore, should object to any of the scientifically-based recommendations of The Plant Programme. So why is it that when you mention using diet as part of your treatment for cancer, there is normally such a negative or, at best, lukewarm response from orthodox doctors?

I think there are several reasons. First, some people use such extreme diets that they become undernourished at a time when they need all their strength. Frequently, this is because they have been to a type of alternative health practitioner who has recommended a diet typically eliminating red meat and wheat products and processed food containing salt and sugar along with tea, coffee and alcohol. At the same time they are told to consume large quantities of fruit – often grapefruit – to 'detoxify' the body, together with some vegetables, the list of which varies according to the practitioner. The diet recommended may be poorly balanced and not nutritious, with too few available nutrients. To make up for these deficiencies, synthetic vitamin and mineral supplements (sometimes the practitioner's own label marketed at excessive prices) are recommended. Sometimes, the diets are developed by asking patients to hold or even think about a piece of food. Their muscle strength is then tested by pushing against the arm of the practitioner to determine their 'food allergies'. Some of my friends with a range of illnesses have ended up with the most ridiculous diets as a result. Often, when they have become undernourished or even more ill, a husband or family member has asked me to intervene. I have to say that I regard this method of developing a diet as complete mumbo jumbo – certainly, I can see no scientific basis in it whatsoever.

There are other alternative 'health practitioners' who use methods that are ill-founded. For example, I remember talking to a homoeopath that I met at Charing Cross Hospital (she did not work there) who was visiting a patient with stomach cancer whom she was 'treating' with ground up granite. She was doing this on the basis that rates of stomach cancer are high in Wales where the rocks are granite. Hence, she argued, small quantities of ground up granite would help the patient to ward off its effects in causing cancer. The homoeopath was somewhat abashed when I pointed out to her that there is almost no granite in Wales and certainly not in the area where the rate of stomach cancer is high. I even brought the geological map of Wales into the clinic to prove the point! I hope her patient's health was not made too much worse by her ministrations. I was also concerned to learn that some homoeopaths prescribe preparations of radioactive salts such as radium bromide to prevent the side effects of radiotherapy. Even if these chemicals are highly diluted the use of such preparations goes against all my scientific training, which seeks always to minimise exposure to radioactive substances.

But it's not only uninformed alternative health practitioners who sometimes give advice that is cause for concern. Several anti-breast-cancer books published recently also contain dubious advice. For example, one book implies that having more children at a younger age and breast feeding them would protect against breast cancer. The suggestion that childbirth *protects* against breast cancer goes back to the observation that nuns in Italy suffered high levels of the disease. However, this observation doesn't prove that pregnancy and lactation can shield you from breast cancer, any more than celibacy might increase your risk. It is important to remember that many convents and monasteries housed very well-fed people: my speculation is that the nuns affected were consuming a rich diet containing lots of dairy produce (and meat). In any case, I can find no evidence that statistical tests were carried out to see whether or not their rates of breast cancer were higher or lower than those of their host community. As discussed previously, modern statistical evidence suggests that being childless or postponing childbearing until later in life may increase risks *slightly*; but this could be just another index of women following a Western lifestyle and diet, since career women in particular tend to delay child bearing.

The strongest evidence on the cause of breast and prostate cancer suggests it is linked to our consumption of dairy food – which is not designed for adult humans and which we have not evolved to eat – especially now it is produced by intensive industrialised methods. Also, our intake of pollutants, including endocrine-disrupting chemicals from the environment – many of which are fat-soluble and accumulate up the food chain – become particularly concentrated in milk. Growing population pressure is one of the drivers of the industrialisation of agriculture and chemical pollution. Hence, increasing pregnancy rates would exacerbate, not alleviate, the burden of breast and prostate cancer for society as a whole.

Nor do I think that the factors such as using mobile phones, deodorants or wearing incorrectly fitting bras cause breast cancer. Breast cancer has been a feature of Western societies long before these relatively modern inventions. Clearly we should not wear bras that are too small to the extent that they stop circulation, but do women, especially middle-class women, really go around wearing such tight bras? The idea that we should all buy new bras may be good for bra sales but I suggest it has little to do with breast cancer. Mobile phones may be implicated in causing problems with the head and brain although existing research is inconclusive, but breast cancer rates had been rising for a long time before the use of mobile phones. In one recent article in the Canadian press, a group of women made the case for breast cancer being caused by their working in an office equipped with computers and other electronic equipment. The main advocate of this idea is pictured drinking a large milkshake! In the case of the contraceptive pill, young women taking it do not have an appreciably increased risk of breast cancer. Any small increase in relative risk disappears ten years after they stop using it. There is, however, evidence of increased numbers of breast cancer cases in women who have used 'the pill' until their early 40s.[2]

Many anti-breast-cancer diets which appear in magazines seem to have no scientific basis or even logic. For example, in a magazine published recently by a health food shop, the same article that promotes the use of soya as part of an anti-breast-cancer diet recommends *against* chick peas and lentils. Did the author not know that these foods are all legumes and contain similar isoflavone chemicals? Moreover, the same author includes soya, oat and rice milk under the heading of dairy products along with goat's milk! A national newspaper recently published a serialisation of an anti-breast-cancer diet book which claimed that parsnips, potatoes, broad beans, pumpkins, honey, watermelon, pineapple, couscous and muesli (all of which I believe to be good foods and of which I eat masses) increase the risk of breast cancer because they stimulate 'excess insulin' production. These foods were lumped together with processed foods such as commercial, refined breakfast cereals, chocolate bars and jelly beans! This is certainly advice I shall choose to ignore. Yet another recent breast cancer diet book enthusiastically recommended consuming live yoghurt as a chemo-preventive food – again, with no scientific basis. A recent article on bowel cancer in a magazine which is linked to several cancer charities advocated consuming 'high calcium foods, i.e. dairy produce (choose low fat cheese and semi-skimmed milk), which are thought to help protect you'. Calcium has been shown to be a factor in bowel cancer, but in the context of malnutrition.[3] And of course, it can be obtained from sources much healthier than dairy (*see* pp. 135–136). No wonder people are confused about healthy eating.

Most other recent anti-cancer diets are based on the principles first set out in the Max Gerson diet published in 1953. Dr Gerson's basic precept was that cancer is a symptom of a diseased body in which the organs – especially the liver – are out of balance. So he reasoned that most animal products, salt and caffeine should be banned to take the pressure off the liver and immune system, and the body should be detoxified and rebalanced using organic fruit and vegetables in order to cure cancer. In his book entitled *A Cancer Therapy* the following substances are forbidden: tobacco, salt, sharp spices, tea, coffee, cocoa, chocolate, alcohol, refined sugar, refined flour, candies, ice cream, cream, cake, nuts, mushrooms, all soy products, pickles, pineapples, berries, avocados and cucumbers, water (you are supposed to drink only fresh juices), canned, preserved or sulphured food, smoked or salted vegetables, dehydrated or bottled juices, all fats, oils, salt substitutes and all sources of fluoride. Butter, cheese, fish, meat, eggs and milk were forbidden during initial treatment although confusingly, cottage cheese, buttermilk and yoghurt are mentioned in the specific section on cancer therapy and are included in the sample menus. Unfortunately, Gerson also recommended raw calves' liver juice as a source of nutrients (not recommended in the post-BSE era) and the use of coffee and castor oil enemas. Gerson published his diet well before the level of industrialisation of agriculture of the present time, but he foresaw the dangers of degrading our environment, particularly of depleting soils of nutrients and polluting them with chemicals.

Gerson's regimen as a treatment for cancer is outlawed in most American states, which his daughter Charlotte blames on 'the lucrative drug industry'.[4] The Gerson method is rigorous, lengthy, time-consuming, demands absolute commitment and includes preparing and immediately drinking fresh organic juices every hour (twelve times a day). Many British doctors are sceptical about the value of the Gerson method. Dr Slavin of St Bartholomew's Hospital, London is quoted in *The Times*, 2 November 1999 as saying 'I would like to say I had seen improvement in even one patient I know of who has taken the therapy, but I have not.' Nevertheless many people do attest to the Gerson method having worked for them although such cases are generally dismissed by doctors as 'anecdotal'.

The Gerson diet was my starting point but I have made many modifications including removing some 'allowed foods' and encouraging the consumption of some 'forbidden' foods such as soya products and berries based on modern scientific research findings in order to develop a diet specific for breast and prostate cancer. I have also eliminated suggestions for which I can find no scientific basis especially those which make the diet unnecessarily difficult to follow and keep to. The Bristol diet developed by Dr Alec Forbes is based on principles similar to those of the Gerson diet to which Dr Forbes refers, but there are variations in the list of good and bad foods and a star system is used to indicate the proportion of foods to be consumed and a black dot system to indicate those which should be avoided. As indicated earlier, following the Bristol diet did not help me (please see Author's Note, page viii).

One of the main reasons that many Western doctors find it difficult to accept diet as part of cancer treatment is that they are trained to administer chemicals which are pure substances in measurable doses with a defined (stoichiometric) formula. The chemicals have usually been tested on cultures, animals and finally humans using statistically designed studies. We have all seen old movies, especially Westerns, where some charlatan or quack is peddling a cure for something which is just a way of making money. Modern clinical medicine is designed to prevent this type of thing happening. Nevertheless, many Western doctors could be given better training in the nutritional and environmental factors that can promote disease. In the case of breast and prostate cancer such an understanding is essential if diets are to be used in the same way as they are in treating coronary heart disease or diabetes, for example. I believe that the Programme described here provides a sound basis to help doctors and other health professionals to help their patients. I used it to recover from what would otherwise have been terminal breast cancer and observed on a day-to-day basis the effect it had on a large visible cancer in my neck. The Programme also helped prevent any hair loss during chemotherapy. I have lived on the Programme for seven years with no sign of under-nourishment despite what many people would describe as a punishing work schedule with lots of responsibility and long hours of work and international travel. On the contrary, most people think I look very healthy and that I am much younger than my fifty-six years. I have not had a day's serious illness since my treatment for cancer ended. Indeed many irritating problems which had troubled me for years such as cold sores, throat infections, thrush or candida, brittle nails which often had infections around their base and recurrent cystitis have all cleared up. Also since adopting the Plant Programme my rate of tooth decay has decreased markedly. I have given the diet to 63 women, all of whom remain cancer free. These women range from the 70-year-old mother of a Canadian friend, with advanced breast cancer which had spread to her bones; to a young English woman whose breast cancer was diagnosed when she was breast-feeding her first baby. The five women who refused to use it or 'cheated' have all sadly had recurrences or have died.

Undoubtedly, the best anti-cancer diet would be completely vegan and I was living on a completely vegan diet at the time my cancer disappeared and for about eight months afterwards. If you can become a vegan (someone who lives entirely on food of plant origin) – so much the better, but you must ensure you don't become deficient in essential nutrients such as zinc and selenium and vitamins such as D and B12. However, do not confuse being vegan with becoming a vegetarian. Vegetarians sometimes consume far more dairy produce (to replace meat) than other members of society and some processed, pre-packaged vegetarian foods can have particularly high contents of dairy produce. If you want to reduce your risk of breast (or prostate) cancer become a vegan **but on no account become a dairy-eating vegetarian**. If any anti-cancer diet includes any dairy produce of any kind, ignore it.

For a long time many middle-class women I know have been substituting cottage cheese and yoghurt for red meat in their diet, partly influenced by health and lifestyle magazines and partly by animal rights activists such as Linda McCartney, who recently died of breast cancer. For many busy women, eating yoghurt or cheese is simpler and therefore less time consuming than creating balanced vegan meals to reduce meat consumption and I suspect an overall increase in dairy consumption has been the result.

Many women have been persuaded they need to consume dairy products for the calcium they contain – especially to ward off osteoporosis, a skeletal disorder of progressive bone mass loss and demineralisation causing increased risk of fracture. Milk and milk products do indeed contain significant amounts of calcium, but calcium is most definitely not synonymous with dairy. In any case, ingesting large quantities of calcium does not, in itself, seem to eliminate bone loss:

- A 1987 Mayo Clinic study, which examined dietary calcium intake and actual rates of bone loss in women, determined that 'these data do not support the hypothesis that insufficient dietary calcium is a major cause of bone loss in women'.[5]
- Many populations with high intakes of calcium also have high rates of osteoporosis.[6]
- The Inuit, for example, consume twice the amount of calcium found in the average Western diet (about 2,000mg

daily). This does not prevent them from suffering from high rates of osteoporosis, and it has been estimated that compared to US Caucasians, the Inuit have an average of 10 to 15 per cent less bone mass. This is probably due to the Inuit's considerable intake of protein (250 to 400 grams daily) from fish, whale and walrus.[7]

- On the other hand, Bantus living in Africa on low-calcium (400mg daily) and low-protein vegetable diets (47 grams daily) are essentially free of osteoporosis.[8]

The World Health Organisation confirms that countries which have relatively low intakes of calcium do not have an increased incidence of osteoporosis. Indeed, they note the suggestion that dietary calcium levels not too different from those proposed to prevent osteoporosis can cause a number of adverse biological effects.[9] The British Government's own nutritional advisory panel confirms this paradox: 'Several populations of the world consume calcium at levels lower than the current RDA for the UK yet show no evidence of adverse effects.'[10] Careful scientific studies into calcium absorption (using radioactive labelling techniques) have shown that only 18 to 36 per cent of the calcium in milk is taken up by the body.[11] This is taken into account by the authorities responsible for setting recommended nutrient intakes, who generally assume that something in the range of 20 to 40 per cent of the diet's calcium content is actually absorbed, and therefore have to build a 'safety factor' for this into their figures.

Some nutrition textbooks, perhaps without always checking to see if the effect is more theoretical than real, argue that certain plants contain chemicals which bind with calcium in the gut so that only a small proportion is absorbed. The American Dietetic Association comments on this question: 'Calcium absorption appears to be inhibited by such plant constituents as phytic acid, oxalic acid and fibre, but this effect may not be significant. Calcium deficiency in vegetarians is rare and there is little evidence to show that low intakes of calcium give rise to major health problems among the vegetarian population.'[12] Dr Neal Barnard, president of the Physicians Committee for Responsible Medicine, summarises the evidence thus: 'The amount of calcium in your bones is very carefully regulated by hormones. Increasing your calcium intake does not fool those

Table 3 Age	Calcium intake requirement (mg)
Normal adult	800
Adolescent growth	1100
Pregnancy	1000
Lactation	1200
Elderly with HRT	1000
Elderly without HRT	1500

hormones into building more bone, any more than delivering an extra load of bricks will make a construction crew build a larger building. . . . For the vast majority of people, the answer is not boosting your calcium intake, but rather, limiting calcium loss.'[13]

The wisdom of these words contrasts with the prevailing recommendations of other authorities. Currently, the adult recommended daily intake for calcium is about 700 milligrams a day. Yet a recent experts' conference on osteoporosis in Virginia, USA put the recommended level as high as 1,500mg per day for women,[14] and a British symposium on osteoporosis has proposed the following intakes for women (Table 3 above).

At the upper level, an intake of 1,500mg of calcium a day would have to be supplied by nearly half a pound of hard cheese, four cartons of yogurt or five cups of milk!

Many plants contain large quantities of calcium. Good non-dairy sources of calcium are: dark green leafy vegetables (such as kale, collards, turnip greens and broccoli). One study shows that 27 per cent of the calcium in watercress can be absorbed. Another study has demonstrated that calcium absorbability is actually higher for kale than for milk, and concludes: 'greens such as kale can be considered to be at least as good as milk in terms of their calcium absorbability'.[15] Other calcium-rich vegetables include: artichokes, cabbage, carrot, celery, celeriac, chick peas, chinese leaves, chives, cress, dandelion leaves, fennel, french beans, horseradish, leeks, onions, parsley, parsnip and spinach, although the exact quantities they contain vary. The fruits that are richest in calcium include: rosehips, raspberries, oranges, kiwi, figs, blackcurrants and blackberries.

Other good sources are: almonds, tofu, soya flour, haricot beans, oatmeal and wholemeal flour, pumpkin, sesame and sunflower seeds, seaweed and dried fruit. Using soya produce provides calcium and magnesium together with iron and in a better balance than milk. Moreover, some soya milk has calcium added to it. Houmous (made from chick peas and sesame) is also a rich source of calcium. Some beers also contain concentrations of calcium – many breweries, for example those of Burton-on-Trent, were set up in areas where the level of gypsum, the most soluble bioavailable form of mineral calcium, is naturally high in the water used for brewing. Other beers are rich in magnesium and phosphorus.

Of equal importance is the need to reduce calcium loss from your body. Here are some points to remember:

- A diet high in animal-based proteins increases the amount of acid in the body. This triggers a buffering mechanism, which releases stored calcium from the bones. The body would normally reabsorb the calcium released, but the animal protein inhibits the parathyroid function that controls this reabsorption. The body then excretes the calcium, causing bone loss. One researcher who put this theory to the test concluded: 'This study suggests that a diet higher in vegetable protein might actually be somewhat protective against osteoporosis'.[16]
- Reduce caffeine consumption. A study of women aged 36 to 45 found that those who drank two cups of coffee a day suffered a net calcium loss of 22 milligrams daily. Reducing this to one cup daily reduced the loss to just 6 milligrams daily.[17]
- Reduce alcohol consumption. Alcohol speeds bone loss because it interferes with the way your body absorbs calcium. When you drink, drink mainly beer as many beers contain high levels of calcium and have lower alcohol contents than most alcoholic drinks.
- Get some sun. Sunlight reacts with dehydrocholesterol in your skin to produce vitamin D, which is essential to the proper absorption of calcium and a deficiency will cause you to lose bone mass.
- Magnesium works with other vitamins and minerals, including calcium, to promote bone growth and the healthy

functioning of nerves and muscle tissue. A deficiency of magnesium can affect the manufacture of vitamin D, so it is important in preventing osteoporosis. Magnesium is a constituent of chlorophyll and so is abundant in green vegetables. Other excellent sources are whole grains, wheat germ, molasses, seeds and nuts, apples and figs.

- The trace mineral boron helps to prevent calcium loss, and is thought to help in the manufacture of vitamin D in the body. Foods naturally rich in boron are easily obtained and include most fruits, particularly apples, berries, grapes, pears, prunes, dates, raisins, tomatoes, almonds, peanuts and hazelnuts.
- Get some exercise. Weight-bearing exercise is also important in building and maintaining bones of integrity.
- Above all, increase your intake of phyto-oestrogens and phyto-progesterones by following the Programme described below.

Below are the seven Food Factors which, together with the five Lifestyle Factors discussed in Chapter Six, comprise The Plant Programme. If you are using The Plant Programme to prevent cancer I suggest that you incorporate the factors into your life at your own pace, proceeding from one to the next as you feel ready and able to do so. If you have active cancer, I suggest you should try to make all of the adjustments as quickly as possible. Before you begin, it is worth making the general point that adding good foods that contain anti-cancer agents to a diet that continues to include other potentially harmful components will not, in my experience, help. For this reason and as explained fully in Food Factor Two, below, I recommend that all the foodstuffs you consume should, as much as possible, be organically produced.

FOOD FACTOR #1: FULL OF BEANS

One of the first and most essential things you can do to reduce your risk of breast cancer and probably prostate cancer is to substitute soya products for dairy products (whether from cows, sheep, goats or other animals) in your diet. Replace milk with soya milk and cheese with tofu and use soya ice cream (or water ices or sorbets) instead of dairy ice cream. There are no half measures here and as discussed previously, using skimmed milk or low fat yoghurt is irrelevant and will not help to reduce your risk of breast cancer or your recovery from the disease, because some of the most likely cancer-causing agents are proteins not fats. Indeed, recent research suggests that any protective factors against breast cancer contained in milk are likely to be in the fat not the protein. Conjugated linoleic acid (CLA) which is created by bacteria in the stomachs of cattle and which is found in milk fat has been suggested to inhibit the growth of cancer. Hence removing fat from milk could make the risk of cancer from consuming dairy products *worse*. Work at Utah University in the USA is aimed at increasing the CLA levels of milk but, of course, it will not increase the CLA content of skimmed milk. However, as discussed in Chapter Six, man-made endocrine-disrupting chemicals are concentrated in the fat.

All dairy produce should be avoided and replaced by soya products. By making this group of changes to your diet you will immediately and dramatically reduce your body's exposure to a powerful cocktail of hormones shown in experiment after experiment to promote breast and prostate cancer cell growth in cultures and/or experimental animals. You will also be reducing your exposure to antibiotic residues and other powerful biologically active chemicals (including man-made endocrine-disrupting chemicals, which can become particularly concentrated in milk – *see* Chapter Six). You will be reducing your cholesterol and triglyceride intake with great benefits for your heart and circulatory system thereby helping to deliver anti-cancer agents derived from plants (*see* Food Factor #2) to the site of the tumour faster and more effectively. And you will reduce the possibility of developing thrombosis. Patients undergoing chemotherapy for breast cancer are especially susceptible to this. For example, the risk of thrombosis increased five-fold in a group receiving cyclophosphamide methotrexate and 5-fluorouacil, precisely the treatment I was given.[18]

Recent dietary studies into the effects of exchanging soya for animal products indicate a reduction in cholesterol levels of more than 20 per cent. Moreover, it is the levels of the 'bad' cholesterol – low-density lipo-proteins or LDLs – which are reduced. However, simply adding soya to a typical Western diet may not be sufficient to counteract high plasma cholesterol and platelet aggregation.[19] You must replace – not supplement – dairy with soya produce to achieve the benefits. Remember that soya also contains plant oestrogens which protect the breast in the same way that Tamoxifen does and one of the plant oestrogens – genistein – seems to prevent cancer through multiple mechanisms: not only is it phyto-oestrogenic, it is anti-angiogenic too, meaning that it actually prevents tumours from developing their own blood supply.[20] It is also a powerful antioxidant, increasing the activities of protective anti-oxidative enzymes in various organs with an important role in the removal of free radicals and, in particular, oxygen radicals which have been particularly implicated in cancer. The vast majority of experimental studies into soya and cancer have shown that soya beans and soya products prevent the growth of a range of cancer cells.[21]

There is only one problem with buying soya now: it has often been genetically modified. One of the reasons this has been done is so that it can withstand being treated with pesticides including herbicides to destroy insects and weeds. So read labels carefully and buy only organically grown soya.

The soya bean is one of the most nutritious vegetables known. It is said that the soya bean was a gift to all generations of mankind from the sages and wise rulers of China. When the very first specimens of the soya bean reached the West, at the end of the eighteenth century, their arrival coincided with the dawn of the industrial revolution. So it was the industrial uses of the soya bean that captivated the entrepreneurial minds of those who came to inspect the first specimens grown in London's Royal Botanic Gardens. Consequently, the first commercial use for the soya bean was as a source of oil to be used in the manufacture of soap, and the remains of the bean, after the oil had been extracted, were fed to cattle. This pattern of usage, so different from that in Asia, is at last beginning to change as more and more people appreciate the extraordinary health-giving properties of soya.

The soya bean is an environmentally-friendly crop, too. One acre of land cultivated by conventional Western agricultural practices will feed an average adult for 77 days if it is used to raise beef. This may seem impressive, until you learn that the same acre can feed an adult for 527 days when it is devoted to growing wheat. However, if soya beans are grown on the same land, then it will yield enough protein to feed a person for over six years! This phenomenal productivity is caused in part by the ability of the soya bean, which is a legume, to fix atmospheric nitrogen into the soil through the action of bacteria on its roots. The protein content of the bean when harvested is about 40 per cent, which rises to 50 per cent after it has been processed. Soya also contains a full range of proteins whereas other plant foods contain only some. Hence vegans depend on combining cereals and pulses to obtain the full range of twenty amino acids necessary for good nutrition. The traditional Jamaican dish of rice and peas, of which I eat a lot when I work there, is a good example. It is delicious.

Most of us are familiar with soya milk, which can be purchased from all supermarkets. However, that's just the tip of the iceberg: there are many other traditional soya products which you will enjoy discovering and experimenting with. Let me introduce you to some of them.

Tofu or fromage de soja (soya cheese) as it is known in France, is made from soya beans (you can make it yourself at home quite easily). It has a higher percentage of protein than any other natural food in existence, is very low in saturated fats and is entirely cholesterol free; at the same time it is inexpensive. It has been a staple food for millions of people in Asia for over four thousand years. Tofu is very good for everyone, from very young children to the elderly because it is so full of good nutrients, so low in bad nutrients and it can be easily digested. In their book *New Tofu Recipes* Christopher and Jean Conil suggest that puréed carrots and leeks with tofu can be used as a nutritious, easily digested food for babies and invalids. Also, for those short of time tofu requires no lengthy cooking and it can be simply stir fried or simmered in soup. It is made by precipitating soya milk, normally using calcium or magnesium sulphates so it is also high in some of the most bioavailable forms of calcium or magnesium. In their classical treatise on the subject, William Shurtleff and Akiko Aoyagi explain its revered status:

Along with rice, wheat, barley and millet, soya beans were included among China's venerated *nuku* or five sacred grains, as early as the beginning of the Christian era . . . the sense of the sacredness of soya bean foods is still alive in Japan today; here the words tofu, miso and shoyu are commonly preceded in everyday speech by the honorific prefix 'O'. Rather than saying tofu, most people say 'O – tofu', meaning honourable tofu. Today, the soya bean has become the king of the Japanese kitchen. Indeed, the arrival of tofu, miso and shoyu in Japan initiated a revolution in the national cuisine. Now when Japanese connoisseurs speak of these foods, they use many of the same terms we employ when evaluating cheeses or wines; traditional tofu masters often say that the consummation of their art is but to evoke the fine flavours latent in the soya bean. And when the new crop of soya beans arrives at tofu shops late each autumn, ardent devotees sample the first tofu with the discrimination and relish of French vintners.[22]

In fact the Chinese Emperor, Shang Nung made the soya plant one of the five holy cultivated sources of protein in his celestial empire in 2838 BC.

Commercially, tofu is available in either 'silken' form (suitable for making low fat, high protein dressings and sauces) and firm, which can be utilised in an infinite number of ways: scrambled, marinated, smoked, barbecued, crumbled into salads, in burgers, sandwiches and soups, or even used in a dessert. Start to use it, and you'll be dazzled by its potential! Tofu may not taste good to you on its own but as described in *New Tofu Recipes* by Christopher and Jean Conil 'It has magical properties of absorbing almost any flavour or colour and so can be introduced in a wide range of dishes.' There are many ways to flavour tofu. I usually use a base or marinade of miso, garlic, ginger and onion for savoury dishes. Tofu also works well with onion and celery and is ideal as a replacement for dairy cream or milk in many potato dishes. It can also be liquidised with a wide range of fresh or dried fruit previously soaked in juice to which honey has been added to make delicious sweets and puddings, to replace yoghurt or ice cream, for example.

Tempeh (pronounced 'tem-pay') is a fermented soya bean product, made in the traditional manner for centuries throughout Indonesia where it is a basic food for millions of people. You can buy it in every health-food shop and a growing number of supermarkets. Like cheese, yoghurt and ginger beer, it is made with a cultured 'starter'. It is highly digestible, smells like fresh mushrooms and tastes remarkably similar to chicken or veal cutlets. Since the protein in tempeh is partially broken down during fermentation (the mould is called rhizopusoligosporus) it is a particularly suitable food for young children and older people. Tempeh is typically sold in six-inch squares which are approximately one inch thick. The easiest way to serve it is to cut the square into half diagonally, and then cut each half into three thinner, wedge-shaped slices. These should then be pan fried until crisp and golden brown on both sides, and then served with rice and a selection of vegetables. Shoyu or tamari sprinkled over the top will give it a little extra flavouring; alternatively, mix with lemon juice for a truly sensational marinade.

Miso is a fermented mixture of soya beans, and other cereal grain, such as rice or barley, and is paste-like in appearance and texture. It is an important component of oriental-based macrobiotic diets. It has subtle, aromatic flavours and comes in many different colours including orange, brown and yellow. It is one of the staples of every Japanese and Chinese kitchen, it is made by inoculating the basic ingredients with a mould (*koji*) and is then aged in cedarwood kegs for at least one year. It is most commonly used as an ingredient in soups, sauces, dressings, spreads, casseroles and other vegetable dishes. The miso industry is among the largest food industries in Japan today, and synthetic misos, which would include various colourings and additives, are quite widely available. Buy only traditionally made miso since it is not only free of additives, but the complex fermentation process produces a wealth of substances such as enzymes and beneficial bacteria which have a positive effect upon human health. Also buy only good reputable brands of miso because fermentation in unhygienic conditions can cause high concentrations of the micro-organisms thought to be responsible for stomach cancer to occur in foods. I buy miso only in waxed cartons, never in plastic (*see* p. 201). The valuable mineral nutrients in miso and other cereals are far more accessible to the body after fermentation than in raw cereals. (The banning of fermentation of cereals by well-meaning missionaries trying to prevent alcohol consumption is one of the contributors to malnutrition in grain-based societies in Africa today.) In Japan, miso is commonly respected as a food that is also a medicine. The various types of miso include:

- Hacho miso – soya bean miso, the heartiest and thickest of all, having a rich, almost chocolate-like flavour.

- Mugi miso – barley miso, made with a combination of soya beans and barley, a mellow-tasting miso whose colour can range from almost white through yellow to red.
- Kome miso – rice miso, made from a combination of soya beans, rice and sea salt, the most commonly consumed in Japan, with a light and almost sweet taste.

A simple miso soup can be made by lightly sautéing a selection of sliced vegetables (onions, leeks, turnips, potatoes) in a small amount of oil. Water is then added, and the vegetables slowly simmered for about half an hour. Finally, turn off the heat, and add a good dollop of miso to flavour. Add a strip of kombu or wakame seaweed before serving. On no account should the soup be boiled with the miso in it, because this will destroy many of the beneficial, health-giving substances including vitamins which live miso contains, while boiling the seaweed would drive off the iodine.

Soy Sauce This is an ancient and traditional Japanese seasoning which has achieved prominence and acceptance the world over. It is a dark, rich sauce with a savoury, salty taste as well as a deep, mellowing background flavour. Very little is required within a dish or serving. There are three types:

The first is the commercial, accelerated production type which is widely available and usually sold as soy sauce. It is made in a very short time by speeding the process of fermentation using chemical additives. It usually contains colourings and preservatives as well. I do not recommend this.

The second is called shoyu and is made by fermenting wheat and soya beans together for at least three years. During this time, the flavour develops making it a delicious addition to most savoury meals; the amino acids present in the ferment aid digestion. It is easy to find in health-food, macrobiotic or Japanese grocery shops.

The third is tamari which is made by fermenting just soya beans and salt over a long period of time, between two and three years. It is less widely available than shoyu as, traditionally, much less of it is made. It is not used so often in cooking or as a table condiment as shoyu as its flavour is much stronger.

Both shoyu and tamari are fermented with koji, a mould which grows at the temperature of the human body and which develops enzymes helpful in the digestion of proteins and starches, similar to those found in our saliva.

Natto Though less readily available than tempeh at the moment, natto can generally be found in Chinese or Japanese grocery stores. Like tempeh, it is made by fermenting soya beans, but in this case, for less than 24 hours. It has an intriguing gossamer-like quality, and is one of the most unusual foods you will ever eat. The fermentation process makes the high quality protein of the soya beans particularly easy to digest. Serve natto in a small bowl beside a serving of freshly steamed rice, stir-fried vegetables and your favourite dipping sauce.

FROM DAIRY TO SOYA

Good soya and tofu products are widely available not only in specialist health-food shops but also in supermarkets so there is no difficulty in buying them. Since there are so many different types and flavours, it is worth experimenting until you find the flavours you enjoy. As described above, I also use tofu to make delicious puddings and ice cream or yoghurt substitutes based on whisking or liquidising tofu with fruit and honey. Your brain will adapt to the change in taste quickly and you will soon find you do not want to go back to dairy produce. Even the smell of milk is nauseating to me now – it smells of cows udders! It reminds me of when I gave up taking sugar in tea. Before I did it, I thought the tea would taste horrible without sugar but within a week of giving it up I found tea with sugar tasted disgusting, and tea with sugar and milk: Ugh!

So what about yoghurt and all those healthy lactobacillus acidophilus bacteria it contains which are so good for us? There is evidence that taking these bacteria increases immunity, prevents infections and increases vitamin production. Actually, giving up dairy products doesn't mean that you have to sacrifice acidophilus, because it is easy to buy capsules of the bacteria and put them in soya milk or other cold drinks. Hence you have the health benefits of the bacteria without the risk that consuming dairy products carries. Moreover, following The Plant Programme will favour the growth and survival of these helpful bacteria in the digestive tract.

It is also worth remembering that soya contains phyto-oestrogens and steroids that are progestogenic and can prevent menopausal symptoms. I carry a small jar of dried soya (WySoy) or a small soya milkshake with me everywhere I go – otherwise within a few hours of not taking it I have appalling hot flushes. I have helped many friends with their menopausal problems by persuading them to drink soya milk and they are all amazed to find out how easy it is to eliminate hot flushes within days.

If you do only one thing to cut your risk of breast cancer (and I believe also prostate cancer), please make the change from dairy to soya products. Remember that soya products reduce breast cancer in laboratory experiments, while milk and the growth factors and hormones it contains have been shown in experiment after experiment to promote the growth of breast and prostate cancer cells. Of the people who have followed my Programme, only those who have 'cheated' on this aspect have ever had a return of breast cancer. When I asked one of my friends – who has recently had to have her second breast removed and now faces six months of chemotherapy – if she had kept to my diet (because if it does not work I do not want to give people false hope) she said 'well I just couldn't resist cheese and I am sure yoghurt is good for you – everyone says it is'.

There is one concern about eating food full of phyto-oestrogen that some men have expressed to me: that is that eating the phyto-oestrogens in soya will feminise them. Despite exhaustive studies, there is no evidence of this.[23] Moreover a lack of male potency and reproductive capacity does not appear to have been a problem in China or other oriental countries over the many centuries they have used soya. Rather the reverse.

MAKING THE BREAK: HOW TO PUT MORE BEANS INTO YOUR LIFE	
If You Used To Do This . . .	*Now Do This!*
Take cows' milk in your tea or coffee	Use soya milk in tea, straight from the carton. In coffee, heat the soya milk first to avoid curdling. Avoid dry 'creamers' and 'whiteners' without first reading their labels: many contain dairy milk proteins and/or fats

Put cows' milk on your breakfast cereal	Use your favourite soya, rice, oat or coconut milk, or pour fresh fruit juice over your cereal instead
Tuck into a bowl of ice cream	Enjoy high-quality sorbets or water ices. Or try one of the growing range of soya ice creams now on the market
Douse your desserts in cream or custard	Most supermarkets sell small cartons of a brand of soya 'cream'; to make your own whisk soft, plain tofu with a little honey or malt extract for a thick, rich topping. One of the oldest brands of custard powder is dairy free! Simply prepare it using soya milk instead of dairy. Or try one of the custard-like soya 'puddings' or 'desserts' now widely available.
Drink glasses of milk or milkshakes	Many producers offer a range of flavoured or naturally sweetened soya, rice, oat or coconut milks in various carton sizes. Or make your own ultra-thick shake at home! See the recipes below.
Use dollops of butter in cooking or served onto bread or vegetables	Use organic, first- and cold-pressed extra-virgin olive oil in cooking. Try herb flavoured olive oil drizzled over toast or baked potatoes and lift your sandwiches with a spread such as tahini (sesame seed paste) to take the place of butter and to enhance your nutrient intake.

Eat masses of hard, soft or cottage cheeses	Several brands of dairy-free hard 'cheeses' are currently available in health-food shops and these may be used in cookery as well as simply grated or sliced. Double-check the labels to ensure the product is free from casein, lactose and other 'hidden' dairy ingredients. Soft soya 'cheeses' abound – available as tofu dips, spreads or patés, for instance. My favourite option is either tofu (smoked, marinated, braised or plain) or houmous! I know it's not soya, but it has similar benefits.
Dive into a daily dose of yoghurt	Soya yoghurt is widely available in plain and fruit flavours and in a variety of carton sizes.
Eat dairy (made from cow) meat products such as burgers, sausages, luncheon meats, patés and pastes	A huge variety of products are now widely available to replace meat in all its guises. Look for these products in the dry mix, freezer, tinned or chilled food sections of your health-food shop or supermarket. Although some of these products are based on nuts, most are based on soya i.e. various tofus, tempeh, and TVP (texturised vegetable protein) in mince or chunk form and in various savoury flavours.
Cook with dairy products	Soya milk or cream readily substitutes for dairy milk in recipes as varied as Béchamel

sauce and creamed soups to rice pudding and quiche. Most recipes calling for butter succeed as well with olive oil or Granose soya spread. The meat replacements mentioned above serve well in traditional recipes, as do the cheese substitutes.

Here are some sensational recipes by my friend Peggy Brusseau which are quick, easy and very tasty! Use them to effortlessly boost your intake of the soya bean.

Chilli without Carne

This dish was originally made with meat that was heavily spiced with chilli peppers. The flavour, texture and aroma of this meatless version is authentic and irresistible. Aim for a level of spiciness at the borders of your tolerance and cook until this sauce has the consistency of ragout: thick and gloopy. Red beans are included here as an option; they are often included in the Americanised version of this dish.

Serves 4
Preparation time 45 minutes

1 tbsp olive oil
5 cloves garlic, finely chopped
2 medium onions, thinly sliced
½–1 tsp chilli powder
100g (4oz) TVP mince
570ml (1 pint) water
140g (5oz) tomato purée
1 × 400g (14oz) tin tomatoes or 6 medium tomatoes, chopped
1 whole chilli pepper, to taste (optional)
450g (1lb) cooked red kidney beans (optional)
2 tsp soy sauce
1 tbsp vinegar

Heat the oil in a saucepan and sauté the garlic and onion until clear and tender. Add the chilli powder and sauté for a further

1 minute. Stir the TVP into the sauté to absorb all the oil and juices then add the water, tomato purée and chopped tomatoes. Stir well and leave over a medium heat. Add the chilli and/or red beans at this point and add a little more water if necessary to ensure the right consistency. Cover the pan, reduce the heat and leave to simmer for about 20 minutes. Add the soy sauce and vinegar about 5 minutes before serving. Serve hot in small bowls with a plate of fresh tortillas nearby and, if you're really keen, a small dish of fresh, hot chillies!

If you like milkshakes, try

Banana Shake
Serves 4
Preparation time 10 minutes

1 litre (2 pints) cold soya milk
4 very ripe bananas, peeled
50g (2oz) ground almonds
½ tsp ground nutmeg

Turn all (or half at a time) of the ingredients into a blender and whisk to a thick, frothy consistency. Pour into chilled glasses and serve immediately with a garnish of flaked almonds or a single banana chip floating on the surface.

How about a stir-fry? Try

Tofu Sukiyaki
Serves 4
Preparation time 45 minutes

100g (4oz) ramen noodles
570ml (1 pint) water
2 medium carrots, cut diagonally into thin slices
2 stalks celery, with leafy tops, cut diagonally into thin slices
100g (4oz) mushrooms, thinly sliced
4 spring onions, trimmed and thinly sliced lengthwise
100–170g (4–6oz) fresh bean sprouts
225g (8oz) fresh spinach, washed and sliced
25g (1oz) fresh parsley, finely chopped
2 × 285g (10oz) blocks tofu, cut into cubes or strips

FOR THE SAUCE:
200ml (7fl oz) vegetable stock
60ml (2fl oz) soy sauce
2 tbsp rice vinegar
1 tbsp barley malt syrup

Break the ramen into a mixing bowl. Measure the water into a saucepan and place over a medium heat. Place the carrots in a steamer over the water. Bring the water to the boil and steam the carrots for 3 minutes. Remove the pan from the heat: arrange the carrot slices in the bottom of a deep frying pan and dissolve the miso in the carrot water. Pour this water over the ramen in the bowl and leave for 10–15 minutes.

Carefully arrange, in the order in which they are given, the remaining vegetables in layers over the carrots. Drain the ramen and place over the vegetables, arrange the tofu on top. Place the frying pan over a high heat and, at the same time, combine the sauce ingredients in a small saucepan and heat to simmering point. Immediately pour the sauce over the ingredients in the frying pan, bring to the boil, cover the pan and reduce the heat from high to medium. Simmer for 5–7 minutes. Serve hot with steamed rice.

Marinated Tempeh
Serves 4
Preparation time 1 hour 30 minutes plus 6–8 hours marinating

2 × 225g (8oz) blocks tempeh, defrosted
5 cloves garlic, finely chopped
2 medium onions, chopped
1 tart apple, quartered, cored and chopped
200ml (7 fl oz) olive oil
200ml (7 fl oz) cider vinegar
juice of 2 lemons
60ml (2 fl oz) soy sauce
25g (1oz) fresh ginger, sliced
2 tsp black peppercorns, crushed but not ground
1 tsp mustard seed, slightly crushed
12 whole cloves
one 3-inch piece of cinnamon

Cut the tempeh into one-inch cubes and arrange in an oven dish. Mix the remaining ingredients together in a large jug. Stir well then pour over the tempeh. Cover the dish and leave to marinate for 6–8 hours (ideal for making in the morning and cooking when you get home from work). You may, if you choose, let the tempeh marinate for up to 24 hours. Preheat the oven to 190°C/375°F/Gas Mark 5 and bake the tempeh for 1 hour. Serve hot over rice with steamed greens and sautéed carrot to accompany.

FOOD FACTOR #2: DON'T HESITATE TO VEGETATE

The second essential component of The Plant Programme is to increase the amount of vegetables and fruit you consume, noting that vegetables are even more important than fruit. The official recommendation of five portions a day, especially when each portion can comprise a glass of (commercial) fruit juice and a tablespoon of dried fruit or a small bowl of stewed fruit,[24] is in my view completely inadequate. The evidence is over-whelming that an abundant intake of fruit and vegetables can play an important role in reducing cancer incidence.[25] You must be careful, however – especially if you are on chemotherapy – to avoid too much fruit containing strong acids such as citric or oxalic acid. Do not eat too many oranges, lemons, grapefruits, limes, rhubarb or berries or you can develop cystitis or other symptoms of excess acid including sore and painful joints. Use apples and pears (which are especially good for the digestive tract and hence colon cancer), melons, peaches, apricots and bananas which are much less acid. Make sure they are fresh and ripe.

In the case of vegetables, do not eat too much spinach, beetroot or too many tomatoes at one time for the same reason. Otherwise eat as many vegetables, including salad vegetables, as possible. The list of anti-cancer chemicals identified in vegetables and fruit just keeps on growing. The investigation of plant chemicals pioneered by Lee Wattenberg of the University of Minnesota in the USA has identified many agents that protect against cancer in laboratory studies.[26] Perhaps this is hardly surprising. I have always wondered why I have never seen or heard of a plant with cancer despite all the chemicals we pour on them, so perhaps in the same way that mankind discovered some substances such as honey contain natural antibiotics because they do not readily 'go rotten', we should have realised long ago that plants contain anti-cancer agents. Indeed some of the latest chemotherapeutic agents such as the taxanes which are derived from Yew trees are effective against both advanced breast and ovarian cancers (but do not attempt to eat Yew directly as it is poisonous).

Most fruit and vegetables include such vitamins as beta-carotene (the precursor of vitamin A) and other carotenoids such as lycopene (especially rich in yellow and orange vegetables such as carrots, saffron, red and yellow peppers and peaches), vitamin C (most fresh fruit and vegetables) and vitamin E (most fresh fruit and vegetables). All these vitamins act as antioxidants; removing free radicals, which can damage cell walls and cell DNA, from the body.

Free radicals are highly reactive molecules that typically have very short lifetimes. The best way to think of the effect of free radicals, which are powerful oxidising agents, in our body is to imagine a pat of butter or a piece of meat or some nuts going rancid. This occurs because of a chemical process called oxidation. The chemicals in vegetables and fruit help to prevent oxidation – they stop our tissues going rancid. The pigments in red, orange and yellow fruit and vegetables – such as beta-carotene in carrots and peaches and lycopene in tomatoes (especially 'baby' ones) pink grapefruit or red grapeskins – are powerful antioxidants and may have other cancer-preventing properties. Garlic and Brussels sprouts are especially rich in antioxidants.

Beta-carotene has long been suggested to be protective against several forms of cancer. Research reported from Israel in 1995 suggests that lycopene (the main tomato carotenoid) is a more potent inhibitor of human cancer cell proliferation than beta-carotene.[27] In addition to its powerful antioxidant properties, it suppressed IGF-1-stimulated growth of mammary cancer cells. Research reported from Japan also showed that lycopene significantly suppressed breast tumour development in genetically susceptible mice, partly because it suppressed serum levels of prolactin and free fatty acids.[28] (Reading some of these papers strongly suggests to me that many scientists know the factors that promote breast cancer. Why have we not been told? See Chapter Seven for further discussion on this point.)

Plants, especially green leafy vegetables and newly sprouted shoots such as bean sprouts and alfalfa also contain folic acid, which is involved in making the copies of the chromosomes carrying our gene sequences when cells divide. This is the very point at which mistakes which could cause cancer are likely to happen. A great deal of evidence suggests that most Americans' diets are deficient in folic acid.[29] Deterioration in the elderly has also been attributed to folate deficiency.[30] Indeed, throughout the West, women wishing to become pregnant are advised to take folic acid pills to avoid birth defects such as spina bifida in their babies. Surely we should *all* be eating a diet that has adequate quantities of folic acid without having to resort to taking pills. As discussed previously, some of the chemotherapeutic drugs used to disrupt breast cancer cells replace folic acid in cell division. I believe that it was drinking fresh juices high in folic acid as soon as I was able to after chemotherapy that helped me to recover so quickly and saved my hair from falling out. I drank about half a pint of green Bramley apple with fennel juice, about 50:50 apple-fennel, and about half a pint of carrot juice each and every day. I also ate lots of melon which is especially rich in folic acid. People who were treated with me who took folic acid pills still lost their hair, but all the people I have persuaded to use juices have kept theirs.

I have mentioned plant oestrogens in the context of soya several times in the book because of their protective effect on breast tissue. Plant oestrogens are found in almost all fruit and vegetables and cereals. Vegetables such as soya, lentils, peas and beans are all legumes capable of fixing nitrogen from the air to make proteins and are rich sources of isoflavones. Typically Oriental, Mediterranean and Latin American diets include large quantities of legumes and it has been calculated that a typical Western diet provides only about 3mg of isoflavones a day compared to the 30–100mg a day in oriental diets.

Red clover has particularly high levels of coumestans and, like chick peas (the basis of the Greek food houmous) and lentils, it contains all of the four important dietary isoflavones. Red clover, which can be bought from herbalists, is something I have started taking recently because I believe it to be protective against breast cancer. Sunflower seeds and alfalfa sprouts also contain substantial quantities of phyto-oestrogen compounds.

Phytoprogesterones in the diet may also be important in protecting against breast cancer. In his book *Natural*

Progesterone, published by John Carpenter Publishing in 1996, Dr JR Lee argues that breast and other problems including premenstrual tension, fibroids, weight gain especially fat deposition at the hips and thighs are caused by oestrogen dominance over progesterone which can become worse as women approach the menopause. Dr Lee suggests the problem is mainly the result of poor nutrition. He recommends including plenty of fresh vegetables, whole grains and fruit eaten as unprocessed as possible and uncontaminated by insecticides, artificial colouring agents or preservatives or other toxic ingredients. One of the richest sources of natural progesterone is wild yam or sweet potato, and soya and fennel contain both phyto-oestrogens and phytoprogesterones. Flaxseed, because of its high content of lignans, which are converted in the digestive tract into substances that help to regulate endocrine function, has been shown in experiments to have a significant and specific role in sex steroid action by improving the progesterone/oestrogen ratio during menstrual cycles of women.[31] Much research on flax has been carried out by the US Food and Drug Administration (FDA), the National Cancer Institute and the Canadian Food Protection Branch.[32] The recommendation is to take about one tablespoon a day of flaxseed in your diet for each 100 pounds of body weight (but be prepared to go to the loo more often!).

I also eat sprouted seeds including soya, pumpkin and sesame (both rich in zinc), sunflower, sesame, alfalfa and lentil. They are rich in vitamin C and other vitamins and minerals and high quality proteins. Here's how to do it:

- Use a container with some sort of drainage, such as a colander, strainer, mesh tray, or even a flower pot with a cloth net over the hole. A jar with a piece of cheesecloth or muslin held in place around the top with a rubber band is perhaps the simplest and most effective. The size of the jar depends on how many seeds you are sprouting, but it should hold at least half a litre.
- Seeds can be bought from health food stores, where they are usually labelled 'organic', and some supermarkets. Do *not* buy seeds from agricultural merchants – they may well be contaminated with seed dressing chemicals which might be fatal if consumed. Use only the clean, whole ones and throw out the rest.

- For every 100ml the jar holds, use between two and three tablespoons of seeds. First, they must be soaked in four times their own volume of water, ideally filtered or mineral water, until their bulk is doubled. This normally takes about eight hours, or overnight. After this time, pour off the water.
- The sprout container should be kept in darkness – just throw a tea-towel over the jar. The seeds must be rinsed two or three times a day through the muslin mesh of the jar. Make sure you drain them thoroughly each time by turning the container upside down, or the sprouts will rot.
- Throw away any seeds that have not sprouted after two days. The rest will be ready to eat after four or five days. On the last day they can be put into the light, but only for a few hours or they will become bitter.
- Most sprouts will need a final rinsing and draining before being put in the fridge in a covered container for storage. Some varieties, however, have loose husks which need to be removed. Place the sprouts in a large bowl of water and agitate until the husks float to the top, then you can skim them off.

Vegetables and fruit also contain compounds, or their precursor chemicals, which have no known nutritional value but which have anti-cancer properties. They include indoles, isothiocyanates, dithiolthiones and organosulphur components (some of which are thought to produce natural pesticides). About twenty years ago epidemiological studies showed that consumption of cruciferous vegetables (bok choy, broccoli, Brussels sprouts, cauliflower etc.) which contain dithiolthiones, was associated with a decreased risk of developing cancer. A synthetic dithiolthione called oltipraz has been shown to inhibit the development of tumours of the breast (and lung, colon and bladder) in laboratory animals. Like other beneficial plant chemicals, it interferes with cancer development in several ways including by activating the liver enzymes that remove cancer-causing agents from the bloodstream.[33] Sulforaphane, an isothiocyanate which is also found in cruciferous vegetables and is responsible for their sharp taste, is also thought to prevent cancer by activating detoxifying enzymes in the liver. In rats it blocks the formation of chemically induced breast cancers. In addition a compound called indo-3-carbinol found in cruciferous vegetables has been found to affect oestrogen metabolism and hence to be especially protective against breast cancer. Recently, research at Robert Gordon University in Aberdeen suggests that only raw broccoli offers any protective effect against colon cancer as measured by the amount of DNA damage in colon cells from laboratory pigs.[34] It is suggested that cooking destroys glucosinolates, which are the precursors of isothiocyanates produced in the colon, which are the substances protective against cancer. The degree of cooking of the broccoli is not described however. As indicated in the section on cooking it is best to eat vegetables which are as raw as possible (light steaming or stir frying) although it is important to cook all meat and fish thoroughly.

Garlic and onions, chives and leeks (the allium family – allium sativum is the Latin name for garlic) are important in helping to protect against cancer. They contain chemicals similar to those used in anti-radiation pills (cysteine-like amino acids) and are particularly useful in reducing the effects of diagnostic X-rays and radiotherapy in the body. They contain powerful antioxidants (active against free radicals including those produced by anti-cancer treatments). Allicin, one of garlic's main biologically active components, is created when garlic is crushed; it has been shown to decrease breast cancer and prostate cancer cell proliferation in laboratory studies.[35]

In addition to allicin, garlic also concentrates other powerful antioxidants such as selenium and germanium which neutralise the free radicals which are believed to promote tumour growth and atherosclerosis (clogging of the arteries). Research into cancer at universities in Pennsylvania and Texas in the USA has identified two other compounds active against cancer, in crushed garlic: diallysulphide and S-allyl cysteine. The Weizmann Institute of Science in Israel has identified a molecular mechanism thought to be the basis for some of garlic's therapeutic effects. Current studies at the Memorial Sloan-Kettering Cancer Center in New York on the mechanism of action of chemopreventative chemicals derived from garlic, indicate that it is effective against breast and prostate cancer, especially in the initial phases of cancer development, partly by improving the cell's ability to eliminate carcinogens and reducing the ability of carcinogenic chemicals to bind to DNA. Preliminary studies at the same centre have indicated that garlic also prevents breast and prostate cancer cells from dividing thereby limiting the growth of tumours.[36] Garlic is also a natural anti-microbial agent active against a wide range of fungi, bacteria and viruses and it was used for these purposes in the First World War. Many people worry about smelling of garlic but if everyone eats it, no one notices!

One of the problems if you have active cancer is in consuming the amount of fresh fruit and vegetables needed to deliver adequate quantities of anti-cancer chemicals to the sites of the tumours. The best way to overcome this problem, is to extract juices from the vegetables and fruits. This way, the active compounds are separated from the large mass of fibre that you would otherwise have to chew through and the anti-cancer agents are made more biologically available to your body. Even if you do not like certain vegetables, you can hold your nose and simply drink the juice as if it is a medicine – it is! Naturopaths and some doctors have been treating patients with fresh juices and raw food to improve their health since the nineteenth century. The therapy was pioneered in Germany and Switzerland before being used by health clinics worldwide. Famous pioneers include Father Kniepp, Dr Kellogg, Dr Max Bircher-Benner and Dr Max Gerson. To make the quantities of juices needed you must invest in a juicer (*not a liquidiser*). There are several available but when I had cancer I found that the cheaper ones burned out fairly quickly and I have had a juicer normally used in commercial juice bars for the past five years.

Carrot juice is good but do not drink more than a half pint glass a day or you may turn orange (I did – with orange palms and an orange moustache, which was described grandly by one of my doctors as carotenosis!). Do not have too much cabbage juice either. Cabbage contains substances known as goitrogens which can cause problems with the thyroid gland if taken in too large quantities, especially if it is eaten raw. It increases the requirement for iodine which is essential for good nutrition (*see* p. 165) and for which the main source in the diet is seafood. I made green Bramley apple, celery and fennel with small amounts of watercress, the main green juice I drank every day when I was ill with cancer.

In addition to juices, you should have masses of fresh salads and vegetables. I cook vegetables by lightly steaming them (not by boiling and certainly not by boiling them to death, and on no account add sodium hydrogen carbonate, commonly known as bicarbonate of soda) or just 'sweating' them in a little extra-virgin olive oil (essentially cooked for a few minutes without water). This is an especially good method of cooking spinach which is delicious if a few onions are softened in the extra-virgin olive oil first.

I eat lots of vegetable soups. Again, I just slowly soften vegetables in a little olive oil and then add boiling water and simmer. Finally I add a dollop of miso and some cubes of tofu (optional), some snippets of seaweed (optional) served with cress or lettuce leaves added just before serving.

One of the problems people complain of when they start to eat lots of fruit and vegetables is the number of times they have to go to the loo. Sorry, but that is what is supposed to happen – two to three times a day is normal, not two to three times a week! Also by not suffering from constipation you will reduce your chance of suffering from haemorrhoids (piles) and varicose veins. A good indication that your diet is correct is when your stools float rather than sink. You may also suffer from 'wind' but don't worry, after a few weeks of the diet recommended here the body will adjust and you will have no further problems with flatulence.

If you're thinking of cheating by drinking bottled or frozen juices instead of freshly made ones, there is simply no point. If you cut an apple it immediately starts going brown (because it has oxidised) and you need the green unoxidised juice. The same is true for all juices. If you buy commercial juices they will be far more oxidised and chemically far less potent as anti-cancer agents. Also they may contain some type of preservative or have undergone some type of process to stop them going rotten (just think about it, how else could carrot juice be sold weeks after it is prepared?) so they will be chemically changed. I have discovered people with colon cancer changing the diet I recommend by eating vegetable pills instead of raw vegetables and their juices! Experimental and observational studies have shown that this does not help. For example, in a study beginning in 1985, beta-carotene was included in two large long-term chemo-prevention trials sponsored by the National Cancer Institute in the USA – the Alpha-Tocopherol (vitamin E) Beta-Carotene (ATBC) Lung Cancer Prevention

Study and the Beta-Carotene and Retinal Efficiency Trial. Previous epidemiological studies had suggested that diets high in beta-carotene (for instance, from carrots) had reduced lung cancer incidence. In the trial studies, daily doses of beta-carotene in combination with either vitamin E (alpha-tocopherol) or vitamin A (retinol) were administered for several years to tens of thousands of people thought to be at high risk of developing lung cancer. What happened? The rate of lung cancer in those taking the pills increased in both trials![37]

Whole foods are a complex package of essential nutrients with many benefits that cannot be found in bottles of pills. Whole foods really are greater than the sum of the parts. For example, natural foods contain enzymes that help break down the components of the food. Hence bananas are rich in carbohydrates and contain amylase, a carbohydrate-splitting enzyme. Natural carrot juice contains all sorts of substances that work with beta-carotene. Foods generally contain hundreds or thousands of substances (many of which have yet to be studied) that may be important for health. It has been suggested that the difference between natural vegetables and commercial juices or pills is similar to that between paper and trees. Be like Chinese people and eat everything when it is as fresh and ripe as possible. Unfortunately with the advent of supermarkets, food tends to be much older when we eat it. Also, we tend to make just one shopping trip a week rather than buying fresh food in season every day as we did when I was a child.

ORGANIC FOOD AND PESTICIDES

In the UK, organically grown food has its origins in the work of Sir Albert Howard who published *An Agricultural Testament* in 1940, advocating that Britain preserve the 'cycle of life' and adopt 'permanent agriculture' systems, using urban food waste and sewage to build soil fertility. The first person to apply the term 'organic' to food production was J I Rodale in his 1942 publication *Organic Gardening and Farming*. In 1946 the young Lady Eve Balfour was inspired by Howard to set up the Soil Association, a pioneering organic farming charity that today is the major organic certification organisation in the UK. In 1960 the Soil Association opened the first shop in the UK selling organic produce. Interest in organic farming grew throughout Europe and the USA during the environmentally aware 1960s.

In 1974 the Soil Association established the UK's first set of Organic Food Standards, which formed the basis of the EU regulation 2092/91 which lays down in detail how food must be produced, processed and packaged to qualify for the description 'organic'. The regulation also specifies detailed criteria for the inspection and subsequent certification of food producers and processors. In the USA, organic regulations have been developed on a state-by-state basis – currently there is no national organic legislation. The US Department of Agriculture (USDA) attempted to bring in national organic standards in 1998 but these standards would have permitted the use of GM ingredients, sewage sludge and irradiation in food labelled as 'organic'. These proposed standards were withdrawn for redrafting.

Sometimes, people who advocate organic food are dismissed as middle-class food fanatics, with no rational or scientific basis for their concerns. I'd like to tell you why this caricature is wrong, and why it is so vitally important that you insist on as much high-quality organic food as possible.

Pesticides are chemical poisons used to control a pest or disease, and they include *insecticides* that kill insects, *herbicides* that kill plants, *fungicides* that kill fungal diseases and many other 'cides' designed to kill everything from worms to birds. Pesticides, together with fertilisers and drugs for animals – known as veterinary products as a group, are called agrochemicals. The establishment view is that a relatively small percentage of cancers are attributable to pesticides following epidemiological analysis in 1981 by Doll and Peto, which indicated that not more than two per cent of cancers are attributable to the use of man-made pesticides.[38] If this is accurate, it is still a lot of cancers! However, this estimate preceded our knowledge of the endocrine-disrupting behaviour of certain chemicals, so it is likely to be an underestimate in the case of breast and prostate cancer. The major categories of synthetic pesticides include: organochlorines, organophosphates and triazine herbicides.

Many pesticides are made from organic chemicals. This is where some confusion can occur, because in connection with food, the word 'organic' has a good meaning; but when it is used to describe a chemical pesticide, it has precisely the opposite sense. Indeed, it is the antithesis of life. Let me explain why.

There are just 92 naturally occurring chemical elements on Earth, ranging from light elements such as hydrogen and oxygen (which together form water), to very heavy elements such as lead, gold and uranium. Everything you see around you (and much you can't see) is made up of various combinations of these 92 chemical elements.

Even more remarkably, every living thing, from the simplest of single-celled plants to the most complex species on the planet, is created from compounds of just *one* element – carbon.

Carbon is an extraordinary substance. It can combine with other elements to form a vast number of compounds. Some of the simplest molecules, which we use for food – sugar and starches – are called carbohydrates (the name comes from the fact that carbon is combined with hydrogen and oxygen in the ratio of 2:1 as in water (hydrate)). Carbohydrates are used by life forms mainly for energy and as an energy store. Fats, proteins and vitamins are also organic or carbon-based chemicals. The chemistry of the unique chemical element, carbon, is the basis of all life – and because of their association with life, such chemicals are known as *organic* chemicals.

Organic chemical pesticides are potentially dangerous to us because they are based on the chemical wonder-element, carbon. Although they have been specially designed and configured to kill other animals or plants, the potential clearly exists for serious and profound disruption to occur within our own chemical life processes.

Since the end of the Second World War, industrialisation of agriculture has been achieved by the increasing application of mechanisation, the use of monocultures and of higher yielding, more efficient crops and animals with the application of an enormous range of pesticides to kill small organisms and a plethora of veterinary products to treat agricultural animals. The introduction of DDT during the Second World War marked the beginning of a very rapid growth in pesticide use and other organochlorine pesticides – such as dieldrin and aldrin – were introduced in the late 1940s. Although environmental scientists have warned of the impact of such pesticides on wildlife for many years – for example, their effect on bird reproduction – the potential impact on humans, including of endocrine disruption, is of increasing concern.

The use of DDT was banned in the USA in 1972, but it is still used in many developing countries. Other organochlorines such as aldrin and dieldrin, which are structurally similar to DDT, are no longer in general use in most developed countries. They share with DDT the common characteristics of a high degree of persistence in the environment, endocrine disruption and the suspicion of carcinogenicity. What are we still using today that in the future we shall find evidence to ban?

Organophosphates were first developed as nerve gas agents for chemical warfare in Britain, France, Germany and the USA during the Second World War. They work by affecting nerve junctions. To fire a nerve impulse across a junction requires the body to produce a substance called acetylcholine. This must be broken down immediately after use by another chemical, an enzyme called acetyl-cholinesterase. Organophosphates prevent this substance working properly by locking on to it. Hence the organophosphate pesticide is called an inhibitor. The locking-on is a two-stage process: the first is reversible, but the second – called ageing – is not. So the nerve keeps firing. Organophosphates are implicated mainly in diseases of the nervous system rather than breast cancer, although recent work suggests some of them are endocrine disrupters. Anyway, reducing exposure is desirable especially in minimising depression accompanying breast cancer and its treatment!

According to Lang and Clutterbuck, animal studies have implicated about 50 pesticides as cancer-causing agents.[39] Many other pesticides are suspected of causing birth or genetic defects; and over 60 pesticides have been implicated in causing various reproductive effects. According to McMichael,[40] there has been a 30-fold increase in global pesticide use and a nine-fold increase in chemical fertiliser use since the 1950s. This has increased food yield, but it has also caused widespread chemical pollution, destruction of wildlife and disturbance of ecosystems. As of the mid-1990s, US agriculture used about 365 million kg of pesticides per year, although even more than that, about 900 million kg of insecticides, were used in non-agricultural applications, including forestry, landscaping, gardening, food distribution and home pest control.

Insecticides and fungicides are the most important pesticides with respect to human exposure in food because they are often applied shortly before or even after harvesting. Herbicide use has also grown as chemicals have increasingly replaced traditional methods of cultivating land such as crop rotation, in the control of weeds. Herbicides now account for two-thirds of agricultural pesticides.[41] Atrazine, a member of the s-triazine herbicides, is reported to be the most widely-used herbicide in the world.[42] Exposure of breast-cancer cells in tissue culture leads to an increased production of an oestrogen metabolite and it has been shown to cause mammary tumours when given in high doses to certain strains of laboratory rats.[43] The International Association for Research into Cancer (IARC, a WHO organisation) has concluded that there is limited evidence that atrazine is carcinogenic in animals but it is a possible human carcinogen.[44] Atrazine is on the Environmental Endocrine Disrupters list of the American EPA, and the World Wildlife Fund. Atrazine has been banned in several countries but is well-established as a herbicide and widely used on corn in the USA and Canada with widespread water pollution in corn-growing regions. Another member of this type of herbicide is metrabuzin which is widely used on soya beans, sugar cane and wheat. They both work by inhibiting photosynthesis.

The alternative to this chemical nightmare is to buy organically produced food. Many farms or co-operatives now offer delivery of fresh, organically grown produce. Even in the 1950s my father, who objected to the increasing use of chemicals to grow and process food, taught me to search for fruit and vegetables with grub holes in them on the basis that they would be less likely to contain pesticides. Prior to getting breast cancer, I had forgotten that advice.

If you can afford to do so, buy organically-grown food or at the very least buy organically-grown potatoes and carrots. If you cannot afford organically-grown produce and have a garden or allotment, grow your own. Salad vegetables in particular should be organically grown because they are eaten raw so the chemicals in them are not broken down at all by cooking. Otherwise, remove the outer leaves of cabbage or lettuce, for example, and wash in a weak solution of (cheap malt) vinegar, bought in glass not plastic bottles, before rinsing thoroughly and preparing in the normal way. This will not remove all chemicals now used in agriculture and horticulture (because many are systemic and hence occur throughout the entire plant) but it will reduce those sprayed directly onto the surface. Peel fruit if it is not organically grown (because unfortunately the skin which is otherwise very nutritious is often treated with chemicals and then waxed so the chemicals do not wash off). It is easy to see this from the way water runs off the surface of the fruit 'just as if it were running off a plastic mac'. This is often the case with oranges, grapefruit and lemons and some heavily marketed commercial apples. Of course, it does not matter too much whether or not citrus fruit has been waxed if it is to be peeled, but it does if you are using it to cook marmalade or other food which uses the skin or the rind of the fruit. I avoid eating apples that have been treated in this way. I stick to English Cox's, and Bramleys which I have never found to be waxed. Just one important cautionary note: animal manure and waste is the main fertiliser universally used in organic farming, so pathogens will remain on your foods unless you are particularly vigilant and wash all fruit and vegetables thoroughly before eating them.

Cooking with vegetables the Plant way:

Delicious Curly Kale
Serves 4
Preparation time 45 minutes

1kg (2lb) curly kale
1 tbsp olive oil
5 cloves garlic, chopped
1 large onion, thinly sliced
1 tsp freshly ground black pepper
½ tsp ground nutmeg
1 sweet red pepper, deseeded and thinly sliced

Trim the kale and immerse it in cold, salty water for 5 minutes. Rinse each leaf under cold running water, slice into narrow pieces and place in a colander. Heat the oil in a large saucepan over a medium heat. Sauté the garlic and onion until clear and tender. Add the pepper and nutmeg and stir the sauté for 1 minute. Add the sliced kale and immediately cover the pan. Leave it cooking over a medium heat for 5 minutes. Stir the kale so that the onion sauté is distributed through the greens, add the pepper and cover the pan. Leave to cook over a low heat for 10 minutes. Stir well and serve immediately with rice, tempeh and sautéed carrots or baked pumpkin.

Quick and Gorgeous Parsnip Soup
Serves 4
Preparation time 45 minutes

3 medium parsnips, peeled and chopped
1 large onion, chopped
3 stalks celery, chopped
2 tbsp olive oil
2 tbsp plain flour
1l (2 pints) soya milk
½ tsp freshly ground black pepper
¼ tsp salt
juice of ½ lemon
2 tbsp fresh parsley, chopped

Prepare the parsnips, onion and celery. Heat the oil in a saucepan and add these vegetables to it. Stir well and sauté for 15 minutes over a medium heat. When the vegetables are tender and golden, sprinkle the flour over them, stir and gradually add the soya milk. Cook until the liquid is hot but not boiling then turn the soup through a mouli or food processor and liquidise to a smooth consistency. Return the soup to the saucepan and add the pepper and salt. Bring the soup to a simmer; add a little lemon juice at this stage to provide some sharpness. The consistency of the soup may be adjusted by adding vegetable stock or water. Leave the soup to simmer for 10 minutes then serve hot with parsley to garnish.

Cream of Spinach Soup
Serves 4
Preparation time 1 hour

450g (1lb) fresh spinach, washed, trimmed and chopped
1 tbsp olive oil
3 cloves garlic, finely chopped
2 medium onions, chopped
1 tsp freshly ground black pepper
2 tsp yeast extract
570ml (1 pint) vegetable stock or water
2 tsp caraway seeds + 1 tbsp olive oil to sauté
1 tbsp plain flour *or* cornflour
570ml (1 pint) soya milk
1 tsp ground coriander

Prepare the spinach and turn into a colander to drain. Heat the oil in a large, deep saucepan over a medium heat and sauté the garlic and onion until clear and tender. Add the pepper and stir for 1 minute. Stir in the yeast extract then add the vegetable stock and bring to a low boil. Add the spinach, cover the pan and reduce the heat. Leave to simmer gently for 3–5 minutes. Meanwhile, heat the other measure of oil in a saucepan and sauté the caraway seeds for 2 minutes. Sprinkle the flour over the oil and stir to make a thick paste (roux). Add the soya milk, a little at a time, stirring after each addition to make a sauce. Sprinkle the coriander over the sauce, stir well and remove from the heat. Pour this sauce into the soup, stirring constantly as you do so. Add a little more stock if necessary to create the thickness of soup you enjoy. Serve hot with a garnish of coriander leaf.

Broccoli In Garlic & Almond Sauce
Serves 4
Preparation time 30 minutes

900g (2lb) broccoli, trimmed and cut into florets
1 tbsp olive oil
1 whole bulb garlic, peeled and chopped
1 tbsp fresh ginger, grated
½–1 tsp freshly ground black pepper
115g (4oz) sliced almonds
1 bunch spring onions, sliced into two-inch lengths

Steam the broccoli for 5 minutes; leave the pan covered and put to one side, off the heat. Meanwhile, heat the oil in a large saucepan and sauté the garlic for 2 minutes, until just golden. Add the ginger and black pepper and stir for 1 minute. Add the almonds, spring onions and the steamed broccoli to the sauté, toss together, cover the pan and leave over a low heat for 7–10 minutes. Serve hot as a side dish or over rice.

Arame & Vegetable Sauté
Arame is a Japanese seaweed, available in health-food shops.
Serves 4
Preparation time 1 hour

50g (2oz) dried arame
1 tbsp olive oil

100g (4oz) mushrooms, sliced
5 spring onions, sliced into two-inch lengths
3 medium carrots, cut into fine chunks
1 tbsp soy sauce
2 tbsp sesame seeds, roasted
freshly ground black pepper, to taste

First, wash the arame to remove any grit, then soak it in plenty of water, in a bowl, for about twenty minutes. The arame will swell considerably. Lift the arame into a saucepan and pour fresh water over it. Place the pan over a medium heat, make sure there is sufficient water to cover the seaweed and bring to a boil. Immediately reduce the heat and simmer for 10 minutes, until the arame becomes very tender. Keep a close eye at this stage as a great deal of froth is created initially and it can easily boil over. Meanwhile, heat the oil in a large pan and sauté the thinly sliced vegetables in it. Drain the tender arame and add to the vegetables. Stir the arame and vegetables over a medium heat to mix the ingredients well. Season with soy sauce and cook for a few more minutes before serving hot. Serve over rice, sprinkling each serving with a teaspoonful of roasted sesame seeds and a little black pepper.

This is a delicious dish which is easy to amend according to whatever vegetables you have to hand. You can make it a delicate little dish using one or two sautéed vegetables, or a huge and substantial one with half a dozen vegetables in the sauté. Try it very spicy with plenty of garlic and fresh chilli or subtle and sloppy with a little extra broth thickened with arrowroot.

Classic Walnut & Red Cabbage Salad
Serves 4
Preparation time 30 minutes

100–170g (4–6oz) walnut halves
1 small red cabbage, shredded
2 tart eating apples, quartered, cored and chopped
1 small onion, thinly sliced
1 tbsp fresh parsley, chopped
3 cloves garlic, finely chopped
2 tbsp cider vinegar
3 tbsp olive oil

½ tsp dried marjoram
¼ tsp salt
½ tsp freshly ground black pepper

Mix the walnuts, cabbage, apple, onion, parsley and garlic together in a large salad bowl. Blend the remaining ingredients together in a jar or jug and pour over the salad. Serve immediately, with a dollop of plain soya yoghurt if desired. This salad will keep for 24 hours if chilled and stirred occasionally; its texture and flavour alter during this time. A variation involves finely chopping 2 slices of orange and tossing these in with the salad ingredients.

Roast Vegetables

- Choose a large pan and coat well with olive oil.
- Preheat oven to 220°C (Gas Mark 7)
- Wash and cut a selection of your favourite vegetables into large chunks or slices e.g. aubergine, celery, courgette, fennel, onions (whichever sort you prefer) garlic, squash or pumpkin, different coloured peppers, corn on the cob, tomatoes, asparagus. Place the vegetable pieces in a layer in the pan. Add your favourite herbs e.g. parsley, thyme, rosemary or basil and then gently drizzle a few tablespoons of olive oil over the mixture ensuring the vegetables are coated evenly. Season to taste and put in the oven. Baste a few times and serve with the juices.
- Any leftovers can be used to make delicious sandwiches with the bread dipped or fried in the juices.

VEGGING OUT TO THE MAX: TEN KEY WAYS TO BOOST YOUR VITAL VEGETABLE INTAKE	
If You Used To Do This . . .	*Now Do This!*
Boil your potatoes and cabbages to death	Buy a stainless steel 'universal steamer' for about a fiver, add an inch of water in the pan, put on the steamer and fill it

	with veg. They take about the same length of time to cook and you won't believe how much better they taste!
Think crudités meant only celery sticks dipped in salt	Keep the celery sticks but add raw carrot sticks, florets of raw broccoli and cauliflower, chunks of raw courgette and sweet pepper, cucumber, tomato, spring onions and on and on. Ditch the salt and, if you have any room left on the plate, add a dollop of houmous or soya yoghurt seasoned with chopped chives and herbs.
Turn up your nose at any vegetable except frozen peas	Get real! And get a hand-turned blender. Now lightly cook a huge mound of chopped veg in a little vegetable stock, push the whole lot through the blender, flavour with pepper and herbs and serve. I call it Sneaky Soup because I always sneak great quantities of greens into it.
Think a salad was a careful arrangement of limp lettuce, shrivelled cucumber, a slice of tomato and half a boiled egg covered in 'salad cream'	Aim to create a salad with at least five ingredients. Here is the 'add list' for one of my favourite salads: grated carrot and turnip, chopped spring onion, diced cucumber and courgette, red kidney beans or tiny cubes of marinated tofu, watercress and parsley, rocket, radicchio and Cos lettuce. Mix and serve with sunflower

	seeds and a little walnut or sesame oil and a cider vinegar flavoured with herbs drizzled over each serving.
Throw the parsley garnish away	Make sure it is fresh, then eat it with relish. If you have no relish, make some. Very finely chopped herbs, such as parsley, coriander and watercress, and vegetables, such as tomato, onion and courgette can be prepared quickly, mixed together and served without a dressing. This will add valuable nutrients to your meal as well as a spot of colour to your plate.
Eat precisely one tablespoon of one vegetable at each evening meal	Well, that's a start. I used the Rainbow Rule to help me get into veg; here's how it works: fill one-quarter of your plate with white veg such as potato, parsnip, celeriac or turnip. These can be mashed, baked, roasted or steamed. Fill the next quarter with orange veg such as carrot, sweet potato or pumpkin; another quarter with yellow veg such as swedes, sweetcorn and sweet pepper; and the final quarter with greens. You know what they are! Of course, you don't have to divide your plate into quarters – all these colours can be mixed and made into vegetable kebabs, roasted vegetable platter, salad, casserole, stir-fry and so on.

Think garlic was for rubbing inside the salad bowls	Buy an enamelled garlic crusher and a whole string of garlic. Whatever recipe you are reading, double the amount of garlic listed. Add chopped garlic to soups, stir-fries and casseroles, and crushed garlic to salad dressings, houmous and savoury sauces.
Reach for a dictionary whenever you heard the word 'brassica'	Think of Cabbage Family, then all the edible members of it that can become a part of your diet: broccoli, Brussels sprouts, cabbages of all sorts, cauliflower, collards, kale, kohlrabi. These are the sulphur greens, rich in calcium and secondary components that are known to be anti-carcinogenic. Eat some raw or lightly steamed every day.
Think vegetable juice meant gravy and that a pound of carrots would last a year	Push one half pound of organic carrots, well scrubbed, through your new juicer. Drink immediately and go buy another pound of carrots. Tomorrow, add a couple stalks of celery to the same juicing.

FOOD FACTOR #3: PROTEIN FOODS

I have put this as Factor Three because of the difficulty many will find with living on a vegan diet, especially if they have not had breast or prostate cancer but wish to reduce their risk. I emphasise, however, that if you have active breast, prostate or colon cancer you should eliminate *all animal produce* until you are better.

After about eight months only eating plant foods I began to feel 'low'. My doctors thought this was a reaction to what I had been through, but I realised that I was probably zinc deficient. After iron, zinc is the next most important trace nutrient needed by our bodies.[45] It is involved in more than 200 enzymes in the human body and deficiency in zinc is a common cause of depression. Zinc is essential for healing so it is important you have adequate zinc to help recover from surgery, radiotherapy and chemotherapy. Its value has long been understood by ancient civilisations. When American doctors thought that they had made a major breakthrough in identifying zinc status as a crucial factor affecting recovery from burns and other injuries during the Vietnam war, it was pointed out that the remedy had been known to the Ancient Egyptians and its use was recorded in the Pyramids.

Many French doctors, and every British vet I know, know how important zinc is but I have yet to meet a British-trained doctor who is aware of its importance. In men its highest concentration in the body is in the prostate gland, suggesting zinc is particularly important for its proper functioning. Zinc is also involved in cell division, and in the way IGF-1 is controlled. Researchers at the University of Illinois, USA have shown that a complex interactive set of factors are required to ensure IGF-1 activity occurs only when conditions are right for cell growth, and they describe a discrete role for trace nutrients – especially zinc – in regulating IGF-1 activity.[46] They have suggested that one of zinc's functions is to help to inactivate IGF-1. New research also indicates selenium may play a crucial role in prostate health. In one trial, men consuming higher concentrations of Selenium, 150mcg/day, had three times less risk of prostate problems than men taking 86mcg/day. One estimate suggests that the average intake of men in the UK is less than half that. Garlic is generally a good source of selenium.

Since I do not like taking zinc tablets (they can interfere with copper uptake and cause other problems – for example taking too much can actually suppress the immune system) and because, at that time, I wasn't very knowledgeable about vegan food, I decided to introduce some meat into my diet because I knew that meat was a good source of zinc and selenium, but this was six months after all signs of cancer had disappeared. However, I buy only organically produced meat from specialist organic meat shops, which sell only meat raised using traditional and humane methods of meat production without the use of chemicals such as antibiotics or other growth promoters. I eat only very small portions of 'young' meat such as lamb, chicken, or duck drumsticks and game such as rabbit or venison (organically produced meat from beef herds is also probably fine). Game generally has higher levels of nutrients and far lower levels of fat than concentrate-fed animals which have a sedentary life.

If I were an American, I would never eat beef or pork unless it was absolutely guaranteed to be organically produced. Growth hormone implants based on male and/or female hormones have been used extensively in beef production in America for about thirty years. According to the Institute of Agriculture and Natural Resources, University of Nebraska in the USA, implants are available for all cattle except calves less than forty-five days old and breeding cattle. Some of the most potent hormone implants combine both male and female hormones. Such meat has higher levels of IGF-1 than untreated meat.[47] A genetically engineered pig growth hormone – Porcine Somatotrophin, PST – is also available for purchase in the United States but I can find no evidence of the use of such products in sheep meat production.

In an article in the Canadian press, Dr Sonnenschein of Tufts University School of Medicine, Boston USA, is quoted as saying 'it is very likely that hormone residues in American beef is a factor in the early onset of puberty among girls in recent decades. Early onset of puberty translates into higher risk of breast cancer'.[48] It has been claimed that PST (Porcine (pig) Somatotrophin) is safer than any of the steroid hormones banned by the European Union (but still used in America) because cooking destroys PST. However, this doesn't take IGF-1 levels into account, nor does it address the problem of uncooked or undercooked meat. Although the use of all such hormones is banned throughout Europe, on a BBC Radio 4 programme, British pig farmers recently complained that European farmers were allowed to feed their animals on sewage sludge which is forbidden in Britain! The message is clear. If you wish to eat pork, bacon or ham (which is a good source of zinc), eat organically produced British products especially from traditional rare breeds such as Gloucester Old Spot and Tamworth pigs.

The way the meat is cooked is important. My mother, who is a hearty 91-year-old, and all her generation of British women were taught to cook meat thoroughly and that meant slowly. For all sorts of reasons, including preventing cancer, I will not now eat undercooked meat (however trendy this is supposed to be) under any circumstances. Meat is a poor conductor of heat and if it is not cooked properly hormones in it (whether natural to the animal or introduced by man) will not be destroyed. Even if it is well-cooked, steroid hormones such as those used in the USA including oestrogens, may survive. Cooking meat so that it is burnt on the outside and raw on the inside is bad for health generally. Cancer-promoting chemicals called hetero-cyclicamines (HCA) are likely to be formed in the burnt parts (burnt meat has been implicated in colon cancer) while cancer-promoting chemicals including hormones, will remain intact in the relatively raw meat inside. I never eat meat that could contain ground up dairy animal, such as hamburger or saus-ages. (Remember official figures show dairy cow meat contains even more IGF-1 than milk). The amounts of HCAs range from low in poached, steamed or stewed meat and fish to very high in flame-grilled or pan-fried meat.

Other good sources of protein and essential trace nutrients such as zinc include eggs – zinc is concentrated in the yolks (but eat only organically produced eggs). Eggs also contain high levels of the amino acid cysteine used in anti-radiation pills so, in moderation, egg consumption will help combat the effects of radiotherapy and diagnostic X-rays. The sulphur in cysteine is in a form thought to de-activate free radicals and thus protect cells.[49] I ate one small organically produced egg a day while being treated with radiotherapy; I often eat organic eggs now, but never more than one a day. Otherwise, good sources of zinc include crabs, snails and oysters (especially Atlantic oysters) or, if you are a vegan, sesame seeds (best as tahini – a delicious spread made from sesame seed), pumpkin seeds, sunflower seeds or wheat germ. Brewer's yeast is a particularly good source of many trace elements including selenium, chromium and zinc and B vitamins which are essential for the skin and nervous tissue (remember breast tissue is a specially modified type of tissue related to skin tissue).

Fish and shellfish (ideally fresh, unfarmed and unsmoked) is an excellent source of protein, but only cold water fish such as mackerel and salmon also contain concentrations of 'good fats' known as omega-3 oils (see p. 172). Indeed, a Canadian scientist has recently suggested that the human brain could not have evolved unless we had access to the large omega-3 resources of shellfish and other coastal food sources. (The coastal zone is typically where nutrients become concentrated at the interface between fresh water from land and salt water. It is unfortunate that in Britain and many other industrialised countries the same processes which are designed to concentrate nutrients in estuaries and the coastal zone are concentrating pollutants, so that I no longer feel able to eat nutritious foods such as certain shellfish unless I can be sure they are from an unpolluted source.)

Populations such as the Eskimos living on a predominantly fish diet have long been known to have less breast cancer than those eating other animal fats. If properly cooked, seafood also contains lots of iodine, and iodine compounds (like those of zinc) are involved in ensuring that mistakes (which could cause cancer) do not occur during cell division in the body.[50] After the thyroid, the highest concentration of iodine in human females is in the breast, suggesting that - as in the case of zinc, which is concentrated in the prostate in males - it plays an essential role in the proper functioning of breast tissue. (Indeed, I have helped many of my friends who had sore breasts before a period, to overcome the problem by taking Icelandic kelp tablets). Also, iodine has been shown to lower the incidence of breast cancer in menopausal laboratory rats.[51]

As a chemical element, iodine has very unusual behaviour. It is called a conservative element which means that it prefers to stay in water and hence in the Earth's system it ends up being concentrated in the oceans. This is why one of the main dietary sources is seafood. The distinctive chemistry of iodine means that it is easily lost when growing, processing and cooking food (Chinese people tend to cook fish in sealed containers and use the juices to make soup which keeps levels of iodine intake higher). Pasteurisation of milk destroys up to 20 per cent of available iodine and several components of our diet contain compounds called goitrogens which increase our need for additional iodine. The plant called rape, from which rapeseed or canola oil is obtained, contains goitrogens and I avoid this in my diet and anything that contains unspecified vegetable oils since this could include such oil.

To ensure I have enough iodine I take kelp tablets. All seaweed has high concentrations of iodine and other nutrients but it can also concentrate pollutants including some radio-active isotopes offshore of nuclear plants. I therefore eat only Icelandic kelp (because Iceland has a low population and uses only natural geothermal energy and it is further away from most pollutant sources than any other supplier of seaweed that I can think of). Earlier this century fish, waste and seaweed were commonly used as fertiliser but these have now been mostly replaced by inorganic fertilisers, including rock phosphate, which generally have low iodine content (but which can be rich in the radioactive element uranium and in the potentially toxic element cadmium, depending on the source).

Soils in most Western countries tend to have much lower organic humic matter contents because of industrialised farming, so they cannot effectively trap the iodine delivered to them in rain water. Hence, crops now generally contain relatively low levels of this essential nutrient making a natural supplement such as kelp important. Taking kelp in my diet has improved my skin enormously. If I run out of tablets for any length of time my skin becomes rough, initially around my elbows, knees and buttocks and the roughness gradually extends over progressively larger areas until I take kelp again, when the roughness retreats. Seaweed is also protective against radiation. Alginate, a mucous material extracted from seaweed, is used as a standard protective agent against radioactivity. Hence kelp and other seaweeds help reduce the side effects of X-rays and radiotherapy. Agar-agar, which is widely used to replace gelatine in vegan foods, can also be used in your diet as a source of iodine. Other seaweeds which I use occasionally include: arame, hiziki, dulse and wakame. After softening in cold water for about 20 minutes, add to soups or stews immediately before serving (to preserve the iodine). Nori, which is commonly sold in sheets, can be used to wrap rice balls, sushi and many other foods.

An extra bonus is that iodine is good for the brain. Iodine deficiency is the world's most common cause of mental retardation and brain damage.[52] Indeed, the untreatable condition known as cretinism whereby children are born severely mentally retarded, can be caused by the mother's deficiency in iodine during pregnancy.

Cereals are a good source of proteins and are discussed further under Food Factor #6 (see p. 182).

Another good protein source is nuts. I eat lots of nuts (but never pre-shelled because they quickly become rancid). I avoid peanuts and other groundnuts because they can be contaminated with micro-organisms which produce cancer-causing chemicals known as aflatoxins, and I avoid brazil nuts which can contain elevated levels of the radioactive substance radium -226. When one of my colleagues told me this because he was concerned that I was eating so many of these nuts, I did not believe him. After leaving some of the nuts I had been eating in our detector overnight, I did!

PREVENTION FOR ORDINARY MORTALS
For those without breast cancer but who wish to cut their risk or those who have recovered from breast cancer (like me). Remember to keep total animal produce to no more than fifteen per cent of calories each day.

If You Used To Do This . . .	Now Do This!
Breakfast Processed refined cereals with milk and white sugar	Organic muesli with a tablespoon of flaxseed, moistened with fruit juice previously sweetened with honey, raw cane sugar or molasses, or use rice, soya or coconut milk
Fried sausage, bacon, scrambled eggs and fried bread	1. Grilled organic bacon or vegetarian alternative, tomatoes and mushrooms brushed with, or softened in, olive oil. Toast or lightly fry bread in olive oil, or 2. Haddock poached in 50 per cent soya milk, 50 per cent water topped with a poached, organic egg, or 3. Boiled or poached eggs on wholemeal, organic bread lightly fried in olive oil.

Toasted white bread and butter with marmalade. Commercial orange juice	Toasted organic wholemeal bread with Granose soya spread and marmalade Freshly made melon and raspberry juice or apple juice or any alternative juice you enjoy.
Snacks and nibbles Commercial biscuits especially those containing dairy including whey, casein, lactose, milk powder etc.	Dried fruit, nuts, pumpkin seeds, bananas, dried coconut. Dairy free sesame bars or other snacks from health food stores.
Main meals Meat cooked in butter or lard eaten rare or undercooked	Roast or grill meat slowly and thoroughly using olive oil, sea salt and black pepper and other herbs to flavour, but only small portions. Roast potatoes in the juices and then use juices to make the gravy.
Fast foods Hamburgers, sausage, paté, prepared dishes from supermarkets	Eat veggie burgers or vegetarian sausages. Fish or eggs are the ultimate fast food. Steam or poach fish in water or white wine flavoured with ginger, onions, fennel or dill or simply grill after brushing with olive oil and seasoning with salt, black pepper and herbs.
Tinned peas	Lightly steam fresh peas, mange tout, asparagus, broccoli or any other vegetables and keep the juice to make soup or gravy. Don't add butter, use olive oil flavoured with herbs.

Chips, buttered or roast potatoes. Baked potatoes with butter or cheese	Just scrub potatoes before baking or steaming, then rub in olive oil and garnish with chopped parsley before serving. Eat baked potatoes with houmous or taramasalata instead of butter and cheese.
Milky sauces and cream soups	In sauces replace the milk with soya milk; in soups substitute as in the cream of spinach recipe on p. 155.
Thin soups	Miso-based soups (p. 132), or use simple vegetable broth.
Puddings	Choose from fresh fruit salads, baked bananas, water ices or sorbets, soya ice cream or tofu fruit puddings described in Food Factor #1, caramelised oranges, pears stewed in red wine, baked apples filled with dried fruit and chopped nuts. Use soya cream and adjust the taste with fruit juice, honey or raw sugar and a few drops of organic vanilla essence. A wonderful orange sauce made with the juice of two oranges gently heated with raw sugar (to taste) and a few drops of vanilla (with a teaspoon of Cointreau) can be poured over many puddings before serving, making them even more delicious.
Cheese course	Substitute a salad course with pine nuts, sun dried tomatoes and herb flavoured olives,

	artichoke hearts and marinated tofu.
Commercial mayonnaise, salad dressing or salad cream	Make a base of 3–1 virgin olive oil to wine, cider, raspberry or balsamic vinegar, season with pinch of raw sugar, sea salt and black pepper to taste and use English or French (Dijon) mustard, various herbs and garlic to ring the changes.
Cheesy or yoghurt-based dips	Use houmous, tahini or taramasalata.
After dinner chocolates	Buy the organic, dairy free, dark chocolate version.
Milky tea or coffee	Substitute from lists in Food Factors #1 and #7
Late night milk chocolate or malt drink	Check the label, then make it with soya milk instead of dairy, using raw sugar, vanilla or other flavourings you enjoy.

FOOD FACTOR #4: OILS AND FATS

Many people are confused about the type and quantity of oils and fat they should be eating. Also, we have been persuaded to buy lots of spreads based on (usually altered and processed) polyunsaturated fats. Our bodies do need fats, but only in the quantities and forms which we would have consumed as hunters or gatherers.

Fats are solid at room temperature, oils are liquid. However, scientists often use the term 'fat' to include all oils and fats, whether they're solid or liquid. Chemically, fats are made up of three molecules of fatty acids a nd one of an alcohol called glycerol. The word 'triglycerides' is also used to describe fat – it means three ('tri') fatty acid molecules plus glycerol – triglyceride.

Fatty acids are, simply, acids that are found in fats. There are four major fatty acids: palmitic, stearic, oleic and linoleic. Remember, each molecule of fat contains three of these four fatty acids. It's the *combination* of these acids in the fat molecule that determines whether the fat is saturated, unsaturated, or polyunsaturated – words we've all heard a great deal in the past few years. Let me explain them.

Lipids (fats and oils) which are made from various combinations of fatty acids combined with glycerol, have long tails of carbon atoms (often fifteen to seventeen carbon atoms long) combined with hydrogen. Some fatty acids are chains of carbon atoms attached by single bonds and all their spare bonds are attached to hydrogen. They are called saturated (with respect to hydrogen). Some have double bonds between carbon atoms and are called unsaturated. Unsaturated fatty acids can have one (monounsaturated) or many (polyunsaturated) double bonds between carbon atoms. Double bonds make fatty acids and lipids melt more easily, hence most oils are unsaturated while fats, especially animal fats, which are generally saturated, are solid at room temperature. In nature, fats serve an important role in storing energy (they store more energy than the same mass of carbohydrates) and as an insulator against heat loss. The way the carbon and hydrogen are assembled means that these substances are generally insoluble in water and are said to be hydrophobic.

SATURATED

Palmitic fatty acid has 16 carbon atoms and no unsaturated carbon bonds. So it's called 'saturated'. Stearic fatty acid has 18 carbon atoms and no unsaturated carbon bonds, so it's also called 'saturated'. Saturated fat is known to raise the level of cholesterol in your blood. The more you eat, the higher your cholesterol level, and the greater your chances of suffering a stroke or heart attack. Animal fat – lard, butter and that in meat – contains lots of saturated fat. A few plant fats also contain significant amounts, principally coconut and palm oil. Among all the controversies about fats and oils, the message to minimise saturated fat in our diet has remained unchanged for more than thirty years.

MONOUNSATURATED

Oleic fatty acid has eighteen carbon atoms and one unsaturated carbon bond. So it's called 'monounsaturated'. Ongoing research suggests that monounsaturated fat is much healthier than saturated fat. Experiments on humans show that switching to monounsaturated fat from the saturated kind can not only decrease the risk of heart disease, but it may also be able to lower your blood pressure. A major source is olive oil. This contains more than 80 per cent monounsaturated fats and is naturally resistant to oxidation, which means it is relatively safe for cooking and is also less prone to rancidity than other types of unsaturated fat. Rancidity is believed to promote cancer.

POLYUNSATURATED

Linoleic fatty acid has eighteen carbon atoms and two unsaturated carbon bonds. So it's called 'polyunsaturated'. Early research indicated that polyunsaturated fats lowered total and LDL cholesterol (low density lipoprotein – the 'bad' form of cholesterol) more than monounsaturated fats. The latest research, however, finds no difference in their cholesterol-lowering ability. However, the more polyunsaturated an oil is, the more it can be damaged by heat, air and light. Most polyunsaturated oils should only be used raw because once damaged they form free radicals. Good sources of polyunsaturated fats include sunflower and corn oil. We all need a little linoleic acid in our diets every day because, of the four major fatty acids, this is the only group our bodies cannot synthesise.

Essential fatty acids

The two classes of essential fatty acids (EFAs) which are polyunsaturated and which you will undoubtedly have heard about are named omega-6 and omega-3. They are both necessary for good health because they provide the catalysts for various metabolic functions (e.g. in the synthesis of prostaglandins, which are important as cell regulators and for the proper functioning of the immune system). Through a complicated transformation process, essential fatty acids become biologically active and therefore become useful links in many metabolic systems. They are called 'essential' because the body cannot make them, and they must be obtained from food sources. Most vegetable oils provide the EFAs to a greater or lesser extent, but they are not significantly present in meat.

- Omega-6 fatty acids (e.g. linoleic acid) are found in vegetable seeds and the oils produced from them. Good sources include oils made from safflower, sunflower, corn, soya, evening primrose, pumpkin, walnut, and wheat germ.
- Omega-3 fatty acids (e.g. alpha linolenic acid) are found in cold water fish such as salmon, mackerel and sardines, and are also found in linseed (flaxseed), evening primrose, borage seed and soya bean oil. In addition to being protective against breast cancer, they are considered protective against a range of other conditions including coronary heart disease and high blood pressure, arthritis, eczema and psoriasis and benign prostatic hyperplasia (enlarged prostate).[53] The food supplement spirulina (a microscopic algae) contains both linoleic and linolenic acids.

Japanese researchers have shown that a deficiency of these essential fatty acids leads to an impaired ability to learn and recall information. Gamma linoleic acid (GLA) is a particularly good Omega-3 fatty acid which is enriched in organ meats such as liver (but eat only from organically reared animals) and in evening primrose oil – but do not have this in gelatine capsules (which are made from rendered dead animal carcasses).

It has been suggested that the amount of Omega-6 oils in most Western diets is about twenty times that of Omega-3 oil.[54] The advice now is to take no more than 10 per cent of daily calories in polyunsaturated fats, with about a seven-to-one ratio of Omega-6 to Omega-3. I do eat lots of fish but I am prepared to pay for wild rather than farmed fish since this is less likely to contain antibiotic residues and other man-made pollutants. However, I do not take fish oils because of concern that they can contain concentrations of pollutants such as organochlorine pesticides and PCBs (see p. 219). Fish are also rich in vitamin D, essential for healthy bones and suggested by research at St George's Medical School, London and Harvard University, to help prevent breast cancer.[55] Vitamins A and D may work to reduce risk by lowering blood levels of IGF-1.[56]

I will no longer eat dairy produce in any guise and I rely mainly on first pressed extra-virgin olive oil for everything from cooking to salad dressings. This contains more than 80 per cent monounsaturated fatty acids and is naturally resistant to oxidation which means it is relatively safe for cooking. However, I never re-use the oil and I cook food slowly so that the oil is not damaged and the food absorbs the flavour. I avoid brands of margarine based on olive oil but which also contain dairy produce.

The only oils I use have been organically grown and extracted by cold pressing. There are three methods of extraction:

- Cold pressing. This is the traditional hydraulic pressing process where the temperature is kept low throughout and which therefore preserves temperature-sensitive vitamins. The end product is expensive, mainly because there is a high percentage of waste in the discarded pulp, but the oil is nutritious and tastes and smells good. It may be more expensive but you consume less!

- Screw or expeller. This process involves high-pressure pressing which generates high temperatures. Vitamins are destroyed during this process and although it enables more oil to be extracted it is dark, strong smelling and needs further refining and deodorising.

- Solvent extraction. This is the most common process used because it produces the highest yields. The grains or seeds are ground, steamed and then mixed with solvents. The solvents used are either the petroleum-based benzene, hexane or heptane. The mixture is then heated to remove the solvents and then washed with caustic soda. This has the effect of destroying the oil's valuable lecithin content. After this it is bleached and filtered which removes precious minerals as well as any coloured substances. Finally it is heated to a high temperature to deodorise it. One other aspect of vegetable oils produced by solvent extraction is that they have lost their vitamin E. This vitamin helps stop the oil from going rancid. Rancid oils are damaging because they provide the raw material for producing free radicals in our bodies. Sometimes chemical retardants are added to stop the oil from turning rancid, but it would seem to be much more sensible to stick with the cold-pressed oils which can keep well, if properly stored, for up to six months.

All oils should be stored in dark opaque stoppered glass bottles to minimise oxidation and used cold in salad dressings or by the teaspoonful. I never use oils from plastic bottles since many of the potentially harmful chemical substances in plastics are fat soluble. In keeping with my general philosophy of eating whole unprocessed foods as much as possible, I obtain my oils as part of the total food: for example I eat fish oils as fish and flaxseed for flaxseed oil. The benefits of this approach can be demonstrated in relation to flax: according to Ingram and others[57] it is flaxseed – but not flax oil – that is rich in lignan precursors which are anti-carcinogenic. Flaxseed or linseed may be particularly helpful against breast cancer and is also excellent for avoiding constipation and hence piles and varicose veins.[58] Research by Dr Lillian Thompson of the University of Toronto reported in 1999 showed that lignan precursor from flaxseed reduces the growth rates of existing breast cancer by more than 50 per cent. It has also been shown to be protective against colon cancer. Flaxseed is an abundant source of lignan precursors, which are thought to be changed by the action of bacteria in the human intestine to compounds extremely protective against breast cancer. Lignans are also antioxidants, antibiotic and anti-tumorigenic. The only non-wholefood oil in my diet is cold-pressed extra-virgin olive oil. I eat no butter and no margarine.

In many Mediterranean restaurants it is usual to have virgin olive oil flavoured with herbs to dip bread into. It is so much tastier and healthier than butter. I do this now if I have dinner parties. Usually my guests eat their bread dipped in flavoured olive oil with great relish. I cannot remember anyone complaining or asking for butter. On the contrary, I have noticed many of them have copied the idea. The Spanish, Italian and Greek people I know use olive oil with fish or tomato paste and salad for example to make sandwiches, instead of butter or polyunsaturated spreads on their bread. This is not only healthier but the sandwiches and snacks are much more delicious than those most people in the UK eat.

I avoid rapeseed or canola oil. Canola has been bred from old varieties of rapeseed in Canada, and is reported to contain very low levels of erucic acid suspected to have pathogenic potential in diets high in the original rapeseed oil in experimental animals.[59] Canola oil is now the most widely consumed food oil in Canada and is approved by the US FDA.

I also avoid products containing vegetable oils where the type of oil is unspecified since they could contain canola, palm or coconut oil. I avoid all margarines including those claiming to be high in polyunsaturates because they have been hydrogenated (involving passing hydrogen gas through them under pressure often in the presence of a nickel catalyst). This process can produce 'trans fat' which some nutrition experts believe are unhealthy and which have been implicated in breast cancer.[60] The Western diet typically contains large quantities of trans fatty acids (TFAs) originating primarily from hydrogenated fats which experimental evidence suggests impair essential fatty acid metabolism.[61] The TFAs are somewhat similar in structure and behaviour to saturated fatty acids and the World Health Organisation recommends that manufacturers should reduce the levels of TFA arising from hydrogenation.

OIL YOU NEED TO KNOW: TEN WAYS TO MODIFY YOUR FAT INTAKE	
If You Used To Do This . . .	*Now Do This!*
Spread your toast with a thin layer of butter, wait until it soaked in then cover it with a thick layer of peanut butter	Leave out the butter.
Spread your toast with a thick layer of butter or margarine	Drizzle a little organic, cold-pressed extra-virgin olive oil over your toast instead. It tastes delicious . . . really!
Buy oil labelled canola or unspecified 'vegetable' oil	Buy only cold-pressed extra-virgin organic olive, walnut, sesame or sunflower oils.
Prepare a fondue every weekend	Keep the little forks but switch ethnic loyalties and prepare a platter of raw and steamed

	vegetables surrounded by a selection of Thai, Japanese and Chinese dips and sauces.
Buy a cheese and pickle sandwich from your local Marks & Spencer every lunchtime	Buy a tub of their hoummus instead, along with a salad and a few baby pittas to dip into it.
Buy crackers and snack foods without reading the labels	Read all labels for fat content! And don't leave your spectacles at home. I suggest you buy matzos to put in your cracker barrel and buy fresh and dried fruit instead of snacks.
Insist on making popcorn before you watched that film	Go ahead, but use an air-popper to make it. They make a good gift (£30–£50) and require no fat. Add salt or your favourite spices as usual.
Order the Four Cheeses pizza from your local	Try the Marguerita without the mozzarella, but extra olives, capers, mushrooms, garlic, etc.
Order the baked potato with butter, chilli con carne and cheese sauce	Order the baked potato with baked beans or houmous and a side salad.
Go crazy for any dessert topped with cream	Dig out a recipe for orange sauce (p. 169), or keep a small bottle of organic maple syrup in your cupboard, and drizzle a little over your favourite non-dairy dessert.

FOOD FACTOR #5: SEASONING AND FLAVOURINGS

Healthy food doesn't have to be – indeed, *shouldn't* be – bland food. Until recently the main methods of preserving food were to add lots of salt, especially to meat and vegetables, sugar to fruit, and alcohol to a range of products. It has been said that the British, because they shipped so much food from their overseas territories, developed a particular liking for these tastes. Food naturally contains sodium so we do not need to add any to our food. Overuse of salt and sodium bicarbonate have been linked by Gerson to cancer and it continues to be implicated by some researchers in promoting certain types of cancer, including naso-pharyngeal (nose and throat) cancer.[62]

It is easy to learn to change your taste and you will find food tastes much better with far more subtle flavours when salt is not added. Oriental people, however, consume lots of salt in soya sauce so I do not think it is one of the most critical things to do in combating breast cancer; but it is helpful to your health generally and I recommend you reduce your salt and refined sugar intake as much as you can, as soon as you can.

I grow fresh herbs such as parsley, thyme, chives, marjoram, rosemary and mint in a small patch in the garden and buy others from the supermarket. Herbs are good for you and help to make food taste delicious. I did not use spices when I was ill, but the Chinese do use spices especially in the Sichuan and Hunan provinces. Also, Korean and Thai food is very heavily spiced yet breast and prostate cancer rates there are low. Hence, despite the recommendations in many anti-cancer-diet books, I do not believe that spices are a primary factor in the case of breast or prostate cancer.

On the other hand, I never eat the horribly coloured pink or yellow food now sold as Eastern food in some shops, restaurants and supermarkets; although real saffron made from crocus stamens and traditionally used to colour rice yellow contains carotenoids and has anti-free-radical properties.

I use vinegar (wine or cider, preferably organically produced) with organic extra-virgin olive oil as the basis for delicious salad dressings. I never eat commercially produced mayonnaise or salad creams or other such 'glop'.

Unrefined sugars or molasses are fine (although check that you really are buying raw sugar as some brown sugar is white sugar dyed with caramel (burnt sugar). I also eat honey (preferably wild honey from unpolluted sources). Refined white sugar (called pure white and deadly by some) is just empty calories stripped of nutrients. I never eat it, but molasses or raw brown sugar is fine. Traditionally Chinese and Japanese have eaten very few sweets, their treats, including for small children, were pumpkin seeds or dried fruit.

Here are some spicy ways to enliven any dish!

Garam Masala

This mixture may be changed to suit your tastes. Use a mortar and pestle, a hand-turned peppermill or an electric grinder, such as a coffee grinder, to grind your spices. It is best, and noticeably different in flavour and aroma, to use whole spices grinding them only when you need them. We all have need for little shortcuts now and again, however, so simply store any surplus ground spices in a labelled, airtight jar in a dark cupboard.

Makes 2–3 tbsp, enough for 1 dish
Preparation time 5 minutes

2 tsp freshly ground coriander
1 tsp freshly ground black pepper
1 tsp freshly ground cumin
½ tsp freshly crushed cardamom
½ tsp freshly ground cloves
½ tsp freshly ground cinnamon

If you can, grind these spices individually, measure them, then mix them.

Mild and Fresh Spice Blend

This mixture can be used to flavour soups, stews and other dishes; adjust it to suit your taste. This amount is for one dish.

Makes 3–4 tbsp
Preparation time 10 minutes

1 tbsp caraway seeds
3 cloves garlic, crushed
2 tsp fresh ginger, grated
1 tsp freshly ground black pepper
1 tsp ground coriander
½ tsp salt
¼ tsp ground allspice

Grind all the ingredients in a pestle and mortar until the caraway seeds are slightly crushed. Stir into the dish, either during the sauté or shortly before serving, and adjust to taste.

Warming Spice and Herb Blend

This is a more robust blend which may be used alone or in combination with the above recipe in savoury dishes. The ingredients may be adjusted to suit your taste.

Makes 140g (5oz)
Serves 4
Preparation time 15 minutes

5 spring onions, finely chopped
3 cloves garlic, finely chopped
1 tbsp fresh ginger, grated
1–2 fresh hot chillies, finely chopped
2 tbsp fresh basil, chopped
1 tsp freshly ground cardamom
1 tsp freshly ground black pepper
¼ tsp ground nutmeg

Blend all the ingredients and add to the dish during sauté.

LIVELY SPICES: TEN HEALTHY WAYS TO EXCITE YOUR TASTEBUDS	
If You Used To Do This . . .	*Now Do This!*
Sprinkle everything with salt	Stop cooking with salt. Try seasoning your meal with tamari (wheat-free soy sauce) or gomasio, a mixture of ground sesame and sea salt.
Spread yeast extract on your toast	Good idea, but on alternate days spread miso on your toast for the similar-but-different flavour and the added nutrient value it brings.

Serve boiled carrots with a dollop of butter	Steam the carrots then toss them in a light sauté of garlic and/or freshly grated ginger.
Think black pepper is the only spice	Arrange a small collection of spicy condiments on the table including black pepper, chilli pepper flakes and Tabasco sauce. Visit your local ethnic grocer to explore a new world of spices, then begin to experiment . . .
Use 'salad cream' and nothing else on every salad you are given	Mix finest olive oil with a herb flavoured cider vinegar, freshly crushed garlic and a little mustard. Or drizzle a little freshly squeezed lemon juice and sesame or walnut oil over your salad. A splash of Tabasco will lift the flavour to the roof.
Think boiled cabbage and potatoes were only there to soak up the gravy	Steam the vegetables then toss them gently in a light sauté of caraway seed and chopped garlic. Season with good old black pepper, to taste.
Every soup needed a hefty dose of beef broth and monosodium glutamate (MSG) in order to be tasty	Make your soups with a strong vegetable broth including the seaweed, Kombu, which has flavouring and thickening properties similar to MSG.
All vinegar was white and only good for making your lips pucker	Buy finest organic cider vinegar and organically grown fresh herbs and put the two together in the prettiest bottle you can find. Try tarragon, rosemary, basil or garlic. As well, some delicatessens sell

	raspberry and other fruit vinegars. Now go and make that salad dressing!
Think that rice was a white and fluffy but rather bland way of bulking out the good stuff	First, change your brand of rice! Buy whole grain, basmati or wild rice then zip up the flavour this way: heat 1 teaspoon olive oil in the saucepan and sauté one teaspoon of Chinese Five Spice or Spices for CousCous. Both of these are available at good supermarkets. Now stir in your dry rice, then add the water and do the usual cooking routine. Better?
Roast onions tasted of cooked water	Leave small onions whole and slice larger ones in half. Now press two or three whole cloves into each onion and place in the baking tray with the potatoes, parsnips and half the oil you would normally use. Instead, get taste to the max by dissolving a tablespoon of yeast extract in a little warm water and pour over the waiting veg. *Now* roast!

FOOD FACTOR #6: CEREAL FOODS, SNACKS AND TREATS

Food is one of life's great pleasures, and The Plant Programme is not a hair-shirt regime for masochists! I buy sorbets and soya ice creams and organic dark dairy-free chocolate for occasional treats (now my cancer has gone). Also, I do occasionally eat some of the delicious soups sold in waxed paper cartons now on offer after checking carefully that they contain no dairy products, but I do *not* buy those available in plastic pots (*see* p. 200).

My favourite treat is fish and chips which I eat at least once a week now my cancer has gone, although I remove all the batter unless I buy from my local fish and chip shop, where they are kind enough to make it without milk. Recently I was struck, walking down a high street in Surrey, by two fast food shops, which were advertising 'the great American experience' (cow burgers on white 'bread') and 'the great British experience' (fish and chips), respectively. If I use fast food I always choose the British version on health grounds as well as taste.

I eat masses of dried fruit of all descriptions. Prunes contain anti-cancer chemicals and figs are an excellent source of calcium. Seeds such as pumpkin, sesame (both a rich source of zinc) and sunflower seeds make delicious snacks and are very nutritious. Traditionally, Chinese people give such seeds and small pieces of fresh or dried fruit to their children as treats rather than sugary sweets, cakes and biscuits as we tend to do in the West. Until recently the good state of the teeth of most Chinese people clearly reflected this practice.

Much snack food, such as sandwiches and biscuits, is based on wheat which has a bad name with many alternative health practitioners – although I fail to understand that wheat or other gluten-based cereals such as barley or rye are intrinsically bad for people, except where there is clear evidence of gluten intolerance. Most people in developing countries rely on cereals as one of their main sources of food and have traditionally had low levels of the diseases of affluence, including cancer. Wheat consumption is often suggested to be bad because its consumption is linked to settled farming, but barley, oats, maize and rice were also domesticated from wild cereal grasses at approximately the same time and have been used by farmers for thousands of years, albeit mainly in a labour-intensive not capital-intensive way. Moreover, wheat is generally eaten after it has been processed in some way whereas rice is traditionally eaten whole. Perhaps the increased incidence of the diseases archaeologists correlate with the beginning of settled farming were due to other factors, including milk consumption, and deficiency conditions caused by over-exploitation and degradation of land. I do not believe wheat itself to be involved in promoting cancer, although there is some evidence that the herbicide sprays used to eliminate weeds from wheat crops might promote breast cancer. Perhaps wheat is an example of how industrialised agriculture and food production can convert a good, nutrient-rich food into one that many alternative health practitioners feel they must tell us not to eat.

Wheat is now produced mainly by monoculture methods under conditions as prairie-like as possible with hedges grubbed up and biodiversity reduced, so that a high degree of mechanisation can be used, including in the planting and harvesting of crops and the spraying of pesticides. Soil used for such industrialised agriculture becomes exhausted and depleted of essential nutrients because of a lack of animal manure, and these are only partly replaced by inorganic fertilisers.[63] Processing wheat to make white flour for white bread and many commercial pastries removes much of the proteins, vitamins and minerals which are often used for animal fodder. In order to compensate, inorganic nutrients such as chalk as a source of calcium, iron and vitamins are added back. Despite adding these vitamins, such processed flour has often lost much of its bioavailable vitamin B6, vitamin B5 and molybdenum; nearly all of its vitamin E, cobalt and zinc content, much of its chromium and some selenium content, too. The degradation of nutritional content is made worse by the addition of bleaches and 'improvers' such as potassium bromate, some of which have been shown to be toxic. I always check the list of ingredients carefully when buying bread and ensure that it is free of chemical additives. If I had the time, I would make my own bread with freshly purchased organic wheat or other cereals, using one of the bread-making machines which are now widely available, but my life is far too busy at the moment!

To avoid any potential problems associated with wheat, I use only organic wholemeal brown bread made with stone ground flour. I eat many other types of organically grown cereals including porridge and oatcakes, organic whole brown rice and wholemeal brown organic pasta in my diet, all widely available in health-food stores and increasingly in supermarkets. Despite some recently published versions of anti-breast-cancer diets there is nothing wrong with muesli providing it is based on organic produce and provided it is not the commercial 'muesli' made with sugar or milk-derived components. Also you should use rice, oat or soya milk or fruit juice rather than dairy milk to moisten it. If you are staying in a hotel use the juice from fresh fruit salad or if there is none use the juice from the prunes which are almost always on the buffet. Fibre is used for the workings of the digestive tract and according to some alternative health writers it helps to carry excess female hormones such as oestrogen out of the system. However, many high fibre, especially cereal-based, diets contain high levels of a substance known as phytate. This can bind zinc in the digestive tract and make it unavailable for absorption. (Apparently people living on such diets for long periods of time become adapted and can absorb enough zinc and other mineral nutrients to maintain an adequate status, but I think it is important to eat the zinc-containing protein in your diet at least eight hours after eating food such as cereal which contains high levels of phytates). Interestingly the fibre in flaxseed has been shown in experiments not to bind zinc.[64]

INNOCENT INDULGENCES: TEN HEALTHY TREATS TO KEEP YOU SWEET	
If You Used To Do This . . .	*Now Do This!*
Tuck into a giant bag of crisps while reading the latest novel	Pour a small handful each of sesame, sunflower and pumpkin seeds into a bowl and munch more nutritiously through your book. Or, try roasting the seeds in a pan and sprinkle with soy sauce.
Leave a trail of sweet wrappers around the place	Mix your own blend of organic dried fruits such as figs, dates, apricots, mango, raisins, etc. and place little bowls or cartons of them in handy places: the car, your desk, near the phone . . .
Reward yourself with sweet and sticky desserts layered with cream	Take an organic Bramley apple, remove the core and fill it with raisins, chopped banana, cinnamon and a little maple syrup. Place it in a dish and bake for about 15 minutes. Serve with soya cream or soya ice cream.

Reward yourself with sweet and sticky desserts not layered with cream	Take an organically grown orange, slice it in half and use a grapefruit knife to slice around the segment edges. Sprinkle the sliced surface with a tiny pinch of nutmeg or cloves and the merest hint of maple syrup. Bake for about 15 minutes. Serve hot.
Eat whole variety packs of snack crackers in a single sitting	Buy rice cakes and oatcakes and arrange them on a plate with a little houmous, tofu dip, tahini or home-made salsa.
Get a sweet craving at least twice a day	Soak a mixture of chopped organic dried fruit in mineral water overnight. When you get your sweet attack, serve a small bowlful dressed with a little rose water and chopped pumpkin seeds.
Get a serious snack attack once a day	Fight back with a piping hot baked potato filled with houmous or baked beans. Sometimes a bean salad will do the trick.
Blow out on ice cream and chocolate in any combination	Do it with soya ice cream and dark chocolate instead, or get moderate and serve a home-made chilled fruit soup with a tiny dollop of soya ice cream or soya yoghurt.
Eat a packet of biscuits every day	Pack your own stack of oatcakes spread with jam and made into sandwiches. Sweet, crunchy and very nutritious.

| Eat toast and whatever until the whole loaf was gone | Buy only wholemeal loaves made with organic flour and be fussy about what you spread on them. Try tahini, barley miso, mashed banana or olive paté. |

FOOD FACTOR #7: WHAT TO DRINK

As I mentioned earlier, I drink freshly-made vegetable and fruit juices from organic produce. However, sources of water are more problematical. Before mankind reached the sort of population densities we have now, especially in cities, and before we began to use large quantities of water for washing clothes and cars and in power generation and factories, most people would have drunk water from wells, springs or rivers. Unfortunately the only way of providing adequate water now is to recycle it by treating or reprocessing water at sewage works. Indeed, we joke that when people drink a glass of water in the East End of London, ten people have previously drunk the same water! During treatment the water is filtered through progressively finer material to remove particles, microbes and chemicals and it is often mixed with other water to dilute harmful chemicals so that their concentration falls below legal requirements. Finally, chlorine is added to kill microbes.

In the early 1990s work by Professor Sumpter at Brunel University in the UK showed that in several rivers in the UK downstream of sewage works a high proportion (and in some cases 100 per cent) of the male fish had been feminised with their testes overgrown with eggs. Some of the chemicals implicated include phthalates from soft plastics, nonyl phenols (breakdown products from detergents and plastics) and residues from the female contraceptive or hormone replacement pills. Reprocessed drinking water can contain many other harmful chemicals including benzene and cancer-causing organic chemicals, pesticides and disinfection by-products such as trihalomethanes (THMs) and haloacetic acids (HAAs). More rigorous limits for disinfection by-products are being legislated for in America.[65] For these and other reasons I do not drink water straight from the tap. However, I do not recommend drinking mineral water either, especially from plastic bottles. Moreover some bottled waters can contain such high levels of radioactivity or nitrates that they would be illegal if they came out of the tap.

I use tap water but I filter it through charcoal into a glass jug. I have found it impossible to buy a filtration unit made completely of glass but the plastic is hard and when thoroughly washed is unlikely to release the high concentrations of phthalates associated with soft plastic into the water. After filtering I always boil the water before drinking it to remove or further reduce harmful chemicals and to take out germs not removed by water treatment. These can occur in tap water and bottled water from shallow sources, and I always add tea or herbal teas to try to further remove pollutants (lots of organic plant matter absorbs harmful chemicals onto the surface, removing it from the liquid that you drink). This takes out or reduces many harmful chemical residues because they are often large molecules that are 'hydrophobic', that is they do not stay in water and if they are given the opportunity they will sorb on to something such as charcoal or organic matter instead.

It is particularly important to boil water before drinking when undergoing chemotherapy because the immune system will not be at its best – technically such patients are regarded as immunocompromised instead of immunocompetent (normal with a healthy immune system). Over the past fifteen years or so it has become apparent that a protozoan parasite present in contaminated water supplies (related to the malaria parasite) called Cryptosporidium, can cause severe sickness, vomiting, dehydration and diarrhoea in immunocompromised people, with symptoms which can persist indefinitely (although the gastro-enteritis it causes usually clears up on its own in healthy individuals).

Some of the first diagnosed outbreaks which occurred because of contamination of the water supply were in the USA and the UK; for example outbreaks in Texas in 1984, and in the UK in Ayrshire and Oxfordshire in the late 1980s. In 1993 more than 400,000 people were affected and several people died after Cryptosporidium breached one of Milwaukee, Wisconsin's water filtration plants. Prevention involves boiling (including of bottled water if it is from shallow sources), and frequent and thorough hand washing and bedding changes. Infection has been reported in domestic animals, livestock and wildlife.[66]

I never drink coffee but I drink lots of Chinese green tea with no milk (if you use lemon, remove the peel first unless you are using unwaxed organic fruits). Extracts of green tea have been shown to prevent cancer in experimental animals and more recently similar claims have been made about black tea (but I find this more difficult to drink without milk). The chemicals thought to have anti-cancer properties in green tea are poly-phenols known as cathechins including epigallo-cathechin-3 gallate, an antioxidant that accounts for much of the solid materials in brewed green tea.[67] It is thought that the well-known anti-cancer activity of green tea is because it inhibits one of the most frequently over-expressed enzymes in human cancers, called urokinase.[68]

Drinking fluid this way is exactly what the Chinese do. When I first worked in China, I used to wonder what the jam jars with strange looking bits in the bottom were in the front of taxis. Eventually, I realised they were jars of green tea! Chinese, Japanese and Korean green teas generally contain less pesticides than commonly produced black tea. In China, green tea is valued for its digestive properties and for assisting circulation and regulating body temperature. Preparation of black teas, unlike green teas, involves fermentation.[69] Black tea can contain twice the amount of caffeine (as theine) when compared to coffee; the tannin content of black tea can also inhibit iron uptake, and brewing black tea oxidises the cathechins, thus destroying any beneficial effects.[70]

I drink only green tea (or weak black tea without milk or sugar if there is no other choice). I also use herbal teas, mostly peppermint or camomile with honey (many people do not like the taste of pure camomile at first). I also use fruit teas but sparingly because some are so acid that if I drink too much they give me cystitis. Also some contain chemicals of the kind used to flavour jellies and sweets and I avoid these.

Excess alcohol consumption has long been suggested to be a risk factor for breast cancer. Recent research at the Harvard School of Public Health in the USA indicates that the more alcohol women consume the higher their risk of developing breast cancer, which is increased by up to 40 per cent for those drinking three glasses of wine or the equivalent of 30g of alcohol a day. The findings however were based on studies in the USA, Canada, the Netherlands and Sweden, countries with some of the highest breast cancer incidences in the world. Certainly, alcohol causes problems with the way the liver functions and it has been suggested to increase oestrogen and IGF-1 mobilisation in the body. Studies are being carried out in Sweden to assess the effects of alcohol on IGF-1 and the proteins which can inactivate IGF-binding proteins.[71] I drank very little alcohol before I had cancer and I had none during treatment. I drink some alcohol now, but keep to real ales which are rich in nutrients, especially the important B vitamins, and which contain malt and hops which are soothing to the mind and help me to have a good night's sleep. I never drink wine which is too acid for me and causes me to have cystitis or joint problems. If you must drink wine, have only organically produced wine. Most wine regions produce at least one organic 'label' and, increasingly, supermarkets and high street off-licences stock these at very reasonable rates. I have seen Chinese men drink alcohol – sometimes lots of it – as beer, rice wine or mautai (distilled rice wine, the equivalent of whisky) but I have rarely seen Chinese women drink alcohol. Chinese men suffer very little with prostate cancer and I do not believe moderate alcohol consumption to be a primary factor in breast or prostate cancer. If, however, your diet is rich in animal foods containing the hormones and other chemicals that I believe to be the primary factors involved in promoting these types of cancer, it could make matters worse by increasing levels of circulating oestrogen or free IGF-1, for example.

When I had active cancer I drank no black tea or alcohol and I never drink coffee. One of the benefits of removing these substances from my diet when I was being treated for cancer was that I felt less anxious (without caffeine) and less depressed (without alcohol). Some of my fellow patients who felt the need to drown their sorrows noticeably fared badly and many were clearly depressed.

THIRST QUENCHERS:
TEN DRINKS TO DELIGHT YOU

If You Used To Do This . . .	*Now Do This!*
Start the day with a hot black one	Make it a hot yannoh instead. This is the finest cereal 'coffee' on the market. Try brewing it with 2–3 pods of cardamom and a few whole cloves.
Drink strong tea with milk all day long	If you must have the milky taste, try switching to roibush tea, available at health-food stores. It is strong, caffeine-free and tastes good with soya milk.
Drink black tea with sliced lemon	That's better, but you could try green tea or a strongly flavoured herbal tea such as nettle or dandelion.
Treat yourself to a Starbuck's hot chocolate	Order it made with soya milk. When you make it yourself, try making it with carob instead. This is a chocolate flavoured bean that is tasty and nutritious but caffeine-free
Guzzle cola all day long	Buy sarsaparilla concentrate from a health-food shop or herbalist and dilute to taste with sparkling mineral water.
Swig soft drinks by the gallon	Dilute natural fruit or flower cordials, such as elderflower, with sparkling mineral water. (If you have active breast cancer, prepare freshly made juices.)

Enjoy a jug of iced coffee now and then	Brew the yannoh and cardamom, above, and leave to cool. Pour a little into an ice cube tray and freeze. Blend the cooled yannoh with cold soya milk, whisk and serve with a yannoh ice cube.
Lead a single-handed campaign to double the government recommendations for intake of alcohol	Switch to real beer. Now become a beer historian and expert. Try making your own without a kit. (Your intake will drop but your enjoyment will soar.)
Spend huge amounts on fresh juices from the chill cabinets	Bet you had to shake them first. Make all juices fresh with your own juicer and organic fruit and veg. Try melon, apple and celery, pear, apple and fennel, carrot and parsley, and so on.
Think carrot juice was a cure for sunburn	Make your own with organic carrots. Add a quarter pint of carrot juice to a half pint of cold soya milk, stir well and serve with a straw.

AT A GLANCE: A SUMMARY OF THE MAIN PLANT PROGRAMME RECOMMENDATIONS

Food and drink I never consume

- Milk: Whether organic, whole, skimmed or semi-skimmed or of any other description – from sheep, goats or cows.
- Cheese: Including so-called vegetarian cheese and cottage cheese.
- Yoghurt: Get the good bacteria from acidophilus capsules from health food shops, but remove gelatine capsules before emptying the content into a glass of soya, rice or oat milk, or juice.

- Crème Fraiche.
- Fromage Frais.
- Cream.
- Butter.
- Foods containing any of the above or whey, lactose, milk solids, milk fats or casein. If in doubt ask the shop owner or manager and do not allow yourself to be confused – dairy products are dairy products including when they are used in processed or tinned foods.
- Margarine.
- Beef or pork meat. I also avoid processed meats including paté because I now follow my mother's practice of not eating anything in which I cannot identify the ingredients.
- Commercial refined and processed oils prepared using high pressure or elevated temperatures including unspecified vegetable oils which can be genetically modified soya or maize oil, canola or rapeseed oil or products that contain these.
- Salt, refined white flour or rice, other refined substances such as saccharine, white sugar or foods containing these products including white bread and pasta, which have been chemically altered and depleted of fibre and nutrients.
- Processed food which comes in packets or tins including biscuits, cakes, sweets, carbohydrates, crisps, soups, salted nuts, processed meat products such as ham or corned beef, bottled or commercial pickles, canned or cartoned fruit juices, fruit squashes or fruit drinks containing additives or colour.
- Wines, spirits, coloured or flavoured fizzy drinks.
- Anything sold in plastic bottles or wrapped in soft plastics (*see* p. 200).
- Ready meals containing gums or starches and emulsifiers to thicken and prevent separation of sauces, artificial sweeteners, flavourings or colouring agents.
- Artificial vitamin or mineral tablets (although I did take selenium combined with vitamins A, C and E when I had active cancer, *see* pp. 198–199).

One portion a day food and drink

These foods are fine as part of a cancer-prevention diet or after recovery, but I did not consume them when I had active cancer.

- Organically reared chicken or turkey, preferably drumsticks and dark meat.
- Organically reared duck.
- Organically reared rabbit.
- Organically reared lamb.
- Wild venison or other game.
- Any fish or shellfish from unpolluted sources including tuna or sea bass and cold water fish, such as mackerel, herring, sardines or wild salmon.
- Organic eggs from poultry fed on grain.
- Real ale or cider.

Occasional treats
Once a week but not when I had active cancer

- Fruit sorbet.
- Soya ice cream.
- Dark, organic, dairy-free chocolate.
- Fish (but I take off the batter) and chips.
- Organic bacon.
- Herbal fruit teas (but not those containing artificial chemicals or colour used to flavour jellies and sweets).
- Going out for a meal. I choose Thai, Korean, Japanese and authentic Chinese restaurants; but be aware that some Eastern cuisine available in the West has been greatly modified to appeal to Westerners. I also go to restaurants of any type that sell truly vegan food.

Food and drink I have lots of

- Fruit and dried fruit (organically produced wherever possible).
- Steamed vegetables (organically produced).
- Salad vegetables including sprouting seeds, especially bean-shoots and alfalfa.
- Garlic.
- Freshly prepared vegetables and fruit juices.
- Cereals including organic unrefined wheat, oats, barley, rice and bread, pasta and other products made from them.
- Flavourings made using wine or balsamic vinegar, garlic, herbs such as mint, sage, thyme, coriander, marjoram and

oregano. I use some black pepper, chilli, lemon grass and other spices to make the occasional oriental dish. I particularly recommend Thai flavourings – remember Thai people have the lowest breast and prostate cancer mortality rate on record.

- Nuts and seeds including flaxseed, sunflower, pumpkin, sesame and spreads such as tahini.
- Soya including soya milk, tofu, tempeh, miso and the growing range of organic soya products available. Meals such as rice and peas – a good Jamaican meal which provides a good range of proteins.
- Houmous and taramasalata.
- Molasses and honey.
- Green Japanese, Korean or Chinese teas.
- Peppermint, camomile and nettle herbal teas.
- Olive oil and other cold-pressed oils such as walnut, pumpkin or sesame.
- Organic wine or cider vinegar.

Liane Baldock is a friend of mine who developed breast cancer, follows my diet and kindly offered to tell her own story.

THE STORY OF LIANE BALDOCK

In June 1996 I sought my GP's advice concerning a small lump on the outside edge of my left breast. He considered it of little significance and claimed there was a 3-month wait for appointments at the NHS specialist breast clinic in my area. He did not feel it was warranted to refer me to it. I requested a second opinion and was referred to a private senior general surgeon in July. I was told by him: 'if ever you have breast cancer it will have nothing to do with this lump'. I requested a needle biopsy to be sure, but was told it was too small to locate accurately. I was not informed (and did not know myself) about ultrasound scans at that stage. By November the lump was easily visible when my arm was raised and in December I returned to request the surgeon to remove it privately to avoid another long wait on the NHS as it still 'could not be considered an emergency'. Two days later he removed it under a local anaesthetic and as I slid down off the table he said 'I'd be willing to bet a million pounds this biopsy comes back negative'. Pity I did not take him up on it! Ten days later I returned to have the stitches removed and to be told (by his registrar!) that it was malignant and that I would need further surgery. Finally I was put under the care of a specialist NHS breast surgeon, who pulled out all the stops for me, seeing me within two days and operating himself the following week.

I was deeply shocked and particularly devastated partly because my attempts to do all the right things had not resulted in the early diagnosis I knew to be so important and because my GP and the general surgeon had continually assured me that it was not breast cancer. Neither took it seriously or seemed concerned.

Jane was one of the first people I turned to for advice and support. I had been told to come off HRT at once, and I also gave up all dairy products immediately. I had known about her theories for several years and the research she had done seemed to make sense. I had admired her attitude to her own more serious problems and her scientific approach to alternative therapies that are not yet accepted by the UK medical establishment. At the very least it was something positive I could do to help myself, while the specialist medics took over my life for the next three months with a lumpectomy and lymph removal, followed by radiotherapy. Thankfully no chemotherapy was necessary, as my lymph glands were clear. I refused to take Tamoxifen – to the obvious annoyance of my oncologist. She seemed to want to put everyone on it indiscriminately, without ever going into the rest of their medical history. I had had abnormal uterine cells a year or so before and did know that Tamoxifen might increase the risk of cancer of the uterus.

As I work at a university I had access to medical research papers and obtained a couple mentioned by the Bristol Cancer Centre on work done in Scandinavia.[72] From that research it appeared that high daily doses of Co-enzyme Q_{10} seemed to make breast tumours regress. This has been totally dismissed by the British cancer research teams I have tried to discuss it with. Nevertheless I have been taking it now for three years.

I feel that, at this still relatively early stage (only three-and-a-half years since diagnosis), it would be tempting fate to say any more, but now I have at last got over the effects of the radiotherapy, which left me with what can only be described as crushing exhaustion for almost two years, I do feel pretty fit, although still very wary and on the alert for any potential problem. I also feel that I am doing all I can to reduce the risk of a recurrence by eating a much healthier diet. This includes far more fruit, vegetables and fish, less saturated fats and no dairy products – except for the odd cheese sandwich which I find irresistible at times and which is the only thing I really miss!

If substituting (GM-free!) soya-based or vegetable oil products for dairy produce helps to reduce the incidence or recurrence of breast cancer it is certainly worth it and no great hardship, compared with the alternative.

The update to this chapter can be found on page 334.

6 The Plant Programme – The Lifestyle Factors

There are important things, apart from diet, that you can change to help cut your risk of breast and prostate cancer. In this chapter I explain why you should make these changes and how to do so successfully: from coping strategies for stress, to ways of avoiding harmful substances in your environment.

As well as dietary factors there are lifestyle factors we can change to cut our risk of developing breast cancer. These range from the way we buy and store our food to the way we cope with stress. Here I shall take you through the five most important lifestyle factors.

LIFESTYLE FACTOR #1: VITAMIN AND MINERAL SUPPLEMENTS

In general, I prefer to eat whole foods because, as I have indicated, problems often arise when we try to separate food into constituent parts. Moreover, vitamin/mineral pills are often synthesised from coal or petroleum derivatives. Also, taking too much of one or other man-made supplement, can cause a deficiency elsewhere in our diet. For example, taking the trace element molybdenum blocks copper intake. The body knows how to deal with nutrients from natural foods, but may absorb too much or too little from man-made chemical supplements. Hence I take no man-made vitamin or mineral pills in my diet, although for the six months when I was undergoing chemotherapy I took tablets which combined selenium with vitamins A, C and E.

Selenium status can often be marginal to deficient in UK diets and it is important for immune function generally and as an antioxidant. This trace mineral is essential to health, though only required in minute quantities. In America, the National Research Council has recommended a daily intake of 50–200 micrograms of selenium for adults (a microgram is one thousandth of a milligram, so 200 micrograms equal 0.2 milligrams). However, one authority – Gerhard Schrauzer, Ph.D., of the University of California – says that 250–300 micrograms can protect against most cancers, and that most people consume only about 100 micrograms daily.[1] At higher doses, selenium can be toxic to the human body. Although it is not certain at precisely what level selenium begins to cause adverse effects, it has been found that doses of 900 micrograms (0.9 milligrams) per day can make hair and nails fall out and can affect the nervous system.[2]

Selenium works best in conjunction with vitamin E, since both are antioxidants and can increase the production of antibodies by up to thirty times,[3] thereby greatly enhancing your immune response. Together they help to detoxify your body and prevent the formation of free radicals. Selenium is naturally present in the soil, and the quantities available in our food relate to soil levels of selenium where the food was grown. A study of the health effects of selenium compared its distribution in soil across the United States with a map detailing the national cancer rates. It was found that those areas with high levels of cancer corresponded with places of low levels of selenium in the soil. For instance, Ohio was shown to have the highest incidence of cancer and the lowest levels of selenium; South Dakota had the highest levels of selenium and the lowest rate of cancer.[4]

A study undertaken at the University of Tampere, Finland, involved taking blood samples from 21,172 Finnish men. The samples were then frozen. Eleven years after the samples had been taken, 143 men had contracted lung cancer. The researchers found that the men who eventually developed lung cancer had less selenium in their blood than those who did not. Overall, it was found that people with the lowest selenium levels were 3.3 times more likely to develop lung cancer than those with high levels. The researchers said their results were 'in accord with other studies which strongly suggest that poor selenium nutrition is a highly significant risk factor for lung cancer'.[5]

In West Germany, a study conducted at the University of Bonn has shown that selenium can protect against the harmful effects of ultraviolet radiation. Blood selenium levels were examined in 101 patients with malignant melanoma (a lethal form of skin cancer) and compared to a control group of healthy people. The skin cancer patients showed a significantly lower level of selenium, and the researchers concluded that their results 'strongly suggest that sub-optimal selenium nutrition preceded the onset of the disease and may even have contributed to its genesis'.[6]

Industrialised agriculture and food production may well be leading to sub-clinical deficiencies in vitamins and minerals. Also, obesity can cause deficiency conditions. I am not overweight and I rely on a varied diet of organically produced food to provide most of my needs. If I feel I need extra vitamins and minerals I use freshly-made organic juices which are less likely to cause toxicity or imbalances. I do, however, take kelp to avoid iodine deficiency and also brewer's yeast which is a good source of many trace elements including iron, zinc, selenium and chromium (which is protective against diabetes), and B vitamins which are important if the body is to synthesise important compounds such as co-enzyme Q_{10}. Co-enzyme Q_{10} has been shown to be essential to the optimal functioning of all cell types and there is evidence that supplementation with co-enzyme Q_{10} helps regression of breast cancer.[7] Co-enzyme Q_{10} is also an antioxidant and free radical scavenger. The body is capable of synthesising adequate quantities given a good diet especially one rich in the B vitamins and minerals concentrated in brewer's yeast. Also, soya contains co-enzyme Q_{10}.

Siberian ginseng and parnox or true ginseng are both reputed to help immunity and to overcome tiredness and debility associated with cancer treatment including radiotherapy (although the Bristol diet recommends against them). I use only whole roots or root pieces of ginseng, not teas or extracts. I used them occasionally especially towards the end of my radiotherapy treatment. They are available from oriental shops and some good health stores.

Food supplements I use
Brewer's yeast (six tablets a day),* Red Clover (a teaspoon a day),† Icelandic kelp (six tablets a day).‡ These are all natural and not synthetic substances. Also I took tablets containing selenium and vitamins A, C and E when I had active cancer.

LIFESTYLE FACTOR #2: FOOD PACKAGING
Food packaging is very important. A recent report, on the abundance of chemicals that mimic the female hormone oestrogen, from the authoritative British Institute of Environment and

---

* † ‡ Follow the manufacturer's instructions and do not exceed the recommended amount – the quantity of tablets depends on the brand.

Health (IEH) has suggested that a group of chemicals called phthalates seriously disrupt reproduction in animals (including damaging the testes in males). Scientific experiments suggest that certain phthalates may cause birth defects, cancer, testicular atrophy and sterility.[8] One of the main sources of phthalates identified in the IEH report is soft plastics such as those which may come into contact with food. The chemicals leak from the plastic into the food, and then accumulate in our body fat (remember breast tissue comprises a considerable proportion of fat). Try whenever possible to buy food in good old-fashioned brown paper bags – be prepared to make a fuss if necessary. One of my friends dumps all plastics wrappings at supermarket tills although I must say I have never dared go as far as that. If you find it impossible to buy food not pre-packed in plastic, and this is increasingly difficult, try to wash food as thoroughly as possible or in the case of vegetables peel or scrape off the surface which has been most in contact with the plastic. Unfortunately the chemicals concerned are fat soluble so it is best to avoid them if possible since they are difficult to remove by washing.

LIFESTYLE FACTOR #3: COOKING

Love it or hate it, cooking is an essential part of our diet and lifestyle. In amongst all the aromas and sizzles, it has an effect on the food that can be enhancing or potentially destructive. For instance, it changes starches, proteins and some vitamins into forms that the body can absorb readily as well as releasing nutrients in some foods, which are otherwise unavailable – like the amino acid tryptophan in cornmeal. Cooking of some foods is necessary to destroy toxic substances such as those found in red beans and cooking also makes some foods, like meat, palatable. However, cooking can destroy and leach fragile nutrients in food, although there are ways in which you can reduce this nutrient loss.

I lightly steam vegetables in a stainless steel or bamboo steamer, otherwise I stir fry lightly after first thoroughly washing and dipping vegetables in boiling water like the Chinese do. Fruit and vegetables should be eaten as raw as possible in order to preserve the vitamins and enzymes they contain. Recent research for example suggests that cooking broccoli destroys the anti-cancer chemical that it contains. I use only organic extra-virgin olive oil to soften or gently fry vegetables. Any meat I eat is cooked slowly in the oven or under a grill and the fish I eat is just lightly grilled. I add no additional fat or salt to meat or fish, which I cook slowly with herbs or garlic and occasionally black pepper or other spices, for flavouring. I do not own a microwave and try to avoid food cooked or heated in one. Unlike normal heating, microwaving food works by vibrating water molecules in food. This generates free radicals and I suspect would not destroy as many 'bad' chemicals as ordinary cooking (although I have been unable to find any data on this). Apart from anything, I do not like the taste of microwaved food. There is no comparison between the taste of a jacket potato cooked in the traditional way and the soggy unpleasant-tasting equivalent prepared by microwaving. Here are some general guidelines:

- If you cook with fat don't let it become so hot that it starts to smoke. At this temperature the essential fatty acid linoleic acid is destroyed.
- Fats which have been used for cooking once should be discarded since the linoleic acid and vitamins A and C will have been lost; they may have become oxidised and rancid and hence potentially carcinogenic.
- If you boil food, do so for the minimum amount of time and then use the water for stock afterwards. The fragile water-soluble vitamins as well as some minerals leach into cooking water, which is why soups are so nutritious.
- Don't add bicarbonate of soda to cooking water, even if you see it recommended in cookery books for cooking pulses. It destroys valuable B vitamins.
- Prepare food immediately before cooking – remember that vitamin C is destroyed once cells are damaged in vegetables – and for the same reason try not to chop them too finely. Scrubbing vegetables is better than peeling them.
- Once prepared, immerse the vegetables in ready boiling water straight away.
- Use pans with close-fitting lids and avoid using copper pans which encourage oxidation and vitamin C loss. I use stainless steel pans and bamboo baskets for steaming.
- Once food is cooked, eat it straight away. Keeping it warm will only result in further nutrient loss, which is why eating out too frequently may be less than healthy for you.

LIFESTYLE FACTOR #4: DEALING WITH STRESS

The idea that cancer could be cured by thinking positively had always seemed ill-founded to me. I certainly did not believe that I could be cured of breast cancer simply by thinking positively. One of the particular problems with the 'think positive' approach is that people who do not get better often feel guilty that they are not trying hard enough. Sometimes this is reinforced by their friends and the patients become convinced that they remain ill simply because they are not being positive enough. In the book *You Can Heal Your Life* by Louise Hay, there is a list of diseases and their probable causes. In the case of cancer (all types presumably), the probable cause is given as 'deep hurt, long-standing resentment, deep secret or grief eating away at the self; carrying hatreds; what's the use'. The advice is to develop a new thought pattern as follows: 'I lovingly forgive and release all of the past. I choose to fill my world with joy. I love and approve of myself.' Fine, but I prefer a more rational approach which seeks to remove cancer-causing chemicals from my life!

It has also been claimed that there is a particular personality type that is likely to be affected by breast cancer. Much has been written about the 'cancer personality' especially by Lawrence LeShan, an American psychotherapist who worked with over 200 cancer patients. According to LeShan, the typical personality had an emotionally deprived youth, followed in later life by a period of fulfilment in an intense relationship or through all-involving work, followed by the loss of that relationship or work at which time the cancer occurs. The other main characteristic is the person's inability to express anger, particularly in their own defence, such a person is often described by others as being like a saint. LeShan believed that this pattern fitted 76 per cent of his patients. This is certainly not a description of me or my life and I cannot think of anyone else I know who has had breast cancer who fits this description!

All carefully controlled research indicates that this theory is wrong. The concept is unhelpful, and again tends to lead to feelings of guilt. As indicated earlier, the problem is one of chemistry and is rooted in the Western diet. The book *Wild Swans* by Jung Chang provides a vivid example of the high levels of stress that Chinese women have suffered in the past, yet they retained low breast cancer rates except when they have changed to a Western diet.

Because stress has been implicated as an important factor in breast cancer, people can become worried and hence more stressed by problems so that a vicious circle is set up. When I was ill with cancer I found that as soon as a stressful situation arose I became so worried that the stress would cause my illness to return that my distress about situations increased rather than decreased. Over the last seven years I have faced up to some extremely stressful situations in my family life and at work, and yet my cancer has not returned – because fundamentally it was a problem caused by harmful chemicals from my food and the environment causing problems in my body. Now my diet and lifestyle are sound, I cope very well with stress.

However, for your health and general well-being it is helpful to reduce the stress and distress in your life as much as possible and there is scientific evidence that stress has physiological effects suggesting it is worthwhile working on methods of reducing or removing sources of stress. Folklore and old wives' tales are sometimes based on observation and wisdom passed down from one generation to the next. At the time I was ill I remembered some of the earthy old ladies in the village I grew up in who used to talk about situations 'worrying their tits off'. I wondered whether there could be some basis for this expression! The chemical changes caused by stress would need a book to describe all their effects. Hormones from the adrenal gland as part of the body's 'fight or flight' mechanism increase the amount of blood sugar available, boost heart rate and slow down digestive function to enable us to run or fight. Too much for too long, however, affects the immune system. As mentioned earlier, prolactin levels also increase as a result of stress.

When humans are confronted by an important loss or change in their lifestyle – such as a diagnosis of breast cancer – their emotions are likely to follow a pattern which is well known to counsellors and others trained to help with our emotional well-being. Initially, shock and numbness may be experienced, followed by resistance, gradual acceptance and depression before beginning to let go of the old reality and adjust to the new one. People differ in the intensity of their emotions and the time taken for each part of the cycle. Indeed, in the case of cancer some people simply give up hope and never leave the 'trough of despair'.

In my case, when confronted with problems I tend to move to the 'what can be done about it' stage very quickly and of course one of the frustrations with being confronted with a diagnosis of breast cancer is that according to orthodox medicine the answer is, 'nothing'. If you have heart disease you can follow a diet and exercise plan, if you have an infectious illness you can take tablets and rest, but with breast cancer you are told there is nothing you can do. The conventional risk factors, as we have already discussed, translate into this: it is too late and there was little or nothing you could have done to prevent breast cancer anyway.

As I have explained earlier in the book, *there is a lot you can do to help yourself* with changes in diet and lifestyle which are crucially important. The diet in itself in addition to helping you fight cancer directly will help your state of mental and emotional well-being by providing a better balance of the essential nutrients (including zinc, iodine, B vitamins and the essential fatty acids) your brain needs.

DEALING WITH THE STRESS OF BREAST CANCER

Let us look at some of the emotional problems associated with coping with breast cancer. A large percentage of people become depressed especially after losing a breast. In a recent study at three cancer centres, 47 per cent of those diagnosed with cancer had a level of distress equivalent to that seen in a true psychiatric disorder.[9] One of the things I was very worried about, and I think most women who have had a mastectomy are, is how different people will react to you. Will you become an object of pity or will people make jokes about you? I was particularly worried about going back to work, especially in such a male dominated office. In fact everyone was incredibly kind, sensitive and considerate. Indeed one of my colleagues who had been one of my fiercest opponents professionally was one of the first to write to me. Dr Peter Allen, at the time BGS's chief geologist, sent me a long, carefully thought out, sensitive letter which actually anticipated and addressed all my worst fears. He set out clearly and unequivocally how much everyone valued me as a person and as a scientist and I should not worry too much about my physical appearance: whatever happened my colleagues' feelings and respect for me would not change. It was a truly wonderful letter which I shall always keep with my most treasured mementos. Peter and I still enjoy our professional spats but I count him and his wife Joyce among my dearest friends.

Some marriages and family relationships break down following the wife and mother suffering from breast cancer. Moreover, many women who have developed breast cancer have done so after trying to come to terms with distressing situations in their lives such as the breakdown of their marriage. I shall try to share with you some of the coping strategies I developed with the help of a wonderful psychotherapist whose help was made available to me by Charing Cross Hospital. It was difficult for me to agree to see her initially because of fear evoked by my childhood memories of the appalling treatment my father had received at the hands of psychiatrists, combined with difficult experiences with my first husband, also a psychiatrist. When I expressed my reservations to her, she quickly reassured me. She had trained initially as a surgeon at Cambridge University before becoming a psychiatrist and finally a psychotherapist. She specialised in helping people who have had limbs amputated come to terms with their problems. She assured me that she would not under any circumstances suggest the use of ECT or drugs.

With the help of my psychotherapist I was able to come to terms with the loss of my breast. Also she helped me to address and come to terms with problems in my life and personality and reactions. I learned that unresolved feelings of fear, anger and guilt are especially damaging, negative emotions. With her help, I revisited, reinterpreted and finally dealt with events in my past and memories which generated negative emotions. In some cases I wrote to or telephoned people I had not spoken to for years to try to heal unpleasant situations and reduce my emotional baggage. But in some situations this was not possible and the only way to come to terms with the past was to develop a new perspective.

I will give one example of how I learned to turn an extremely negative situation into something positive. Like many first marriages now, mine ended in break up: in my case, a particularly unpleasant and protracted process which caused me an enormous amount of personal grief and anxiety. My father was ill at the time and my mother was working hard to keep both of them. With no family support of my own I was persuaded to allow my former parents-in-law to care for my son on the basis that my ex-husband and I would stay friends and when our futures were more settled we could decide what was in our son's best interest.

It emerged at the time of the custody hearing that my son had been staying with my ex-husband a great deal, so the court took the view that he should remain in the situation with which he was familiar, and I was merely granted access. An awkward, and awful, situation; and for me, the saddest part has been the almost total lack of contact between me and my son. With my psychotherapist's help, I eventually managed to understand how this situation came about. As I came to understand what had happened, I became more determined than ever that I would survive. I decided that whenever my son feels able to come back to me, I shall be there for him – a strong and worthwhile person who loves him dearly. In this way, I learned to turn a terrible situation of chronic stress full of hurt and anger into a reason to survive. With help, we can do the same with even the most distressing situations. I found psychotherapy helpful even over the few months I worked with my doctor. According to MIND, the mental health charity, psychotherapy may last for several years and is particularly helpful in understanding, and coming to terms with, past events.

With my psychotherapist's help I learned two other coping strategies which I found particularly helpful in dealing with cancer. The first is cognitive therapy. Part of being a creative thinker, which I need to be as a scientist, is that I develop large 'worry castles' from one or two odd bricks. In dealing with cancer it is particularly easy to develop frightening scenarios for the future. Cognitive therapy teaches you to trace the building of the worry castle backwards and stop at the facts. You can then develop a more sensible, rational, less frightening vision. Again according to MIND, cognitive therapy is about learning to think and behave in positive ways. It is a type of behavioural therapy which is helpful in overcoming negative thinking. My psychotherapist also taught me how to be more assertive without being aggressive which helps avoid situations where one is affected by negative emotions. For example if you calmly but clearly state your concerns or dislikes, many situations that lead to negative emotions can be avoided. There are many excellent books on cognitive therapy and assertive behaviour which are well worth reading.

I have to say that I found counselling of the type which was based on trying to release any pent-up emotions far less helpful than the psychotherapy sessions which were intellectual and analytical and gave me new understanding and insights into situations so that I could develop clear, simple coping strategies. The analogy I would use about my counselling sessions is that of a pond in which emotions had settled to the bottom and the water had cleared, and every week I was encouraged to put in a large stick and stir it around until I became upset. Also counsellors are trained never to give reassurances and I found that by repeating answers to 'how do you feel about that' or 'what is your worst fear' I was giving my brain only negative feedback and reinforcing my fears. Others I know have found counselling very helpful – it just did not work well for me. Also I tried self-help and support groups but found these made me feel that I was 'wallowing in breast cancer' and I found them depressing. Again, others I know have found attending such groups helpful.

The person I found most helpful was a lady who has become one of my dearest friends – Peggy Heason who is a trained hypnotherapist. I found sessions with her extremely helpful. Also, having brought up three children in the war, cared for six years for a husband with a stroke, helped see her four grandchildren through school and into university: she has so much common sense and she was prepared to reassure me where she could. But above all she was always there for me. She cared for me but she was not so emotionally involved as my own mother, husband or children so she was better able to help me. If you have breast cancer or any other serious problems in your life, my advice is to find yourself a Peggy Heason. I went to relaxation sessions with her and I also used her relaxation tape a great deal.[10]

The basis of most techniques to reduce stress and tension start with relaxation. First, turn off the telephone, doorbell etc. so you will not be interrupted. Then turn off the light or draw the curtains and lie flat (I do this without a pillow – at most use only one) and make sure you are warm and comfortable. Then systematically relax each part of your body beginning with your toes, then your feet, your lower legs, gradually progressing up through the body. Repeat until you feel totally relaxed. This way you relax each bit of you from toe to top. There are several good relaxation tapes based on these methods but Peggy Heason's was the one that I found the best. At the same time I used diaphragm breathing which is very relaxing. When we are anxious we tend to take lots of shallow breaths by breathing using only our ribcage. Diaphragm breathing is a technique to ensure you are using your full lung capacity by using the large muscle called the diaphragm at the base of the lung cavity to suck in and expel air. You simply place your hands on your abdomen and make sure that they go up and down as you breathe in and out. Used with imagery you can accompany your relaxation by imagining yourself walking through a beautiful calm garden listening to the birdsong or walking along a beautiful beach with waves gently crashing on the sand. It is possible to buy tapes to guide you through imagery and relaxation but do listen to them first, do not rely simply on the promotional statement. I found some voices on tapes that I bought without first listening incredibly irritating. It is important to find ones that you enjoy and find helpful because you will probably use them many times. Many such tapes are readily available from health and new age shops. Some include affirmations (quiet verbal instructions) and subliminal messages to your body. I also learned meditation which I still use, and despite being such a simple method, it clears worries out of the mind and allows deep relaxation. I chose the words candle and crystal and repeat one of them continuously in my mind and visualise the candle gently flickering or the crystal sparkling. After a time one feels truly relaxed. I found meditation difficult at first because I am normally a busy-busy sort of person but the technique really does clear my mind and helps me in my work especially in solving problems. I think yoga would also be helpful although I did not use it. There is a great deal of evidence of the effectiveness of such techniques in reducing stress and tension and the physical symptoms that stress creates in the body, for example several of the methods described lower blood pressure.

Another technique sometimes used for cancer patients is visualisation. Visualisation involves imagining your body killing the cancer, removing the debris from your body and finally visualising situations where you are well and whole again. The visualisation technique was made famous by the Simontons in the USA. It typically involves going into visions of cancer being attacked and cleaned up by the body's defence system. This is how one of the visions begins: 'Your white blood cells are fish swimming in and eating up the greyish cancer cells. Project this image as if it were on a screen that you're viewing in your mind's eye. When you have that image very clearly then *become* one of the fish and lead the rest of the pack into the attack. Feel yourself as the fish eating. At the end of each visualisation, imagine yourself engaging in activities you would pursue if you were healthy. Picture yourself at the healthiest time in your life and create images of the present, feeling just that way.' I found visualisation techniques unhelpful but others feel better for using them.

So far I have not said much about my husband, children or my mother. Perhaps this is because at the time we were all so distressed that we coped badly as a family. My mother was an elderly widow living alone and I am her only child. With Dr John Camac's help I worked hard to shield her from the worst of the situation. John and her local vicar gave her tremendous support and she found great comfort in her Christianity. At all times I told my husband the truth and also told my daughter Emma as kindly and unfrighteningly as possible when the cancer kept coming back in 1993. I was also 'gently truthful' with Tom my youngest son. At the time, my husband was working in Nottingham looking after Tom while I was treated in London. Hence he was hardly ever able to attend clinics or treatment sessions with me and he often found it difficult to talk about my illness. Peter would help me a lot with housework and shopping and other practical tasks but he found it difficult to talk about emotions. At the time I was very resentful about this. I blamed it on his stiff upper lip upbringing at public school and Cambridge. However, having discussed those feelings with Peter since, I realise that his reactions were not because he did not care but because he cared too much. He found the situation extremely upsetting, especially seeing me undergoing chemotherapy. In order to avoid letting me see his distress he preferred not to become involved in discussions because he thought he would break down in front of me.

I began writing this book partly for young women like my daughter Emma. She was deeply distressed from the time I first developed cancer when she was thirteen until I recovered when she was nineteen. She is an extremely clever and capable young woman who had always been good at her schoolwork especially mathematics and science. Shortly before my illness she was one of a few children chosen to represent physics at an evening designed to impress the parents of prospective students at her school. Unfortunately my illness affected her studies and for a long time she appeared to be an angry young woman. Only recently have I come to understand what she went through and how much she suffered because of my illness. When I first became ill in 1987 she had only recently developed breasts herself and there was her mother with a deadly disease in her breasts which it seemed might kill her. Previously Emma had seen me only as someone totally in control, someone who could always explain things, put things right, make things better – probably more than most of her friends' mothers. Certainly she would bring lots of her little friends' problems to me. Suddenly I was transformed from being a secure pillar in her life to a victim of something against which I appeared to be helpless in defending myself. Emma is strong and courageous and has worked hard to recover her life, to 'get back on track', and now has a very successful career as an account manager with a dynamic young advertising and marketing company in London. We are totally devoted to each other. Only recently when we went on a 'shop 'til you drop' trip together, did I notice how often she spontaneously hugged me or put her arm through mine. She sometimes talks in front of me now about how frightened she was that she would lose me. Emma has helped me to write this book by providing information, encouragement and support.

Tom, my youngest son, was six when I was first diagnosed with breast cancer and did not understand what was happening at the time. In 1993 when I had recurrences of breast cancer four times in seven months he was eleven and like Emma, his schoolwork also suffered for a time. Nevertheless he was very supportive emotionally. He was able to help me a great deal without showing his own distress. We were able to talk about this situation a lot and he helped to 'heal' problems that developed between the rest of us. He is now studying medicine at one of the UK's most highly regarded universities. I know he will be a wonderful doctor.

What I learned was how important it is that you understand how distressed your family is, if your relationships are to survive cancer. They will all react differently. They are having to come to terms with their own distress, fears and anxieties about your illness as well as helping and supporting you. They have different personalities with different capabilities and methods of coping. I soon learned not to dump my fears, feelings and anxieties onto them – they were too close and too frightened and upset already and as a family we could quickly enter damaging downward-spiralling emotional situations.

I learned instead to rely on others who cared about me but who were not so close that their fears became amplified and spiralled out of control. I found my women friends, my vicar Julian Reindorp, my former doctor John Camac and Peggy Heason whom I have already mentioned, the best equipped to help me. They knew me well enough to care about me and give me support but there was not the intense emotion that there is in the family. A group of my women friends, all professionals with busy lives, each gave some of their time to take me to hospital and stay with me during radiotherapy and chemotherapy treatments. Somehow they worked together as an efficient team, each giving the help they could and the time they could spare and to provide me with a wonderful cocoon of total care. When they asked me how they could help I managed to shed my typically British reserve and independence and tell them.

Working with your friends is a two-way process and can be so helpful. If you want to do something for a friend with cancer, ask them sincerely how you can help and show that you mean it. All sorts of practical things – helping collect children, doing some shopping, going with them for treatment, means so much at such times. I will give some of the examples of how friends in London helped me (in addition to coming to Charing Cross on several occasions for treatment sessions with me). Edna Lewis, an architect with her own practice and my neighbour in London, was always there for me, often just listening to my fears in her quiet way or getting help for me from my local vicar Julian Reindorp. While my husband was away in China the fifth and last time my cancer came back, she slept at my house and manned the telephone. She also helped by talking to Emma and Tom a lot and being there for them. Vicky Guiton, a talented interior designer with her own business helped me in many ways, from tidying up my kitchen to coming with me to ensure my unnecessary wig looked good after my hairdresser had restyled it. She introduced two of her other friends to me to help provide support – one of them, Sarah Scott a retired social worker was like Vicky herself, a tower of strength. Roberta Stoker, a talented artist, and Choo Simmonds, a mathematics lecturer, made lots of visits and endlessly supported me, often doing shopping for me. Iris Campbell, a brilliant children's fashion designer, kept me endlessly supplied with organic vegetables from her own allotment and was a port in a storm for Tom whenever he was in

London. Jenny Long and Maria Calvert also made lots of visits, took me out and gave me masses of support and encouragement. Sarah Wherry, now a senior publisher took me out a lot, was a second Mum to Emma and when I was at my lowest ebb with the big lump in my neck, forced me to buy myself a new shirt. I still have it. Sarah now agrees that she bullied me into making some gesture to show myself I still had a future at a time when I had virtually given up any hope of surviving. Other friends in Nottingham, especially Penny Tutty gave me lots of practical help by caring for Tom – often having him to stay with her family for days at a time.

Some friends could not cope – they did not visit or telephone and distanced themselves until I recovered. This is a common experience for cancer patients. You should try to understand that these people do care about you, they just do not know how to cope themselves. You should not allow yourself to become bitter. Let them back into your life when they feel able to cope. When I was ill I found on occasions I simply could not talk to anyone with any connection with cancer, let alone breast cancer sufferers. My mind was telling me that I could not take any more but it certainly was not because I did not care, I just had to let go. On one occasion while having lunch with a group of friends at work, someone started talking about a colleague whose wife had cancer, thinking I suppose that I would be able to offer help. Instead of helping or offering advice, I made some excuse and rushed out of the room. All the people there later told me that they understood. (Since 1994, when I first began to realise that my cancer had gone, I have been able to advise other cancer sufferers or their friends who have asked for my help.)

During my illness, I found it helpful to keep working and took the minimum of sick leave, for example four days twice a month when I was on chemotherapy (two days for treatment and the following days to recover from the nausea). This gave me a sense of purpose and took my mind off my problems. Many other friends and colleagues with cancer or with partners with cancer have also found the routine of going to work helpful in coping with the disease. Of course, this depends on the type of work you do, the working environment and your personality and it requires a supportive boss and colleagues. The Head of BGS at the time, Dr Peter Cook, and his wife Norma were wonderful to me, often telephoning and arranging dinner parties to cheer me up. Dr David Morgan, my deputy at the time, went out of his way to ensure I felt involved in decision making. He refused to move into my office but sat there for several hours a day doing my work on the days I was away for treatment. I had left lots of high-heeled shoes under my desk and apparently he put up with much teasing about stepping into my shoes rather than ask me or my husband to move them because he thought this might upset me. We also have a wonderful Welfare Officer at BGS, Reverend Howard Bateson, a former geologist and now a Canon who was immensely supportive and kind. Hilary Heason, BGS's press officer, and my then secretary, Janet Drury, provided female support in my male-dominated workplace. Friends and colleagues showered me with flowers, messages and cards, and they telephoned me a lot – this was very important in maintaining my morale. At the time I thought that the situation was reminiscent of the story of Peter Pan where everyone has to shout Tinkerbell's name if they wish her to recover her health. If you have a friend with cancer do whatever you can – even if you only send a card to contribute to shouting 'Tinkerbell'. The whole episode was a great learning experience for me. Previously I had been highly competitive and ambitious and people and relationships had come second, third or fourth in my list of priorities. Learning to let people into my life made me a much better and happier person and, amazingly, also much more successful!

I think that the best way of coping with cancer emotionally can be summed up by quoting a friend and colleague Dr Chris Evans whose wife, Norma, sadly died of cancer in 1995, 'I learnt during the four years that Norma was ill that we all react differently. There is no right or wrong way. There are people out there who can help and people who are going through the same thing. These people can suggest a range of coping strategies but friendship, openness and love are at the heart of most.'

THE BIG DOS AND DON'TS

- Do not believe the old adage 'cancer equals death'. Today, many cancers are curable; others can be controlled for long periods during which new treatments may become available.
- Do not believe that you caused your cancer. There is no

evidence linking specific personalities, emotional states or painful life events to the development of cancer.

- Do rely on strategies that helped you solve problems in the past, such as gathering information, talking to others and finding ways to feel in control. Seek help if they don't work.
- Do not feel guilty if you can't keep a 'positive' attitude all the time. Low periods will occur, no matter how good you are at coping. There is no evidence that these periods have a negative effect on your health. If they become too frequent or severe, though, seek help.
- Do use support and self-help groups if they make you feel better. Leave any that make you feel worse.
- Do not be embarrassed to seek counsel from a mental-health professional. It is a sign of strength, not weakness, and it may help you to tolerate your symptoms and treatments better.
- Do use any methods that aid you in gaining control over your emotions, such as meditation and relaxation.
- Do find a doctor of whom you can ask questions and with whom you feel mutual respect and trust. Insist on being a partner with him or her in your treatment. Ask what side effects to expect and be prepared for them. Anticipating problems often makes them easier to handle if they occur.
- Do not keep your worries to yourself. If the person closest to you can cope, involve them. If they find it difficult you may need to involve a group of friends so each can give you some support. If all else fails, phone the Samaritans and talk to them of your fears. Ask a close friend to accompany you to visits to the doctor when treatments are to be discussed. Research shows that you often don't hear or absorb information when you are very anxious: a second person will help you to interpret what was said.
- Do explore spiritual and religious beliefs and practices that may have helped you in the past. They may comfort you and even help you find meaning in the experience of illness.
- Do not abandon your treatment in favour of an alternative method, especially those which make no sense and are irrational. But do change your diet and lifestyle in the ways described here to help to overcome your disease and withstand treatment.[11]

LIFESTYLE FACTOR #5: AVOIDING HARMFUL SUBSTANCES IN YOUR ENVIRONMENT

Cancer cells are relatively big and when they spread they usually get trapped in the first network of capillaries – the very fine blood vessels that take blood to and from all the tissues in our bodies – that they encounter downstream of their origin. The first highly vascularised organ encountered by blood leaving most organs in our bodies is the lung, except in the case of the intestine from which the blood supply goes to the liver first. Hence in the case of all types of cancer, the organs to protect from secondary tumours as much as possible are the lungs and liver. This is particularly important in the case of breast cancer. I therefore decided to cut my exposure to all cancer-causing chemicals as much as possible.

The effects of exposure to harmful chemicals depends on the dose, the duration, how you are exposed and the presence of other chemicals. The main task of the lungs is to exchange 'old blood' containing carbon dioxide created by body processes for 'new blood' invigorated with fresh oxygen. They can cope with some dust, particles and bad chemicals but if you overwhelm them with harmful chemicals (for example from tobacco smoke or if you live in a city environment where the air usually contains high levels of car, aeroplane and other exhausts containing benzene, a potent cancer-causing agent, as well as many other cancer-causing agents) they are far more likely to become diseased with primary lung cancer. They are far less likely to be able to fight against invading breast cancer cells trying to establish secondary tumours.

The liver is also an amazing organ responsible for eliminating poisonous chemicals, including those produced by our own metabolism, from the body as well as manufacturing all sorts of important enzymes and other chemicals essential for our bodies to function. The liver detoxifies our system and produces anti-cancer chemicals. My strategy was, and continues to be, to have as many good nutritious substances as possible to help my liver to help me and to keep it as unburdened as possible with pollutants in my food, applied to my skin or inhaled.

One of the main sources of pollutants to try to eliminate is tobacco smoke. It is estimated that smoking tobacco causes approximately 30 per cent of all cancers in the USA alone. Smoking tobacco causes cancer not only in the lungs but it is also implicated in cancer of the mouth, windpipe, oesophagus, bladder and pancreas and probably of the stomach, liver and kidney. It may also contribute to some forms of leukaemia, cancer of the colon, rectum and other organs. Tobacco smoke is the single most lethal cancer-causing agent known. It contains more than 200 cancer-causing agents. These include radioactive substances such as polonium 210, highly poisonous heavy metals such as cadmium and dangerous organic chemicals such as the polycyclic aromatic hydrocarbons (PAHs) which cause serious damage to DNA (see p. 218). Heavy smoking on its own increases lung cancer risk by about 2,000 per cent.[12] I have never smoked. I find the cough most smokers develop, their brown teeth and thin wrinkly skin, not to mention their smell, is all I need to say 'no' and I try to avoid passive smoking. If people ask me if I mind if they smoke in my presence I say 'yes'. If you do smoke and are addicted to nicotine and find it difficult to give up, you can reduce your risks by having nicotine as patches or by chewing nicotine-impregnated gum – it is the tar in tobacco which contains the powerful cancer-causing agents, not the nicotine. I do not blame individual smokers for their habit. Such is the power of advertising and image that increasingly young people are persuaded to spend a lot of money taking up a habit which makes them become progressively less attractive to the rest of us to look at and smell, and potentially seriously ill. I think that the television programme EastEnders is to be congratulated for the Dot Cotton character who is portrayed as over-anxious and is made to look thin, haggard and wrinkly with a hoarse voice. My daughter and her friends who are trying to stop smoking, say one of the reasons that they want to do so is because they do not want to develop a 'Dot Cotton voice'.

I am now going to tell you about some other damaging chemicals in the environment before advising you on how to cut your exposure to them. The concentration of many of them, especially the endocrine disrupting chemicals, can actually be measured by their effects on breast cancer cell cultures. Many are fat soluble and bioaccumulate up the food chain, becoming especially concentrated in milk.

CANCER HAZARD: POLYCYCLIC AROMATIC HYDROCARBONS (PAHs)

These are formed by the incomplete combustion of other hydrocarbons. Because there are so many partial combustion processes that favour production of PAHs, they can be abundant in the atmosphere, soil and elsewhere in the environment from sources that include engine exhausts, cigarette smoke and grilled food and coal and wood smoke. Coal tars and petroleum residues such as road and roofing asphalt also have high levels of PAHs. Many contaminated land sites such as old gas works have high levels of PAHs.

They deserve special attention because as well as some of them acting as Endocrine Disrupting Chemicals (EDCs – discussed, p. 222) some of them cause cancer in other ways. What makes them particularly dangerous is their rather sinister chemical properties. In the environment they are very unreactive, which makes them persistent and difficult to get rid of. When they enter the human body, the liver tries to eliminate them but oxidised PAH metabolites can react chemically and become permanently inserted into the structure of DNA thereby introducing mistakes into it. It is the ability of PAH metabolites to become *intercalated* in, or slotted into, the DNA structure because of their limited chemical reactivity in the body, that makes some PAH compounds so carcinogenic.

Their complicated name refers to the fact that they comprise more than one ring of carbon atoms. Benzene, which is the basic single ring structure of carbon atoms with hydrogen atoms attached from which PAHs are built up, is itself a very powerful carcinogen. Some PAH compounds, including benzo(a)pyrene, the molecules of which comprise an arrangement of five benzene rings and which is concentrated in tobacco smoke, are well known to be the precursors of cancer-causing metabolites.

Benzene has special regulations for its use in laboratories in order to meet Health and Safety regulations. So it always strikes me as strange that we are allowed to be exposed to this dangerous chemical every time we fill our cars with petrol or walk down the street and breathe in car exhaust fumes or our own or other people's cigarette smoke.[13] Typical tests on exhaust fumes from cars show that they emit about 10mg of benzene for every kilometre travelled.[14]

CANCER HAZARD: DIOXINS

The major source of dioxin in the environment (95 per cent) comes from incinerators burning chlorinated wastes. Dioxin is formed as an unintentional by-product of many industrial processes involving chlorine, such as waste incineration, chemical and pesticide manufacturing and pulp and paper bleaching. Dioxin pollution is also associated with paper mills which use chlorine bleaching in their process and with the production of Polyvinyl Chloride (PVC) plastics. Dioxin was the primary toxic component of Agent Orange, was found at Love Canal in Niagara Falls, New York and was the basis for evacuation at Seveso, Italy, and the Bhopal disaster in India.

Dioxin (Polychlorinated Dibenzo-para-dioxins and Dibenzofurans) is a general term that describes a group of hundreds of chemicals that are highly persistent in the environment. The most toxic compound is 2,3,7,8-tetra-chlorodibenzo-*p*-dioxin or TCDD. The name dioxin is also used for the family of structurally and chemically related polychlorinated dibenzo-para-dioxins (PCDDs), polychlorinated dibenzofurans (PCDFs) and certain polychlorinated biphenyls (PCBs). Some 419 types of dioxin-related compounds have been identified but only about 30 are considered to have significant toxicity, with TCDD being the most toxic.[15]

TCDD dioxin is, in fact, one of the most toxic chemicals known. According to the September 1994 report of the US Environmental Protection Agency (EPA), not only does there appear to be no 'safe' level of exposure to dioxin, but levels of dioxin and dioxin-like chemicals have been found in the general US population that are 'at or near levels associated with adverse health effects'. The EPA report confirmed that dioxin is a cancer hazard to people; that exposure to dioxin can also cause severe reproductive and developmental problems (at levels 100 times lower than those associated with its cancer-causing effects); and that dioxin can cause immune system damage and interfere with regulatory hormones.

Short-term exposure of humans to high levels of dioxins may result in skin lesions, such as chloracne and patchy darkening of the skin, and altered liver function. Long-term exposure is linked to impairment of the immune system and reproductive functions. Chronic exposure of animals to dioxins has resulted in several types of cancer. The International Agency for Research on Cancer [IARC] – part of the World Health Organisation – announced on 14 February 1997, that the most potent dioxin, 2,3,7,8-TCDD, is now considered a Class 1 carcinogen, meaning a 'known human carcinogen'.

According to the USA EPA's Health Assessment report, dioxin is hydrophobic, fat-soluble and bioaccumulates up the food chain; it is found mainly (97.5 per cent) in meat and dairy products.[16] The North American intake based on a total exposure of 119pg (picograms)/day is as follows: dairy products and milk, 34 per cent; beef 32 per cent; chicken 11 per cent; pork 11 per cent; fish 7 per cent and eggs 3 per cent. Milk in the UK also contains dioxins and PCBs.[17]

Extensive stores of waste industrial oils with high levels of dioxins exist throughout the world. Long term storage of this material may result in dioxin release into the environment and the contamination of human and animal food supplies. Dioxins are not easily disposed of without contamination of the environment and human populations.

Incineration is the best available method of destruction although other methods are being investigated. The process requires high temperatures over 850°C. For destruction of large amounts of contaminated material, even higher temperatures – 1,000°C or more – are required. Further information on dioxin is available on several websites including http://www.enviroweb.org/issues/dioxin/index.html and those of the WWF, the WHO and the US EPA.

CANCER HAZARD: POLYCHLORINATED BIPHENYLS (PCBs)

The abbreviation PCB refers to polychlorinated biphenyls, a family of man-made chemicals that contains 209 individual compounds with varying toxicity. Commercial formulations of PCBs enter the environment as mixtures consisting of a variety of PCBs and impurities. They have very high chemical, thermal, and biological stability; low vapour pressure and are good electrical insulators and fire retardants. Between the 1930s and 1970s these properties led to the manufacture and use of PCBs as coolant-insulation fluids in transformers and capacitors; for the impregnation of cotton and asbestos; as plasticisers; and as additives to some epoxy paints. The same properties that made the extraordinarily stable PCBs so useful also contributed to their widespread dispersion and accumulation in the environment. The manufacture of PCBs was discontinued in the US and their uses and disposal were strictly controlled after 1976.

It has been estimated that since 1929, a total of 1.2 million tons of PCBs have been manufactured.[18] Of this total, 31 per cent (370,000 tons) has so far escaped into the general environment. An estimated 4 per cent of original production has been fed into incinerators, in the hope of destroying it. However, 780,000 tons of PCBs are still in use in transformers and capacitors, or have been sent to landfills. Thus the amount that could potentially be released into the environment is approximately twice as large as the amount that has already been released.

PCBs enter the body through contaminated food and air and through skin contact. They are particularly found in fatty food including milk.[19] Fish have been implicated but a survey of fish products reported in 1997 indicated that fish liver oils contained higher concentrations of PCBs and dioxins than fish body oils, so fish is safer than fish oils.[20] Exposure from drinking water is minimal. It is known that nearly everyone has PCBs in their bodies, including infants who drink breast milk containing PCBs.[21] Animal experiments have shown that some PCB mixtures produce adverse health effects that include liver damage, skin irritations, reproductive and development effects and cancer. Some PCBs cause mutations in cells and they are endocrine disrupters (see opposite). Therefore, it is prudent to consider that there may be health hazards for humans.

While the risk of PCBs in producing cancer, reproductive and developmental effects in humans cannot be clearly defined, the suggestive evidence provides an additional basis for public health concern about humans who may be exposed to PCBs. The complexity of relating the specific mixtures for which data are available to exposures in the general population has resulted in a tendency to regard all PCBs as having a similar health hazard potential, although this assumption may not be true.

The American Food and Drug Administration (FDA) specifies PCB concentration limits of 0.2 to 3 parts per million (milligrams PCB per kilogram of food) in infant foods, eggs, milk (in milk fat), and poultry (fat). The American Environmental Protection Agency guideline for drinking water ranges from 0.005 to 0.5 micrograms of PCBs per litre of water, which also reflects the risk of a person developing cancer in populations of one in 10,000,000 to one in 100,000 people.

In Britain, levels of PCBs in soils peaked in the late 1960s but have now fallen to 1940s' levels and the estimated UK dietary intake of PCBs has declined to about one third between 1982 and 1992.[22] Disposal of PCBs from discarded electrical equipment and other sources remains a problem.

CANCER HAZARD: ENDOCRINE DISRUPTING CHEMICALS (EDCs)

One of the ways in which many pollutants are now implicated in causing cancer is in the way they have been shown to mimic hormones, hence they are called Endocrine Disrupting Chemicals (EDCs). (There is a move to call these chemicals endocrine modifiers, presumably because this plays down to the public the potential hazard that these chemicals represent). Because breast and prostate cancer have been suggested to be hormonally controlled cancers, EDCs are of particular significance.

Residues from many pesticides, plastics and household chemicals such as detergents that mimic hormones – including oestrogens – leach into our food and water. They are fat soluble and in the case of oestrogenic EDCs have an oestrogenic effect on the body because the body cannot distinguish the molecules from those of natural oestrogen. In addition to oestrogen-mimicking substances, other endocrine disrupters are thought to block oestrogen, mimic or block androgens (male hormones) and possibly also mimic or block thyroid hormones. Because EDCs are related to hormones an infinitesimal quantity can have a negative effect.[23] In the case of derivatives of persistent organochlorines and herbicides which have high residence period, they can accumulate in the body and be passed from one generation to the next.

The following substances, some of which we have discussed above, have been identified as environmental endocrine disrupters by the World Wildlife Fund and/or the American EPA:

- persistent organochlorines (usually called polychlorinated dibenzo-p-dioxins/dibenzofurans (PCDD/PCDFs) or dioxins and furans and PCBs)
- pesticides such as dichloro diphenyl trichloroethane (DDT), lindane and malathion

- some polycyclic aromatic hydrocarbons (PAHs)
- lead and mercury
- some industrial chemicals such as butyl benzenes-P
- polymers such as polyurethane
- phthalates (used as plasticisers)
- alkyl phenols (surfactants or detergents)
- steroid hormones from natural sources, the pill and HRT
- tributyl tin (antifouling paint used on large ships and as a wood preservative)

Although EDCs are of great interest to agencies responsible for determining their potential effects on humans and wildlife, it is expensive and difficult to monitor most of them in the environment. Some of the new methods designed to measure their concentrations and distribution in the environment and in biological samples, actually use bioassay methods which depend upon the ability of the chemicals to stimulate cultures of breast cancer cells. For example, Shin and co-workers have used genetically modified human breast cancer (MCF-7) cells to show that nonylphenol – a breakdown product from detergents and plasticisers, bisphenol A – a plasticiser, pentachlorobiphenyl – a PCB and DDT cause the breast cancer cell cultures to respond in a dose-dependent manner, i.e. the ore EDC that is added to the breast cancer culture, the more the culture responds.[24] Also, A M Soto has shown that combinations of commonly encountered chemicals in the environment can have more than multiplicative effects on cultures of breast cancer cells.[25]

Xeno-oestrogens ('stranger' oestrogens) in addition to altering oestrogen metabolism can produce direct genetic damage throughout the cell cycle.[26] Some xeno-hormones or their metabolites can produce free radicals or otherwise indirectly modify DNA structure or function.

Some researchers have suggested that xeno-oestrogens are unlikely to cause harm because we are already exposed to phyto-oestrogen chemicals. Humans are likely to have evolved defences against harm from phyto-oestrogens however. Moreover bioaccumulative persistent xeno-oestrogens and other endocrine disrupters accumulate in body tissues to much higher levels than phyto-oestrogens.[27] All of the epidemiological and other research I have read suggests that phyto-oestrogens are protective against breast cancer while xeno-oestrogens are potentially harmful.

The situation has not been helped by the fact that many doctors take little or no interest in the environment and they often do not know much about the chemicals used in industry, agriculture or even in the home environment, or their effects. For example, an article in the October 1999 issue of the *British Medical Journal* implied that crop yields would go on increasing but there was no mention of the input of chemicals that this would require.[28] The article stated:

> Since 1945 the United States and Canada (with Australia) have been the world's most important exporters of cereals. The average growth of yields in these countries has been and remains strong. For example in the United States the average cereal yield rose from 4.58 tonnes per hectare in 1989–1991 to 5.04 tonnes per hectare in 1995–1997. There is no reason to believe that average yields will not continue to rise at a reasonable absolute rate.

There is no mention in the article of the pesticides and other chemicals that have been used to achieve the increase in yield. I have served on committees or attended many meetings concerned with the environment and health. At one meeting I recall that all of the environmentalists sat through the presentations given by the medical specialists. However the doctors all left before any of the papers on the environment were presented. Thank goodness for doctors such as Professor A J McMichael at the London School of Health and Tropical Hygiene, author of the book *Planetary Overload* (CUP 1993), who has developed a broader vision of the causes of ill health related to the environment – including as a result of industrialisation of agriculture – and pollution.

According to a European Environment Agency (EEA)/United Nations Environment Programme (UNEP) report published in 1999 entitled 'Chemicals in the European Environment: Low Doses, High Stakes' there are now many thousands of (man-made) chemicals on the market, and little is known about their fate or impact on people or the environment. The EEA/UNEP report states that such chemicals are widespread in the air, soil, water and stream, river and coastal sediments of Europe following the marketing, use, disposal and degradation of about 100,000 novel substances since the 1950s. Monitoring of a few of these substances is required by law in the US and Europe. However, since much of the monitoring involves analysis of water samples and since many of the compounds of concern are fat-soluble, not water-soluble, the monitoring schemes are likely to underestimate their true impact and presence in the environment. This means that, for many of these chemicals, we have no systematic data on their concentration or distribution in the environment. We also know next to nothing about methods of exposure, about their effect on the environment, and about their effect on human health. And we know nothing about the chemicals as they break down in the environment or in the body (metabolites).

In some cases, for example that of pesticides, release to the environment has been deliberate (although the consequences were often not foreseen and not recognised for many years). In other cases releases have been an unfortunate side effect of the use of substances by the manufacturing industry. In addition, harmful organic chemicals have accumulated in the environment because of energy generation, especially the combustion of fossil fuels. In some cases chemical releases have caused major incidents, for example the release of dioxins at Love Canal in Niagara Falls, New York and Seveso, Italy – but contamination is usually a more insidious process.

Let me quickly summarise how I and many other earth and environmental scientists see the situation.

Life on Earth has evolved in a complex interrelationship with the environment for at least 3,500 million years. Modern man, whose body chemistry has developed over that period of biological evolution, has appeared in the last ten-thousandth of the planet's history (equivalent to the last ten seconds on the 24-hour clock). In the past fifty years or so (much less than a fraction of a second on the 24-hour clock) we have set about dramatically changing the types and proportions of chemical molecules in the environment.

In particular, we have reconfigured organic chemicals, which were the basis of all life, into new 'organic' substances to use in industry and industrialised agriculture. In some cases the new 'organic' substances, which range from plastics to pesticides, their by-products or their metabolites are the *antithesis* of life. Some of the new chemicals and their by-products are implicated in causing cancer. Chemicals which disrupt the endocrine system whereby chemical messengers or hormones control our physiological function are of particular concern in breast and prostate cancer.

MAKING SENSE OF IT ALL – THE PRACTICALITIES

I try to have as few man-made chemicals in my life as possible. I cannot live without my make-up but I use Boots' hypo-allergenic range (Boots are very helpful in providing information on their products). In America in 1990 (the latest figures available) 38,000 patients had cosmetic-related health problems including contact dermatitis, asthma and nausea requiring medical attention. One of the most extreme cases involved a woman whose bone marrow was affected by chemicals in hair dye, to the extent that the level of her blood platelets dropped (not very helpful, especially if you are on chemotherapy).

I do not wear perfume and I use unperfumed simple soap and unperfumed deodorant. I recently read the label on some expensive shower gel marketed by a prestigious company, to find that it actually listed phthalates – one of the main groups of endocrine disrupters implicated in the feminisation of fish – among the chemicals it contained. Research by Professor John Sumpter of Brunel University, London, now suggests that parabens (a very common preservative in cosmetics) could be an oestrogen-mimic (EDC – see p. 222).[29] With cosmetics, as with all other products: read the label, and remember simpler is better.

I do not add chemicals other than simple salts such as Epsom salts to my bath water. Even familiar man-made chemicals are often eventually shown to cause problems. A recent report in the magazine Nature suggests that a commonly used anti-bacterial agent, Triclosan, may work by causing mutations in bacteria.[30] Triclosan is used in many antibacterial soaps, lotions, mouthwash, toothpaste, plastic toys, socks and cutting boards. I prefer to use good, old-fashioned simple soap which will bind with dirt, fat-soluble chemicals and 'germs' and wash them away.

I do not use chemicals to stay young artificially. I do not and would not take hormone replacement therapy especially based on unopposed oestrogen. Some doctors in America and at some London clinics are reportedly providing their patients with human growth hormone (the human equivalent of BST or BGH-1) to prevent ageing. A study published in the British Medical Journal in 1998 reported that high natural levels of the hormone could lead to premature death from cancer. Also, growth hormones available to athletes and body builders must be of concern.

Many other cancer-causing agents have been identified mainly as a result of occupational exposure – of, for example, factory workers, painters and decorators and hairdressers – to high levels of particular chemical substances. Some of the most dangerous chemicals implicated include benzene (used in the manufacture of some furniture and rubber and emitted from some types of fresh paint and car exhausts); formaldehyde (often used as a preservative for example on fabrics in new cars, clothes and furnishing and in some cosmetics and shampoos); hair dyes; and polychlorinated byphenyls (PCBs) in transformers, hydraulic fluids, some paints and varnishes, lubricants, some inks, adhesives and insecticides.[31]

I have my hair streaked but this does not involve having chemicals applied directly onto the scalp, I would avoid using hair dyes especially certain dark coloured ones, some of which contain chemicals suggested to cause cancer, when applied directly to the scalp. Discuss this with your hairdresser and ensure they have checked the information on the carcinogenicity of any chemicals they use.

One of the alternative therapies I question as a treatment for cancer is aromatherapy, especially if you are undergoing chemotherapy. Your liver already has a massive job to do to clear out all the unwanted chemicals and dead cells and other debris from the treatment without having to deal with other powerful chemicals. The skin is the body's largest organ and a proportion of many of the things we put on it are absorbed into the bloodstream.

In aromatherapy a carrier oil such as almond oil (thought not to be absorbed by the skin) is used as a base and an essential oil which normally evaporates (and has molecules that can pass through the skin), is added to achieve particular effects. Some of the oils absorbed through the skin (transdermally) are concentrated extracts of powerful chemicals. Many people wrongly believe that because the essential oils used in aromatherapy are extracted from plants and flowers they cannot be harmful, despite being delivered in high concentrations through the skin. In nature they are at low concentrations as part of a total fruit, flower or leaf. Many of the 'essential' oils have never been tested scientifically for their side effects but medical research has shown that camphor, hyssop and sage oils can have such serious side effects as causing fits. Limonene – the lemon smelling aromatherapy oil – is known to be capable of causing kidney damage. Basil oil which is said to lift mood, and tarragon oil also contain a chemical called estrogole which causes cancer in rodents. Dr Sharon Hopkiss of The Department of Pharmacology and Toxicology at St Mary's Hospital Medical School in London has been quoted as saying that many oils used in aromatherapy are extremely potent natural agents.

The only car I drive is an old Land Rover of 1972 vintage with an engine converted to use lead free petrol. If anything goes wrong we simply buy a new part and put it in. Any volatile organic chemicals used in manufacture or sprayed on its interior will long since have evaporated. Even so, I try to use it as little as possible and to travel by public transport. The chemicals emitted by cars, even when well tuned and running optimally, include many hazardous substances such as benzene (see John Pearson's book *The Air Quality Challenge*). If you paint your house or have it painted, ensure it is well ventilated (some of the oil-based paints used in Britain are now banned in Scandinavia). Also, new furniture, curtains and upholstery can be important sources of formaldehyde and benzene and benzene is given off by many fast drying glues. Vinyl chlorides (PVCs) should also be avoided as much as possible. In an article in *The Times* of 11 November 1999 by Martin Fletcher, it was reported that the European Commission had called for an emergency ban on soft PVC (polyvinyl chloride) toys, including rattles and dummies which babies suck. It is claimed these contain dangerous chemicals. Again, the dangerous chemicals concerned are phthalates. The report claims that eight EU states have already banned phthalates from toys but Britain is not among them. It goes on to point out that phthalates are used for softening the plastic.

If some plant in my garden is going to die, so be it. I will feed it with composted household waste to help it survive but I minimise my use of chemicals around the house or in the garden. My garden has lots of different wild bird species, butterflies, ladybirds, toads and hedgehogs. The degree of bio-diversity in my garden compared to those of many friends who use chemicals says a great deal about the damage our use of chemicals does to the animals, so why do we think that we will be unaffected? We have already discussed problems associated with pesticides implicated in breast cancer. Although I know of no evidence that organophosphates are carcinogenic they are damaging to the central nervous system. Aside from sheep dip and shampoos to kill headlice, many familiar products are based on organophosphates. They include many insecticides, sprays and treatments for lice or fleas on pets including flea collars. I avoid all these products. I never use aerosol sprays for hair, deodorants, cleaning, gardening or any other purpose because of the increased risk of inhaling man-made chemicals.

I use wood, glass, ceramics and natural mineral materials in my home and stainless steel, enamel or toughened glass for cooking and aluminium foil to wrap food. I use natural materials for clothing and furnishing whenever I can, with as few plastics or man-made fibres or other chemicals in my life as possible. Also, I always wash and thoroughly rinse new clothes before wearing them to remove preservatives. I also minimise my use of detergents and ensure they are thoroughly rinsed from crockery and clothes before use. You might find it strange that someone who has spent her professional career working in chemical laboratories should try so hard to avoid them in everyday life. Like many of my colleagues, I have a healthy respect for what chemicals can do to biological processes and so minimise my exposure.

If you have good, nutritious food and reduce exposure to pollutants, you will find your skin and general appearance improves without the need to add polluting man-made chemicals to your body or the environment. We can all reduce our personal risk from hazardous chemicals and by doing so we help the environment generally, with cleaner water and soils and hence more wholesome food. To most natural scientists this is all just common sense and is very easy to live with.

It is impossible to entirely eliminate risk from man-made chemical substances, but you can reduce your personal risk by following the guidelines above and whenever your read or hear a new advertisement for a new beauty product, man-made fabric or garden spray for example, think very carefully whether you really need it. Almost certainly you do not. People who avoid such products are frequently portrayed as odd especially by those wishing to sell us products that we do not need in order to make money. No one looking at me, spending time with me or visiting my home would think I was a crank. Unless pointed out to them they probably would not notice anything is missing or different. Indeed, most people comment on how normal I am (presumably despite being a scientist)!

All of the factors described in Chapters Five and Six are easy to control in your own surroundings. I travel a lot internationally and here are a few tips to help you maintain The Plant Programme while on your travels.

AWAY FROM HOME

1. When travelling, allow plenty of time for every aspect of the journey. Do not allow yourself to become stressed or upset by delays. If flying, try to fly at night to cut your exposure to cosmic radiation.

2. Count out the number of kelp, brewer's yeast and red clover tablets to cover you for your entire time away and take a small pot of dried soya milk (normally sold in cans for babies and infants). Take herbal tea bags and enough fruit to see you through until you can find a local supply.

3. When flying, ensure you order a vegan meal and check that the travel agent uses the code VGML, as other codes can include dairy. Drink lots of boiled water flavoured with your own herbal tea bags to avoid dehydration. Drink beer to make you sleepy.

4. Travel only on 'No Smoking' flights or in 'No Smoking' train compartments.

5. When you arrive at your destination, locate the nearest fruit and vegetable stall or shop and buy fresh supplies daily. In many countries these must be washed in boiling water before eating. This is really a brief immersion (use the hotel sink) similar to the blanching process used in cooking.

6. Before you travel, look up key words in a dictionary and jot them down in the language of the country you will be visiting. For example, in France 'soya' is 'soja': having a small number of ready-translated words to hand will greatly ease your visit. Ask your hotel where to buy the items you need using the written version if necessary. There will usually be a supermarket near your hotel where you can buy supplies, including beer, and thus avoid using the hotel's expensive minibar.

7. Research the local cuisine and check which dishes you will be able to eat without problem or fuss.

8. Tell everyone you are terribly allergic to dairy produce and insist that you have none at all. (I have found this is most difficult in France). If all else fails you can remove the

cheese, or scrape off the yoghurt or cream etc. – I do so ostentatiously!

9. Be inventive in avoiding dairy produce. For example, at the breakfast buffet use prune or other fruit juice to moisten your cereal.

10. If you have trouble sleeping in a different time zone, camomile is soothing and beer always makes me sleepy.

The update to this chapter can be found on page 369.

7 Reflections from West to East

In this chapter I explain why 'the system' has failed to protect us from, or even inform us of, many avoidable risk factors in breast and prostate cancer. It explains why I have come to the conclusion that women must to a great extent rely on themselves in matters of health. Your life really is in your hands. You become empowered by knowledge. The facts and scientific insights provided in this book are intended to reduce risk – as an individual and as a society. In conclusion, there are ten Golden Guidelines for you to follow.

I believe that, in this book, I have put together compelling evidence on the likely causes of breast and prostate cancer, and then developed methods for modifying diet and lifestyle that have the potential to greatly reduce the threat that these diseases represent.

But one thing still greatly puzzles and disturbs me.

All of the information, scientific experiments, epidemiology, surveys and research you've just read have been published in respected, peer-reviewed scientific journals. In many cases, this information has been available for years, even decades.

Why haven't we been told about it?

As a scientist, I read quite widely: numerous general scientific journals, as well as specialist journals in my own field. And I read the usual newspapers, watch television programmes, and generally keep as up-to-date as most people do. And yet, before contracting breast cancer, I'd never heard of any of this vital information.

Why not?

True, the media are full of information and advice on breast cancer: but most of it is either simplistic, unscientific or conflicting. I have *never* seen anything about the case against dairy food which is set out here, or much about the connection with endocrine disrupting chemicals. Who else has made these connections – and why has no one in authority acted on them?

Let us consider what has happened in other situations that involve commercial products that affect our health.

Many elements of the Western diet are known to cause ill health; for example, the high levels of cholesterol and triglycerides in butter, cheese and meat have been linked to heart disease for a very long time. Yet the public has never been given a clear explanation of the risks. In presenting the results of the China study we examined earlier in Chapter Three, Campbell and Junshi showed that even small intakes of food of animal origin are associated with significant increases in plasma cholesterol concentrations, which are associated, in turn, with significant increases in chronic degenerative diseases (cardiovascular, diabetes and several types of cancer including breast and colon cancer).[1] They noted that in the West, reduction in fat consumption was being achieved by using lower-fat foods e.g. low-fat dairy foods, leaner cuts of meat, less added fat: while the fruit–vegetable–cereal recommendation appeared to have received little attention – even though these foods contain virtually *all* of the individual constituents known to prevent chronic degenerative disease. Concerned by this highly-selective distortion of their important message, the scientists speculate that pressure from food industry lobbying groups has influenced both the media (and hence public perception) and also those who set official policy. I have to say that this seems to be the most likely explanation.

Instead of developing good risk communication methods aimed at disease prevention, we continue to treat disease with pills and potions, surgery or other expensive invasive methods to suppress symptoms. Communicating problems in our diet and lifestyle that affect our health is typically done poorly – or not at all – and usually without proper, clear advice on how to change our behaviour.

This whole approach avoids antagonising special interest groups, and it maintains the material wealth of (and jobs in) sectors such as farming, agrochemicals, the food industry, pharmaceutical research and the manufacture of medicines and medical equipment. But would it not be better to communicate facts as they are known, clearly and simply so that people can make their own choices and prevent disease? Would it not be better to create jobs in sectors working for the well-being of society and the environment, for example, in growing wholesome, nutritious organically produced food, with medical professionals being concerned more with health education, disease prevention and monitoring than dishing out pills?

WHERE DOES THE FAULT LIE?

I believe that much of the problem is the genuine lack of understanding of science among politicians. Very few politicians are scientists. Most of them have degrees in law, politics or economics, and many frequently appear more concerned that Britain retains its competitive edge economically than with public health or the environment. Wealth creation generally takes precedence over quality of life, and, I suspect, reflects the views of most of their constituents.

A perfect, and very public, example of the problem MPs face occurred a few years ago when health minister Edwina Currie famously spoke out in the interests of public health to warn people about the danger from eggs contaminated by Salmonella. She was promptly sacked for being so direct and outspoken. The public didn't want her to lose her job; neither did the media. Indeed, almost everyone applauded her courage. However, she had upset some powerful economic interests and her head had to roll.

Of course, politicians are often only as good as the advice they receive and in this, we are also frequently poorly served. The tradition in Britain has been to use generalists as administrative civil servants: 'mandarins' to advise ministries. The character known as Sir Humphrey in the television series *Yes, Minister* and *Yes, Prime Minister* plays the part of such a 'mandarin'. In Britain, of the twenty senior civil servants who are Permanent Secretaries, *none* has a scientific degree.[2] Most of the senior administrative civil servants I have met are ancient historians or classicists who graduated from Oxford or Cambridge, and who are unlikely to have a proper grasp of anything scientific. In my own experience, I have met senior administrative civil servants in the former Department of Energy who did not know what a kilojoule or joule (the basic units of energy) were, and mandarins concerned with coal who had never heard of even the most basic mining terminology.

I remember on one occasion attending a meeting at a government department with a senior British scientist, Professor

Janet Watson FRS, of Imperial College, London. Janet had a gift for putting her finger on the nub of a problem. When we left she expressed her concerns about the difficulties associated with 'the system' for dealing with scientific and technical issues I remember her saying, 'The trouble is that they do not know what they do not know'.

Traditionally in Britain, administrative civil servants have relied on the scientific civil service and public sector research establishments, and to some extent on autonomous universities for authoritative, impartial, scientific advice. Since the end of the 1970s when Margaret Thatcher came to power, however, there have been progressively fewer impartial, independent scientific civil servants to advise on policy. According to evidence given to the House of Commons Science and Technology Committee in 1998, by the Institute of Professionals, Managers and Specialists (IPMS) Union, 'the total number of people engaged in scientific Research and Development (in government) had declined by more than 33 per cent between 1986/7 and 1997/8.' According to David Packham, a senior scientist from the University of Bath who has published widely on the impact of commercialisation on science in the UK, 'The run-down of the scientific civil service and of public sector research establishments must, at the very least, call into question the ability of the remaining resources to provide comprehensive scientific advice over a wide range of government responsibilities. It is important to remember the importance of continuity and stability in building up a reservoir of scientific expertise – it cannot be turned on and off like a tap'.[3]

The increasing commercialisation of science, too, is all too often a limiting factor. In Britain, former scientific civil servants are now working mainly in privatised research organisations with funding increasingly having to be sought from the private sector. The Atomic Energy Agency, the National Physical Laboratory, the Laboratory of the Government Chemist, the Building Research Establishment (BRE), the Transport Research Laboratory and the National Resources Institute have all been sold off or privatised and much government scientific advice is now bought from the market on the basis of short, often three-year contracts. At the end of the contract they are renewed again, usually by tendering operations in which cost can be as important as soundness and quality. There is an increasing drive for commercialism in the research organisations that remain. The same is true of university research. Again since the 1980s funding on a 'per student' basis for the universities has been driven down dramatically. In England and Wales the amount of capital spent per student has been approximately halved. As a consequence, in universities, a higher proportion of traditional research aimed at publication and higher degrees is now sponsored directly by industrial and commercial interests.[4]

This has happened also in the USA. According to Derek Bok, until recently President of Harvard University: 'Universities are constantly pressed to accept questionable arrangements with industry [which may include] provisions prohibiting academic scientists funded by one company from collaborating with investigators funded by another. A few institutions have even agreed to clauses that require them to keep faculty members from speaking about their commercially funded research at academic meetings without first submitting their remarks to their industry sponsors'.[5]

Many industries have sponsored university research as part of a policy of blunting the impact of adverse findings associated with their products. The most fully documented example is the use made by the tobacco companies to mislead the public over the risks associated with smoking. The tobacco industry kept secret its own findings, dating from the early 1960s, that nicotine was addictive and that smoking probably caused cancer. To protect its commercial interests it funded special 'public science' contracts with universities in Britain as well as the USA. These were designed to carry out research in areas where evidence might be found which showed tobacco in a better light and which could then be used to create controversy over 'alleged' dangers of smoking. The source of funding for this research was not publicly disclosed. When eventually in 1994 the details of this campaign became known, the tobacco industry used all the weapons available to a powerful industry to try to suppress their publication. This included attempting to stop a university library from holding the documents in stock, seeking to obtain from the library a list of all the readers who had consulted the documents and using party political influence in an endeavour to cut off the research funds of the academic involved.[6]

Even government-funded research – which should be conspicuously in the public interest and surely, freely available to every citizen – all too often seems to be regarded as a tool of policy. If the research supports the existing or proposed policy, fine. But if not, then it may typically be subject to any or all of the following:[7]

- No press release or press conference
- Not published through usual departmental channels
- Only duplicated copies of typescript available in minimal numbers
- Release timed to coincide with the Friday before the August bank holiday.

The BSE (bovine spongiform encephalopathy) or 'mad cow' crisis was a prime example of the way in which public-interest science can be concealed, distorted or misrepresented. Problems included secrecy of 'scientific' meetings, partial publication of research results, the implied threat to future research funding and the vilification of critics or, indeed, any concerned scientist.[8] According to Sheila Jasanoff, Professor of Science and Technology Studies at Cornell University in the USA, 'What made the news so appalling was not just the thought that beef, a staple of British diets, could be fatally contaminated. It was not even that CJD struck without notice, was incurable, and caused a horrifying death. It was that, since 1988, the government and some of its advisers had repeatedly stated that beef was safe, a formulation widely taken to mean that transmission of BSE from cows to people was impossible. If government officials had deliberately misled the public, then how could anything they now said be trusted?'[9]

Scientists are increasingly concerned about the poor image they have in Britain following fiascos such as the BSE crisis, for which they are unfairly blamed by politicians and public alike. But their image will only improve when we adopt official policies which have far greater transparency, and when public scientists regain the public's respect for forthright and straightforward impartiality.

Clinical doctors, too, must develop far more awareness and interest in diet, lifestyle and the environment. The fact that many of the doctors I know do not eat healthy diets suggests they do not know the importance of good nutrition. Let me describe what happened to John Camac. John was so impressed by my recovery that he put many of his patients suffering from breast cancer, including a close friend of one of his daughters, in touch with me and strongly suggested that they followed my advice. However, he could not bring himself to do this. He lived on a traditional Western diet with very few vegetables. He refused to eat any cruciferous vegetables, the only green vegetables I ever persuaded him to eat were peas. He suffered progressively from a series of degenerative diseases – diabetes, arthritis, coronary heart disease, which was treated with a heart bypass, and he finally died of liver cancer. To deal with his symptoms he took an increasing range and quantity of pills prescribed by what he described as 'top specialists in their field' to treat his ailments. The only foods or drink he used to help his health was red wine for his heart, which Western medicine seems to believe in. By the time he was prepared to listen to me it was far too late, although shortly before he died he was drinking juices and eating soya. I still recollect visiting him in hospital after his heart bypass operation when he was offered a choice of several drinks by a nurse. I urged him to choose orange juice but he drank a large glass of milk. He died of liver cancer six months after his heart bypass operation.

Very few of my friends who are medical professionals seem to know much about food chemistry and I have often seen consultants and junior doctors at Charing Cross Hospital buying junk food. It is my impression that they are all so busy that they do not have time to eat a proper lunch, probably because they work such long hours under intense pressure. All my observations tell me that most doctors are unaware of the likely connections between the food we consume, chemicals in our environment and breast and prostate cancer. Instead, much of their knowledge is based on the literature they are bombarded with about new drugs and procedures. I think it is unrealistic to expect clinical doctors, who are incredibly busy trying to meet targets imposed on them by politicians to assuage public concern, to root out all of the scientific literature on breast cancer that I have found. Anyway, even if I am right and we now know the cause of breast cancer, will we change our behaviour or will we still expect to consume what we want and then expect doctors to pick up the pieces? Experience of what we have done with our knowledge of the dangers of smoking, which we have had for at least 40 years, suggests that this is most likely. Some people still expect to smoke regularly throughout their lives, despite knowing the risks, and then expect doctors to treat them for the range of cancers, including lung cancer and other diseases caused by smoking tobacco.

My answer to the question of 'whose fault is the breast and prostate cancer epidemic?' is that it is all our faults – especially the relatively well-educated women and men in society. It is also my view that we are the ones who must make the changes that will reduce both our personal and societal risk of suffering from these diseases.

OUR LIVES IN OUR HANDS

It was thanks to a particularly unusual set of circumstances that I was able to join up many of the pieces of research into the causes of breast and prostate cancer and develop methods of preventing and treating the disease. These included my experience of working in China and Korea and to a lesser extent with Japanese, Taiwanese and Thai colleagues; my good fortune on being given *The Atlas of Cancer Mortality in the People's Republic of China* and having many opportunities to talk to Chinese and other oriental scientific colleagues. I am grateful to have had the scientific training to fight my way through the scientific jargon, and to have found the strength to withstand the disease, develop methods of treating it and finally cure myself. Even the controversy about the use of BST (bovine somatotropin, *see* p. 95) in milk production helped my understanding of problem chemicals in milk.

Timing was also important. I was lucky enough to travel to Hong Kong, Beijing and Seoul when the Western influence on their diets was less marked. Had I been only recently, I would not have realised the traditional differences between the oriental and Western diets. I always used to enjoy eating in China, Japan or Korea because I could relax knowing that the food was safe for me. Lately I have become very concerned when I have revisited China and Korea to see the amount of Western junk food that is now consumed there, especially by young people. They have been persuaded by advertising and marketing that it is sophisticated to drink strongly promoted Western fizzy drinks, and to eat burgers made from processed dairy cows, butter, and salads covered with pale yellow or pale pink 'glop', which is usually dumped over salads and sandwiches in North America unless you insist beforehand that you do not want your food covered in this stuff. Increasingly, oriental people now eat chocolate puddings covered in cream and end their meals with chocolate and coffee with cream. (They still do not appear to eat much cheese.) Food shopping and eating in Beijing used to be a great pleasure for me but when I last visited my favourite supermarket, it was full of typical Western processed junk food and I had to search very hard to find even soya milk! In Hong Kong last year it was difficult to find truly traditional Chinese food in the area around my hotel. No wonder rates of breast and prostate cancer are rising in Eastern countries.

In this book I have given information to reduce individual risk of breast and prostate cancer, but the only long-term, final and lasting answer to these scourges of our Western lifestyle is to *change* that lifestyle. We have to develop greater awareness of, and sensitivity to, the impact of our lifestyle choices on our own health, that of our fellow beings, and that of our planetary home. Let me quote from Professor McMichael from the London School of Tropical Hygiene and Health and Dr Powles of Cambridge University; their paper in a recent volume of the *British Medical Journal* states:[10]

Population size and the material intensity of our economies are now so great that, at the global level, we are disrupting some of the biosphere's life support systems. These systems provide the natural processes of stabilisation, replenishment, organic production, cleansing, and recycling that our predecessors were able to take for granted in a less populated, less disrupted world. We no longer live in such a world. We are changing the gaseous composition of the atmosphere: there is a net loss of productive soils on all continents: we have overfished most ocean fisheries: we have severely depleted many great aquifers on which irrigated agriculture depends; and we are extinguishing at an unprecedented overall rate whole species and many local populations. These changes to Earth's basic life supporting processes pose long term, and somewhat unfamiliar, risks to human health. Meanwhile the accompanying increases in local environmental pollutant levels, especially urban air pollution, exacerbate more familiar risks to health.

The authors could also have mentioned the industrialisation of agriculture requiring the use of many chemicals to produce ever-increasing crop, milk and meat yields and the future risks posed by genetically modified organisms if full risk analysis is not carried out for each product and their combinations. They conclude:

Overall the larger potential threat is not from the increase in human numbers in itself but from today's globally averaged, mildly environmentally disruptive humans becoming highly disruptive – that is, from attempts to generalise production and consumption patterns typical of today's rich countries. Recent attempts at 'full cost accounting' estimate that the demands of the current world population already exceed global carrying capacity by approximately a third.

The 'living planet' index is one of the first systematic attempts to quantify the effects of human activity on natural ecosystems. It gives equal weight to three contributing indices: forest ecosystems (area of natural forest cover) and freshwater ecosystems and marine ecosystems (trends in the population of 70 and 87 indicator species, respectively). Set to 100 in 1970, it was estimated to have fallen to 68 by 1995 – an unsustainable rate of decline.

Accordingly, a shift of emphasis from income to other types of wealth, especially stocks of human resources, improves the scope for enhancing health at any given level of income which is particularly important if we are to maximise human well-being while minimising consumption which leads to degradation and pollution of the planet.

What they are saying is that, if we are to survive as a healthy species, we must change our values and emphasis from materialism to other measures of well-being. We need increasingly to put more value on good food, education, the arts, beautiful unspoilt environments populated by diverse species other than man, friendships, social interaction and health than on 'things'.

Looking back, I realise that I have changed my diet and lifestyle from that of a middle-class, ambitious career-minded Western woman to a woman with a more traditional Eastern diet, lifestyle and values. So here are some simple, practical guidelines that we can follow to help us as individuals and as a society to cut our risk of breast and prostate cancer and probably many other non-communicable or degenerative diseases, and improve our health at the same time.

MY TEN GOLDEN GUIDELINES

1. Make good food ingredients your top priority when it comes to spending money. Keep as closely as you can to The Plant Programme and wherever and whenever possible be prepared to pay extra for organically grown food produced as naturally as possible or grow your own. This sends the clearest possible message to government and the food industry.

2. Eat only those foods which human adults have evolved to eat. Most crucially leave out dairy produce which is designed for baby calves, goats or lambs. Also refuse to eat food depleted of nutrients or otherwise altered by food processing, including food which contains artificial chemical additives such as colouring and flavouring agents, preservatives and emulsifiers or food which has been chemically altered, for example fats which have been hydrogenated. Refuse to be bamboozled by marketing and advertising, look for the 'weasel words' and separate them in your mind from the underlying facts. Be suspicious – check labels and demand information.

3. Make eating good nutritious meals based on wholesome nutritional ingredients your top priority when it comes to your time. Saving money to acquire material possessions to demonstrate a sophisticated lifestyle and saving time to further your career ambitions are probably two of the fundamental causes of breast cancer in career women. One of my favourite novels is George Eliot's *Middlemarch*, and I continually strive to become more like Dorothea and less like Rosamund!

4. Be concerned and take action to improve the environment for everybody. There are many chemicals being introduced that we can do nothing about as individuals. Collectively, we *can* reduce the impact of chemicals on the environment by reducing our use of materials such as perfumes and cosmetics, soft plastics, detergents, cleaning products and house and garden chemicals, and man-made fibres. Remember how in the past we were sold 'wonder' chemicals such as DDT and PCBs which have turned out to cause serious problems to the health of man, animals and the environment and which are still with us. What

chemicals are we using today that scientists will have a similar view of in the future? Press for more research into the environment, nutrition and human health, with more medical research on epidemiology aimed at prevention.

5. Try to understand some basic science. Usually it is *your* money that scientists are spending directly or indirectly and you need to understand what they are doing. Ensure scientists contribute more to the public understanding of science by asking questions. If you do not understand the answer do not be embarrassed to repeat your question until you get a satisfactory answer. If a scientist cannot explain their work properly it is their problem, not yours. Women in particular frequently throw up their hands at the very mention of science and say how unscientific they are – as if to admit knowing anything about science is unfeminine. It is essential that a well-informed body of opinion exists if science is to be directed for the benefit of humankind rather than lead to our downfall. It is vital that women in particular are involved in the direction of science for the good of society. Books that will 'fire you up' are *Silent Spring* by Rachel Carson, *Our Stolen Futures* by Colborn, Dumanski and Myers and *Planetary Overload* by A J McMichael. If you want to become more involved as lay members of the boards of scientific organisations, write in and offer your services.

6. Learn to understand your basic anatomy and carry out self-examination of your breasts at least once a month. Use books about the human body (there are some good, clear books aimed at children) to learn about your body and ask the nurse at your local health centre practice to show you how to examine yourself thoroughly. Do a thorough examination once a month, a few days after your period ends, to ensure you know how your body looks and feels when it is normal so that you will learn how not to bother your doctor with non-problems, but you will get attention as soon as possible if there is a problem. This is particularly important if you are over forty. Also, if you are over forty try to arrange a check of your breasts by a doctor or nurse once a year at a Well-Women clinic which most good practices in the UK run.

7. If the worst happens and you are diagnosed with breast cancer – use all the tools at your disposal to fight back. For

your orthodox treatment ensure you are treated at a centre of excellence which uses a specialist cancer team led by a surgeon, radiotherapist and chemotherapist. Work with your doctors and be an involved and constructive participant in overcoming your illness, not a passive victim.

8. Follow my diet and the lifestyle recommendations aimed at avoiding man-made chemicals as closely as possible. This includes minimising the use of prescriptions available from doctors and pills from pharmacists. If you are prescribed or recommended drugs, demand to know precisely how they work and what the side effects are. Take them only if you are satisfied with the explanation and convinced there is no alternative. If your physician cannot explain how the drugs work and give examples of their successes and failures, be sceptical.

9. Use methods such as meditation, hypnotherapy and visualisation and yoga to cope with any emotional distress to develop the most positive approach possible. But do not rely on positive thinking alone. It is changing your body chemistry by changing your diet and lifestyle that is the crucial thing to do. Talk to your friends and family members and allow their help and support into your life, but if they find difficulty in coping, understand that they are distressed. Forgive them and allow them back into your life as soon as they feel able to return.

10. Breast cancer is NOT an automatic death sentence. Keep reminding yourself that IT IS possible to overcome even advanced cancer. Believe me. I did it.

Knowledge is power. In this book I have tried to empower *all* women to deal with breast cancer, individually and as a society, by trying to share with them the knowledge that I have gained on the subject of breast cancer as a scientist and as a five-times breast cancer sufferer.

Before my first diagnosis of cancer I was a go-getting career woman, acquiring material possessions and although I always made time for my children, I was something of a 'lifestyle' wife and mother. I had become ill-nourished because of reading food industry (so called health) propaganda literature. I had survived on what was marketed and advertised as health food, albeit low fat and high fibre with high quantities of dairy food: cottage cheese and yoghurt and dishes made using mincemeat from slaughtered dairy cows, washed down with milky tea or commercial orange juice. I ate lots of fruit and cereals but few salads or vegetables. I simply took high dose vitamin C pills and multivitamin multi-mineral pills to cover any deficiencies.

I am now kinder to myself and to other people. I ensure however hurried I am, however simple my meals, that they are based on sound nutritional values. I now make time for family and friends and – amazingly – I seem to be even more successful in my work and my life. I am no longer a 'fashion victim' in my clothes, home, garden or car and I try to be as unmaterialistic as possible.

Instead, I am increasingly concerned with the environment and the sustainability of the surface of the beautiful blue planet called Earth as a place to live. Breast cancer changed me: from being insecure and easily persuaded by authority to a stronger woman who is her own person.

It made me stop.

And smell the (wild) roses . . .

The update to this chapter can be found on page 401.

Update to Chapter 1. Keeping Abreast

Conventional medical treatment and management of breast cancer has changed over the last fifteen years, and there has been a significant decrease in mortality reported in the UK, USA and many other Western countries. The trend to find the most breast- conserving methods of treatment has also continued. In this update to Chapter One, some of the new options for conventional diagnosis and treatment of breast cancer and ovarian cancer are considered. Mortality from ovarian cancer, although somewhat lower than a decade ago, remains high, mainly because the disease is often not diagnosed until it is at an advanced stage. The conventional treatment and management of ovarian cancer are discussed.

THE GOOD NEWS IS . . .

The death rate from breast cancer has declined in most Western countries in recent years, falling by about 1 to 2 per cent a year.[1] The UK has seen the highest reduction in the world in the rates of death from female breast cancer and male lung cancer.[2] The fall in deaths from breast cancer is attributed to better diagnosis and treatment, while the fall in lung cancer deaths is attributed to a decline in smoking – interestingly the decline in one type of cancer is attributed to treatment and the other to prevention. If there is one message I hope people will take away from this book, it is that we can do much more to prevent breast and ovarian cancer and other cancers such as cancer of the womb and colorectal cancer by following the dietary and lifestyle factors described in Chapters Five and Six which make up the Plant Programme.

TO SCREEN OR NOT TO SCREEN

It seems almost self evident that all middle-aged and elderly women should be screened for breast cancer, but the whole subject remains controversial in a way that seems at first to defy common sense. The argument against screening is that some cancers are detected that would not, in the past, have been detected at all and would not have caused problems during the patient's lifetime. Another argument is that, at a population level, mortality is not reduced by early detection. There is also the concern about the cumulative dose of ionising radiation from a lifetime of mammograms, X-rays and other scans, and that the money spent on screening, in a limited-budget health service like the NHS in the UK, could be put to better use. The argument in favour of screening is based on the evidence from randomised trials that early detection reduces mortality, which means that any additional cancers detected must include ones that would both progress during the patient's lifetime and be curable by earlier treatment.[3]

It has been said that 'Few topics in medicine have been the subject of so much debate and controversy as breast screening by mammography.'[4] The falling death rate from breast cancer is attributed by some experts to early detection (involving routine screening mammography) and treatment (including early surgery, hormone therapy and better chemotherapy).[5] Other experts, including Professor Michael Baum[6] and Dr Steven Goodman of Johns Hopkins School of Medicine in the USA,[7] have been more sceptical of the contribution from screening mammography and attribute any decline in death rate to better characterisation and optimisation of treatment in relation to different types of breast cancer.

The controversy is reflected by conflicting findings in scientific publications. For example, one study showed that Canadian women in their 40s receiving annual mammography screening did not have a higher survival rate from breast cancer, after an average 13-year follow-up, than the control groups of women who had physical breast examination by their doctors and instruction on breast self-examination.[8] A different study, however, concluded that teaching women breast self-examination is not cost-effective nor does it lead to improvements in survival from breast cancer.[9] More recently, the rate of over-diagnosis of breast cancer 15 years after the end of a mammographic screening trial in Malmo, Sweden has been shown to be 10 per cent in women between the ages of 55 and 69.[10] The latest addition to the debate is a report published in February 2006 by the Advisory Committee on Breast Screening summarising the results of the English breast screening programme. The findings are summed up by the *BMJ* as 'time to accept that despite limitations screening for breast cancer does save lives.'[11]

The purpose of screening is earlier identification of the tumour, allowing for earlier treatment, although it continues to be essential that a biopsy, where a small portion of the suspect lump or tissue is removed for examination, is performed before a firm diagnosis of cancer can be made. It is important that, when cancer has been confirmed, the patient should have time to recover from the initial shock and to review the options for treatment fully with their doctors without being rushed into a decision. I have already described (see p. 33) how I had an unnecessary mastectomy because I panicked. The prevailing view at the time was that diagnosis and excision of cancer was of the utmost urgency. This was misguided. In a letter to the *BMJ*,[12] R. Paul Symonds concluded that although diagnostic delay is highly undesirable, in most cases the type of cancer the patient is suffering from is more important to remission and survival than short delays in diagnosis.

The US Preventive Services Task Force recommends screening mammography, with or without clinical breast examination, every one to two years for women aged 40 or over.[13]

In the UK, the advice is for screening at intervals of three years for women aged 50 and over.[14] Advice to women to undertake breast self-examination was abandoned over ten years ago in the UK.

There continue to be concerns about errors and misdiagnosis associated with national screening programmes. The UK Government Health Service's watchdog, the Commission for Health Improvement, has recommended that the NHS breast-screening programme requires a greater degree of standardisation, including notation and improved quality assurance and follow-up.[15]

A common concern following mammography is when women are told that they have calcification, which in some cases can indicate cancer or a precancerous condition. Breast calcification can occur for many other reasons, however, including the fluid in cysts, as a result of previous injury to the breast, as a result of inflammation or mastitis, or as a result of radiotherapy for breast cancer.

My advice remains that the common-sense thing to do is to learn about your body and maintain a regular monthly check of your breasts so that you can identify problems as soon as possible and seek medical attention (see p. 243). A DVD explaining how to do breast self-examination, together with a special glove that increases sensitivity, is now available from one chain of pharmacies in the UK. I think that all women should be educated to be breast aware, ideally when they are young and healthy. Premenopausal women should examine their breasts routinely every month, one week after their periods have finished.

I also continue to recommend that all women over 40 attend for a physical examination at least once a year by a trained specialist health professional at a clinic or general practice. Young women (under 40), in particular, should bear in mind that mammography involves irradiation of the breast and should discuss the risks and benefits fully with their physician before proceeding. It is worth recalling that about 14 per cent of the average dose of ionising radiation to a UK citizen is from medical diagnostic procedures and treatment, compared with less than 1 per cent from the nuclear industry (including weapons fallout); the remaining 85 being from natural sources, including food.[16]

Frequent mammograms have been used to monitor women with mutations in genes associated with a high risk of breast cancer, but MRI scans which do not involve the use of ionising radiation are now being used increasingly.[17]

It is worth repeating that most breast lumps turn out to be benign. Benign breast masses include

Cysts – fluid collections caused by hormonal factors that are rarely malignant

Fibroadenomas – solid, benign tumours that may be multiple and occur in both breasts and are commonest in younger women

Fibrocystic masses – combinations of cystic and connective tissue changes

Abcesses – local collections of pus, frequently associated with breast feeding.

DETECTING OVARIAN CANCER

Ovarian cancer can affect one or both ovaries. It may be present for some time before it is discovered, and is often discovered unexpectedly during an operation such as a hysterectomy. Early symptoms of ovarian cancer are often open to other diagnoses, and may not be recognised as signs of cancer. They include: pain in the lower abdomen, which may be diffuse and difficult to pinpoint; low back pain; abnormal menstrual cycles; vaginal bleeding; weight loss; increase in girth; general abdominal discomfort; increased urinary frequency; non-specific gastro-intestinal problems, including changed bowel movements; and constant tiredness. Most of these symptoms can also reflect the presence of non-malignant conditions that are readily treatable.

It is easy to understand why they are often discounted by patients or their physicians, especially when ovarian cancer is a relatively uncommon disease. It is worth having any persistent symptoms checked out, especially if they are gradually worsening. Urinary frequency, for example often reflects a simple infection that can be treated easily with antibiotics following a culture of a urine sample to ensure that the correct drug is selected. Women should ask for a thorough examination if such symptoms develop gradually, persist despite the absence of infection, and are accompanied by other symptoms, even if they are subtle.

Ovarian cancer affects between 1 in 50 and 1 in 70 women in most Western countries, but it is the leading cause of gynaeco-logical cancer death. The age of diagnosis is generally over 60 but some women suffer from the disease at a much younger age. Efforts are in hand to identify a simple cost-effective screening test for ovarian cancer. There is a tumour marker, CA-125, that is used to monitor treatment, but this is not considered suitable for routine screening.

SOME FACTS ABOUT BREAST CANCER

There are several different types of breast cancer (Table 1.1).

Although the ultimate goal of orthodox medical treatment remains improved survival, increasing emphasis is now put on treatments that are considered to have less drastic side effects, with more emphasis on maintaining quality of life.

Decisions on treatment depend not only on the type of cancer but also on the stage it has reached. The stages are as follows:[18]

Stage 0 – non-invasive cancer (carcinoma), or cancer *in situ*.

Stage 1 – cancer cells have not spread beyond the breast, and the tumour is less than 2 cm across.

Stage 2 – the tumour is less than 2 cm across and has spread to the lymph nodes under the arm; or the tumour is between 2 and 5 cm, with or without lymph-node involvement; or the tumour is larger than 5 cm but has not spread.

Stage 3 – the tumour is more than 5 cm across and has spread to the under-arm lymph nodes and/or to other lymph nodes or tissue near the breast. Stage 3 cancer also includes a condition called inflammatory breast cancer.

Stage 4 – the cancer has spread from the breast to other parts of the body. Unlike many other cancers, even Stage 4 breast cancers have responded to medical intervention.

Table 1.1: The most important types of breast cancer[19]

Non-invasive (usually early cancers)	**Invasive** (when cancer cells have spread into the underlying connective tissue in the breast, which is rich in blood vessels and lymphatic channels capable of carrying cancer cells beyond the breast)
Ductal carcinoma *in situ* (DCIS), consisting of cancer cells in the lining of ducts. A non-invasive early cancer, that if left untreated may progress to an infiltrating ductal carcinoma	Infiltrating ductal carcinoma, accounting for 70–80 per cent of all breast-cancer cases
Lobular carcinoma *in situ* (LCIS), a marker for an increased risk of invasive cancer in both breasts, which can be either lobular or ductal	Infiltrating lobular carcinoma, accounting for 10–15 per cent of all breast cancers; may sometimes be widespread in both breasts

There are other less common breast cancers, which are not included here.

Breast-cancer cells are now classified routinely as hormone-receptor-positive cells (*see* 'The Wrong Knitting Pattern,' page 57) if they have receptors or binding sites for hormones such as oestrogen or progesterone. Women with such tumours are considered to have a better prognosis than those with receptor-negative cells, because receptor-positive cells are considered to grow more slowly and there are more treatment options.

Several chemical markers are being researched as a means of predicting the likelihood that a cancer will spread. For example, the HER-2 protein, which is high in 25–30 per cent of breast-cancer patients, is being used to select those patients considered likely to benefit from chemotherapy combined with Herceptin. Research suggests that women with HER-2 positive metastatic breast cancer have a more aggressive disease, greater likelihood of recurrence, poorer prognosis and approximately half the life expectancy of women with HER-2 negative breast cancer.

Other methods of identifying which patients should be targeted with more powerful drug/chemotherapeutic treatments are being developed based on outcomes of research into the human genome. One example is based on the presence of a form of a chemical known as cyclin E.[20]

Breast cancer risk increases with age in the West[21] and it is the commonest cause of cancer deaths in women over 65 years of age,[22] increasing in incidence up to 80 years of age before levelling off between 80 and 85 years of age.[23] According to both clinical observations[24] and laboratory studies,[25] however, breast cancer, including its secondary tumours, is less aggressive in elderly people. Age alone should not be a barrier to treatment, but the risks and benefits of the various treatment options need to be carefully weighed. Further information is given in an article by Balducci and Phillips in *American Family Physician*.[26]

SOME FACTS ABOUT OVARIAN CANCER

There are three main types of ovarian cancer. The commonest type, epithelial ovarian cancer, accounts for about 90 per cent of all ovarian cancers and develops on the surface of the ovary in epithelial cells. The second type, germ-cell cancer, accounts for about 5 per cent of ovarian cancer cases and affects the cells that would normally develop into eggs. The remaining 5 per cent, known as stromal cell cancer, develops in the tissue of the ovary that holds the structure together and produces female hormones such as oestrogen. In addition, there are Low Malignant Potential (LMP) tumours of the ovary and benign ovarian cysts.

DIAGNOSIS[27]

Breast cancer

Mammography, followed by biopsy, remains the main diagnostic procedure for breast cancer. If cancer is confirmed, chest X-rays and scans should be carried out to detect any spread and optimise treatment strategies based on the type and stage of the disease. MRI scans are now used more frequently, especially where there is a recurrence of cancer. New ultrasound techniques can detect tumours less than 1 cm across. These methods are time-consuming and less effective than mammography, but involve no ionising radiation.

Thermography, which measures an increase in temperature in the breast, can indicate the presence of disease, including cancer. As with mammography, however, the final diagnosis always requires the examination of a biopsy sample of the suspect tissue.

Ovarian cancer

If ovarian cancer is suspected, your family doctor is likely to carry out a thorough internal examination before referring you to a specialist who will first carry out tests including scans. A diagnosis is usually made from a biopsy, which will also identify the type of ovarian cancer and its stage.

SCANS

Since I wrote the first edition of this book there have been major advances in the application of scanning methods, involving the use of computers to prepare detailed images of the body. Since the diagnosis and management of breast cancer and ovarian cancer now frequently involve undergoing many different types of scans, it is worth learning more about which scans are available and their relative advantages and disadvantages.

Remember, some scans such as CT scans and bone scans involve the use of ionising radiation (see p. 249).[28] Also, abnormalities detected by many types of scans, including bone scans, can include arthritis and other degenerative diseases and lesions that may or may not indicate active cancer.[29] The choice of scans normally depends on the physician's preference and the availability of scanners, but I think it is important for patients to be well informed and to discuss alternatives with their doctors, especially if they are being treated by a private clinic. Whichever type of scan is used, patients should be given comprehensive safety information and advice on how to prepare for the tests. Women should tell their health professionals, before undergoing a scan, if they think that they might be pregnant.

Radionuclide bone scan

A bone scan involves injection with a radioactive substance called technetium in a phosphate compound designed to 'stick' to the bones. The radioactivity of the technetium decays quickly and the total amount of radioactivity is low compared with the much higher doses used in radiation therapy, and generally does not cause side effects. The radioactive substance is attracted to diseased bone cells throughout the skeleton and can therefore be seen on the bone-scan image. These concentrations of technetium may suggest that metastatic cancer is present, but other bone diseases can give the same pattern.[30] If you have one of these scans, do follow instructions carefully so that the procedure does not have to be repeated, exposing you to more ionising radiation.

After the test, drink several glasses of a well-known cola which contains phosphoric acid to try to encourage your body to exchange the radioactive phosphates for the non-radioactive phosphate compounds in the cola as soon as possible. (Otherwise I never drink colas.)

Computed tomography (CT)

A CT (or CAT) scan uses a rotating X-ray beam to create a series of pictures of the body from many angles. A computer combines the information from the pictures, producing a detailed three-dimensional image of the body and its internal organs which can be viewed from many different angles. The CT scan may reveal abnormally enlarged lymph nodes, which could be a sign of a spreading cancer (or a sign that the immune system is fighting an infection). The CT scan can also detect cancer that has spread to other internal organs, such as the liver, and is frequently performed prior to treatment, especially if there is evidence of lymph-node involvement.[31] CT scans are ideally used for examining tissue such as bone and calcifications or structures artificially enhanced with agents such as barium or iodine which have a high radiological contrast to the rest of the body.

Remember that repeated CT scans can involve significant exposure to ionising radiation, and discuss this with your doctors (some people seem to forget how damaging such radiation is to the body if they repeat scans too frequently). In 2000 and 2001, only 7 per cent of all radiological examinations in the UK were CT scans but they contributed almost 50 per cent of the total dose from medical X-ray examinations.

CT scans are still quite expensive. Several private institutions offer full-body scans. This is highly controversial due to its lack of proven benefit, the increased exposure to ionising radiation and the high cost, especially to the NHS, because 'incidental' abnormalities frequently trigger further investigations.[32]

Magnetic resonance imaging (MRI)

MRI scanning involves the use of radio frequency signals rather than X-rays to create detailed three-dimensional images of the body and its internal organs. It is performed following injection of an intravenous contrast agent, usually a low-toxicity complex of the trace element gadolinium. Images produced by MRI can identify cancer spread, and, as with the CT scan, may be performed if there is evidence of lymph-node involvement.[33] Unlike CT scans, MRI does not involve the use of ionising radiation and it is ideal for non-calcified soft tissue. Some of the other advantages of MRI compared to CT are that many parameters can be changed to improve image contrast and it can more easily generate cross-sectional images in any plane. Safety precautions are nevertheless important, and having a pacemaker generally means that patients cannot have MRI scans. If you are aware that you have any metallic objects in your body such as insulin pumps, cochlear implants or foreign bodies such as shell fragments or dental implants you should inform your health professionals before having an MRI scan. It is worth putting the information in writing so it is with your records and is not forgotten by overworked doctors. It is particularly important to report any possibility of metal fragments in the eye (for example, from a previous accident) so that a check X-ray can be carried out prior to scanning. Titanium is generally considered safe for MRI, but not titanium steel. Other safety concerns include obese patients or those with difficulty in regulating their body temperature who may become too hot.

In March 2007 the American Cancer Society advised women over 30 years of age with mutated BRCA-1 or BRCA-2 genes, those who have been treated for Hodgkin's disease, and those with a strong family history of breast cancer or ovarian cancer to have regular MRI scans combined with mammography. Whereas mammograms detect calcification that can indicate cancer, MRIs were said to be better at showing increased or abnormal blood flow that can be an early sign of cancer and to be more appropriate for those with high-density mammographic breast tissue. MRI scans are extremely expensive (costing up to 20 times as much as a mammogram), and there is a high error rate, leading to unnecessary biopsies and scarring.

Positron Emission Tomography (PET)

PET is a relatively new method of detecting cancer spread. It involves the acquisition of physiological images based on the detection of radiation from the emission of tiny radioactive particles called positrons given off by radioactive isotopes such as fluorine-18. Normally, such isotopes are used to label glucose, which is taken up more readily by cancer cells than normal cells, or sometimes to label ammonia or water. The method depends upon generating detailed computer images, like CT and MRI scans, but in this case the images are obtained from high-energy short-lived particles.

At the time I wrote the first edition of this book, the technique was being used mainly for the early detection of lung and brain cancer. It is now more widely available and is used to detect the spread of several types of cancer, including breast and ovarian cancer. The main advantage of PET is that it identifies centres of unusual metabolism, whereas most other methods can identify only the presence of lesions which may or may not be active cancer. Also it can detect alterations in biochemical processes that suggest disease before changes in anatomy appear. It can give false results, however, especially in diabetic patients or in those who have eaten too near to the time the scan was performed.

PET scans do involve the use of ionising radiation, but because the isotopes used are very short-lived the overall radiation exposure is low. Nevertheless, any woman who thinks she might be pregnant should inform her doctors before having a PET scan.

Sentinel lymphadenectomy

Sentinel lymphadenectomy is increasingly used to identify the spread of cancer into the lymph nodes. It is a minimally invasive method of identifying patients whose lymph nodes are affected by cancer. The sentinel node is defined as the first node to receive drainage from a tumour and is identified by injecting a special substance around the primary tumour and noting its spread via lymphatic channels. This method has been said to have a 95 per cent success rate in identifying cancer spread to lymph nodes.[34] It is replacing removal and pathological examination of lymph nodes and is suitable for many, but not all, patients. This method reduces the incidence of lymphoedema (build-up of fluid due to disruption of normal lymph drainage following surgical removal of lymph nodes). Since only 15 per cent of breast-cancer sufferers are found to have affected lymph nodes, the savings to health-care systems of not having to provide lymphoedema sleeves and other treatment is significant.

Some new techniques

A new advanced technique of high-resolution magnetic resonance computerised imaging is being developed, which uses magnetic nanoparticles to seek out affected lymph nodes.[35] This method should help doctors to distinguish more accurately between normal nodes and those affected by cancer. The studies reported found detectable metastases, confirmed by pathological examination, and also showed that some lymph nodes, which might otherwise have been removed, contained no cancer. Forty-five of the 63 malignant nodes were so small they would not have been identified as malignant by conventional imaging techniques.[36]

Prostascint scan

This is still a relatively new type of test, which, like the bone scan, uses low-level radioactive material to find cancer that has spread. In this test, the radioactive material is attached to a monoclonal antibody, a type of antibody engineered in the laboratory to recognise and stick to a particular marker on cancer cells. The disadvantage of this method is that it often suggests spread when there is none.[37]

TREATMENT OPTIONS

Considerable work has been carried out to evaluate the relative benefits and adverse effects of the conventional medical treatments for breast cancer, separately and in combination. One startling aspect of breast-cancer treatment is that local control of the tumour may have limited impact on survival. When followed up 20 years later, patients undergoing mastectomy or lumpectomy or lumpectomy with radiation therapy have identical survival curves although those having lumpectomy alone had a 25 per cent rate of recurrence.[38]

There are no such studies of outcomes for ovarian cancer. Surgery remains the preferred treatment and is usually combined with chemotherapy. Radiotherapy and hormone treatments may also be used. If you have ovarian cancer, your doctor will discuss the options for treatment with you when all the results of the diagnostic tests are available. The type of treatment usually depends on the type and stage of cancer, your general state of health, other personal considerations and, in premenopausal women, whether or not you wish to have children.

My general advice to all UK patients remains to obtain treatment for serious illnesses such as cancer at NHS centres of excellence, such as the Charing Cross Hospital in London where there is a team of doctors trained in surgery, radiotherapy, chemotherapy and drug and other treatments.

SURGERY

Breast cancer

The trend to minimally invasive surgery to treat breast cancer has continued, with the retention of as much breast tissue as possible. The much-feared Halstead radical mastectomy, which involved removal of the entire breast and associated chest wall muscles and all nodes from under the arm, has been abandoned and we can only wonder at the misery and pain that women with breast cancer suffered in the past.

There are still two main types of surgery for breast cancer, lumpectomy and mastectomy. In women with small tumours, less than or equal to 1 cm in size, lumpectomy followed by radiotherapy is now the preferred treatment, regardless of tumour oestrogen-receptor status, and tamoxifen together with radiotherapy is used when tumours are oestrogen-receptor positive.[39]

The benefits of lumpectomy followed by radiotherapy, compared with mastectomy, are now quite clear for most types of cancer. Recently, a 20-year follow-up in America comparing total mastectomy, lumpectomy, and lumpectomy with radiotherapy for the treatment of invasive breast cancer demonstrated that there were no significant differences among the three groups with respect to disease-free survival, metastatic-disease-free survival or overall survival.[40] The risk of a second cancer developing in the same breast was about 40 per cent in women who had had a lumpectomy without radiation and 14 per cent in women who had also had radiotherapy. A similar study in Italy reached the same conclusions.[41] The *BMJ* quotes Dr Monica Morrow of the Feinberg School of Medicine in Chicago as saying that it is time to declare the case against breast-conserving therapy closed and focus our efforts on new strategies for the prevention and cure of breast cancer. In her view, the findings of the two recent studies should convince even the most determined sceptics that lumpectomy is just as effective as mastectomy for treating small breast cancers. Dr Morrow and other experts also said that the two studies indicated that it made no difference whether tiny clusters of cancer cells were removed or left behind.

These results confirm that my experience and subsequent mastectomy, described on page 33, shows I should have listened to my consultant surgeon, who was clearly aware of these early findings.

As discussed on pages 31–37, there are several types of breast cancer that point to the use of mastectomy rather than lumpectomy. Other indications for mastectomy include (1) when a breast contains widespread Ductal Carcinoma in Situ (DCIS)[42] and (2) when there is evidence of exceptionally high risk due to familial and/or genetic predisposition. Again, neither of these factors applied to me.

Modern mastectomies leave the chest wall muscles and lymphatic pathways intact so that movement and lymphatic drainage is retained. The three main types of mastectomy now used include (1) subcutaneous, which removes the entire breast but leaves the nipple and the pigmented area around it in place, (2) total (or simple) mastectomy, which removes the whole breast but not the lymph nodes under the arm, and (3) modified radical mastectomy, whereby the whole breast and most of the lymph nodes under the arm are removed. The subcutaneous and total (simple) mastectomy are the preferred options to reduce the risk of breast cancer for women at high risk (Table 1.2). Mastectomy is now considered very safe, and most patients recover well, with no complications.[43]

Preoperative treatment for breast cancer

Many hospitals now offer preoperative treatment of breast cancer using drug treatments such as tamoxifen, anastrozole or arimidex, alone or in combination, or chemotherapy to 'downstage' large cancers and reduce the need for mastectomy. Another advantage of this approach is that the effectiveness of the drug treatment or chemotherapy regime can be gauged easily, which is not the case after the tumour has been removed.

Breast reconstruction

Breast reconstruction at the time of mastectomy or at a later date can help to restore a normal appearance, though not always when the woman is nude and reconstruction does not restore normal sensation. Techniques for breast reconstruction have advanced greatly, including reconstruction of the nipple and areolar area. Many women choose not to undergo breast reconstruction. Despite being offered such an operation by one of the best plastic surgery teams in the world, every time I attend for my annual check-up at Charing Cross Hospital, I still have not managed to find the time – and I doubt if I ever will.

If you are thinking about having reconstructive surgery, it is a good idea to discuss it with your surgeon and a plastic surgeon experienced in breast reconstruction before undergoing mastectomy. This will allow the surgical teams to plan the treatment that is best for you, if you decide to have reconstructive surgery later.

Following reconstruction, the appearance of the breasts in a bra will hopefully be so similar that you will feel comfortable about how you look. Your body image and self-esteem may improve, but this is not always the case. Breast reconstruction does not remedy pre-existing psychological and personal problems, and some women may be disappointed with how their reconstructed breasts look. You and those close to you must be realistic about what to expect.

Breast reconstruction may require one or more operations. You should discuss the benefits and risks with your doctors before proceeding and give yourself plenty of time to make the best decision for you.

Further detailed information is available on the website of the American Cancer Society.[44]

Counselling and other types of emotional support are increasingly available to help women to adjust to the loss of a breast or following hysterectomy, and to help their partners and families to understand and help.

Ovarian cancer

There are several different types of surgery for ovarian cancer which all require treatment by a specialist gynaecological surgeon. Removing one ovary is called a unilateral oophorectomy; if both are removed, it is a bilateral oophorectomy; and likewise if one or both fallopian tubes are removed the operations are referred to as unilateral or bilateral salpingectomies. If the ovaries and the womb are removed the operation is a hysterectomy. If both ovaries and the womb are removed, pregnancy will not be possible and menopausal symptoms are likely to develop. Most women will be in hospital for a few days but recovery can take several weeks and in some cases months. If it is not possible to remove the entire tumour the surgeon will remove as much as possible.

Treatment for low-malignant-potential tumours generally involves removal of the affected ovary and tube, if the woman hopes to become pregnant, or hysterectomy if pregnancy is not a consideration. Generally there is no chemotherapy or other treatment. Epithelial cancer usually involves removal of one or both ovaries and other organs depending on the extent of spread; with removal of as much cancerous tissue as possible if the tumours cannot be removed completely, followed by chemotherapy. Germ-cell tumours are rare, and treatment usually involves removal of the affected ovary and tube followed by chemotherapy. Stromal cell tumours are usually confined to the ovary and surgery usually involves simply the removal of the affected ovary.

RADIOTHERAPY

As with surgery, the trend with radiation therapy is for the most cosmetically pleasing results possible, with the aim of retaining an intact breast or as much breast tissue as possible. Evidence that lumpectomy alone was likely to lead to a recurrence of breast cancer whereas whole-breast irradiation therapy, even months after surgery, cut this risk drastically led to its widespread use. Re-examination of the evidence showed, however, that most recurrences were at or close to the original tumour site. This means that radiation therapy is required over a much more limited area, and partial breast irradiation has become more widely used. Conformal radiotherapy and intensity-modulated radiation therapy, which concentrate exposure on the tumour but severely restrict the radiation dose received by normal tissue, achieve excellent clinical and cosmetic outcomes with very few patients experiencing problems.[45]

Radiotherapy is not routinely used for treatment of ovarian cancer.

DRUG TREATMENTS

In post-menopausal women, tamoxifen was, until recently, the first-line treatment for oestrogen-receptor-positive metastatic breast cancer. Patients with advanced breast cancer may be prescribed tamoxifen for various lengths of time, depending on their response to the treatment.[46] When used following treatment for early breast cancer, it is generally prescribed for five years. Tamoxifen works by binding to oestrogen receptors and blocking their activation (a new drug being investigated actually degrades and destroys the oestrogen receptors). Patients taking tamoxifen, who have not had a hysterectomy, should have regular pelvic examinations to detect cancer of the womb well before it becomes life-threatening (see Table 1.2). They should be checked promptly if they have any abnormal vaginal bleeding or pelvic pain.

Recently, a class of drugs known as aromatase inhibitors are used as a first line of treatment. These drugs work by inhibiting the conversion of testosterone (and another steroidal hormone) into oestrogen, though only in post-menopausal women. The US Food and Drug Administration (FDA) has approved some of these drugs as first-line treatment after studies showed small but significant improvements in outcome compared with tamoxifen, with lower incidence of blood clotting. No association between aromatase inhibitors and risk of endometrial cancer has yet been found, but longer-term studies are required. Such drugs are also considered helpful for patients who cannot be given surgery or chemotherapy. Studies of combined aromatase-tamoxifen treatment show that it further improves outcome. Some teams will use chemotherapy only when these and similar options are exhausted.[47] Also, a new aromatase inhibitor, exemestane, sold under the brand name Aromasin, lowered the death rate by 17 per cent in post-menopausal women with oestrogen receptor positive cancer who were switched to it from Tamoxifen after 2–3 years rather than keeping to Tamoxifen for the usual 5 years.[48] In June 2006 NICE (National Institute for Health and

Clinical Excellence) recommended aromatase inhibitors as alternatives to Tamoxifen for treating early oestrogen-receptor-positive breast cancer in post-menopausal women following full discussion with the patient that takes account of the side effects of the different drugs as well as their efficacy.

Other drugs being used to prevent the spread of breast cancer, especially to the bones, include drugs called bisphosphonates, which are commonly used to treat osteoporosis.[49] These may be used in combination with Tamoxifen or aromatase inhibitors.

Another treatment which has been more fully evaluated since completion of the first edition of this book is Herceptin, the first humanised antibody approved for the treatment of HER-2 (human epidermal growth factor receptor 2 protein) positive metastatic breast cancer. Herceptin is designed to target and block the function of HER-2 protein over-expression, which occurs in 20–25 per cent of breast cancers.[50]

Herceptin in combination with Paclitaxel is used for treating patients with metastatic breast cancer who have not received chemotherapy. It is used as a single agent for treating patients with metastatic breast cancer, whose tumours over-express the HER-2 protein and who have received one or more chemotherapy regimens. The FDA approved Herceptin for use in September 1998. In evaluating the benefits of Herceptin used in combination with chemotherapy, the median time to disease progression increased from 2.5 (for Paclitaxel alone) to 6.7 months (for Paclitaxel with Herceptin), with median survival time increasing from 18.4 to 22.1 months. In combination with Anthracycline and Cyclophosphamide, the increase in median time to disease progression was from 5.7 to 7.6 months, and in median survival time from 21.4 to 26.8 months.[51]

In addition to many clinical trials with Herceptin for the treatment of metastatic breast cancer, the drug has been studied to evaluate its safety and efficacy in women with HER-2 positive early-stage breast cancer. One trial, which showed that treatment with Herceptin following standard chemotherapy reduced the risk of recurrence by 46 per cent, sparked legal and media pressure in the UK for it to be prescribed by the NHS.[52] NICE now recommends the use of the drug, but no additional funds have been made available. The problem has been discussed by Barrett and others of the Norfolk and Norwich University Hospital trust.[53] These authors pointed out that, although the three published trials showed a significant reduction in recurrence, only one showed any survival benefit – 4.8 per cent at 4 years. The high cost of the treatment (about £26,000 for a single course) means that their hospital trust will be required to spend £2.3 million a year to treat the 75 patients who might be eligible for Herceptin. The cost is almost 50 times that of using aromatase inhibitors to treat oestrogen-receptor-positive cancers. The doctors point out that, without additional funding, choices could mean that other cancer patients' treatment could be affected or other patients requiring 'Cinderella' rather than 'sexy' services could be affected.

The final NICE guidance on the use of Herceptin for the treatment of early-stage breast cancer in women with HER-2 positive disease issued in August 2006 recommends that the drug is provided at three-weekly intervals for a year or until disease recurrence, whichever is sooner, after surgery, radiotherapy and chemotherapy, if applicable; heart function should be assessed before treatment starts and repeated quarterly in women whose left ventricular ejection fraction drops 10 per cent; it should be avoided in women with a left ventricular fraction of 55 per cent or less, heart disease generally (including arrhythmias – i.e. irregular heart beat) or poorly controlled high blood pressure.

A new drug called Tykerb is now being billed as better than Herceptin by the media.[54] Like Herceptin, it is claimed to give 'precious extra months of life to those with advanced breast cancer'. It is less expensive than Herceptin, can be taken in tablets, and targets two rather than the one protein targeted by Herceptin, so that it is claimed to slow the progression of both advanced HER-1 and HER-2 receptor-positive types of breast cancer. In one trial, the life of patients on a drug called Xeloda was extended from 20 weeks to 37 weeks when Tykerb was added to the treatment regime. Tykerb is claimed to be particularly valuable in cases where breast cancer has spread to the brain.

Patients should ensure that they are fully aware of all the potential side effects of drug treatments, in discussion with their doctor, before commencing treatment. Some of the known benefits and side effects of these drugs are listed in Table 1.2.

The US Preventive Services Task Force[55] recommends that clinicians should discuss the potential benefits and risks of drugs such as Tamoxifen to reduce the risk of breast cancer in high-risk

Table 1.2: Benefits and adverse side effects of certain cancer drugs

Drug	Benefits	Side effects
Tamoxifen	Helps to prevent the original breast cancer from returning and/or the development of new cancers in the other breast; lowers blood cholesterol; slows bone loss.[56]	In the short term: hot flushes; vaginal discharge, dryness, itching or irritation or rashes; headaches; fatigue; nausea and/or vomiting; irregular menstrual periods (in pre-menopausal women). Over the longer term: endometrial cancer and a more aggressive type of cancer, sarcoma of the womb (the FDA now requires a 'black box' warning about this in the labelling of Tamoxifen[57]); a higher risk of blood clotting and strokes; cataracts and rarely other eye problems including scarring of the cornea and changes in the retina; effects on liver function; foetal damage in pregnant women. In men: headaches, nausea and/or vomiting; skin rash; impotence.[58]
Aromatase inhibitors[59]	One of these drugs has been shown to have similar disease-free survival to Tamoxifen but with fewer side effects in a major trial of post-menopausal women with hormone-sensitive early breast cancer.	Reduced bone density associated with a small increase in fractures and non-specific joint pain.
Herceptin[60]	Modest increases in time to disease progression and in	Ventricular dysfunction and congestive heart failure, particularly when used in

Table 1.2: *Continued*		
Drug	**Benefits**	**Side effects**
	survival time, when used in combination with chemotherapy.	combination with anthrocyclines (e.g. Doxorubicin, Epirubicin) and Cyclophosphamide; hypersensitivity reactions, including anaphylaxis, infusion reactions and acute respiratory distress. Fever and/or chills are common during the first treatment, and other possible side effects include pain, weakness, nausea, vomiting, diarrhoea, headaches, difficulty breathing, and rashes – all generally less severe after the first treatment.[61]

patients, but recommends against the use of such drugs by women at low or average risk.[62]

A general anti-cancer drug called dichloroacetate (DCA) was also suggested to be a 'cheap safe drug that kills most cancers'.[63] It has been used for years to treat some metabolic disorders and has been found to be relatively safe. It has been shown to kill cancer cells in cultures of breast, lung and brain cancer cells while leaving healthy normal cells undamaged, and it has been claimed that it shrinks tumours in laboratory rats. DCA is thought to work because it interferes with the unique way that cancer cells obtain their energy by an anaerobic process called glycolysis, which takes place throughout the main body of the cell rather than in distinct organelles called mitochondria. Apparently DCA reawakened the mitochondria in cancer cells which then withered and died. The next step is to perform clinical trials, but since the drug has no patent and could be made available at a fraction of the cost of most newly developed drugs it is considered unlikely that pharmaceutical companies will pay for these and it may be left to charities or governments to provide funding.

Unfortunately, within weeks of the story being published, blogs and websites were touting DCA as the answer to human cancer and some people began to locate sources of the drug and self-administer it. *New Scientist* has pointed out that this could cause liver or nerve damage and be dangerous if combined with other drugs. Moreover DCA obtained over the internet could be contaminated or incorrectly buffered for acidity, so that people could be caused burns. Moreover, the chances of DCA becoming a wonder drug are not large. Of the many anti-cancer agents that appear promising in animal tests and also pass their initial safety trials in humans, only 1 in 20 is ever approved. *New Scientist* recommends those who have exhausted conventional treatment to enlist in a clinical trial using the matching service run by Cancer Research UK or the American Cancer Society rather than self-medicating dangerously.[64]

A recent study[65] claims that doctors should be wary of starting their patients on newly approved drugs generally, because of the high rate of adverse side effects which can be undetected until late in the post-marketing surveillance period. Also, new anti-cancer drugs reaching the European market between 1995 and 2000 offered few or no substantial advantages over existing preparations, yet cost several times – in one case 350 times – as much.[66] Four of the drugs considered were chemotherapeutic agents for advanced metastatic breast cancer.

Further discussion of the use of drugs in the treatment of cancer is included in the update to Chapter Seven, which considers some of the political aspects of cancer treatment, especially pharmaceuticals.

CHEMOTHERAPY

Chemotherapy refers to the use of drugs prescribed by an oncologist, usually administered through a vein or as tablets, to kill cancer cells. The treatment is especially useful when cancer has spread beyond the breast or ovary. For ovarian cancer the drugs may be injected directly into the abdomen to increase the effect on cancer cells while limiting the effects on other normal tissues in the body.

Chemotherapy is usually given in cycles of treatment followed by a rest period to allow the body to recover. Side effects depend on the type and dose of the drugs used and reflect damage to fast-growing cells in the body other than cancer cells.

Common side effects reflect damage to cells lining the digestive tract, hair follicles or red and white blood cells and platelets, and include:

- loss of appetite, nausea and vomiting
- hair loss
- rashes, especially on the hands or feet
- mouth sores
- increased likelihood of infection, bleeding or bruising
- tiredness

Most side effects go away after the treatment ends, although menopause and infertility are likely to be permanent.

On pages 20 and 50 there is much advice on coping with chemotherapy. One of the commonest observations of patients following the diet in this book and *The Plant Programme* when undergoing chemotherapy is how well they are able to withstand treatment, and this is often noted by their health-care professionals.

Additional advice from the National Cancer Institute (NCI) of America[67] includes telling your doctor about any side effects of the treatment, asking before you take any other medicine or supplement, and talking about your feelings (to counsellor, friends or family). Some further tips for eating if your appetite is badly affected by your treatment include:[68]

- Eating frequent, small meals or snacks whenever you want, perhaps four to six times a day, rather than three regular meals.
- Keeping snacks (such as seeds, nuts, and fresh and dried fruits) within easy reach, so you can eat something when you feel like it.
- If you do not want to eat solid foods, trying to drink soup, juice and herbal or green tea.
- Varying your diet by trying the new foods and recipes from *The Plant Programme* and *Eating for Better Health*.
- When possible, taking a walk before meals to stimulate your appetite.
- Eating with friends or family members, or, when eating alone, listening to the radio or watching TV.

In the case of adjuvant chemotherapy (chemotherapy given after the tumour has been removed by surgery) to treat breast cancer, significant survival benefit has been demonstrated in women younger than 70 years old, especially in younger women.[69] This is thought to reflect their higher incidence of grade III and hormone-receptor-negative cancers. In the case of oestrogen-receptor-positive breast cancer, chemotherapy may cause ovarian failure which might reduce oestrogen levels and hence be protective. Hormone treatments such as Tamoxifen and aromatase inhibitors were found to be as effective as chemotherapy in high-risk women older than 50, except where the tumour is grade III and HER-2 positive and several lymph nodes are affected.

PHOTODYNAMIC THERAPY (PDT)

Photodynamic therapy has recently become available for the treatment of breast cancer. It uses laser or other light sources, combined with a drug that is activated by light, called a photosensitising agent, to destroy cancer cells. The types of drugs used are ones that are preferentially taken up by cancer cells and which, when they are activated by light, destroy cells. Clearly it is essential that the light reaches the cancer cells. Hence PDT was used initially to treat skin cancers or those on or near the lining of internal organs, such as cancers of the lining of the mouth or the lining of the bladder which could be easily reached using lasers or light probes. Fibre-optic cables are now being used to treat solid tumours such as breast cancer. If the cancer is confined to the breast, the aim will generally be to cure the cancer but for advanced metastatic breast or ovarian cancer the aim of PDT is usually to reduce symptoms by shrinking the tumours that can be reached by light. PDT treatment can be given in hospital, although it is more frequently used in outpatient clinics.

The first stage of treatment involves an injection of the drug, or it may be given as a drink or in tablets. The second stage involves shining light directly on to the cancer. This may involve a laser or non-laser light delivered through flexible tubes to ensure that it is taken as close as possible to the cancer. The interval between the two stages of treatment allows the drug to accumulate in cancer cells; this depends on the type of drug used, and can vary from about 90 minutes to four days. Healing after PDT generally causes much less scarring than surgery; the time taken to heal depends on how deeply the light has penetrated, and can be several weeks. The method offers particular hope in the case of breast cancer because of the breast's importance to self-image. It may be particularly helpful in poor areas of the world because of its low cost and simplicity.

The results for PDT treatment of breast cancer suggest that it is important in the control of recurrent breast cancer that has failed conventional therapy.[70] Evidence that partial breast irradiation following lumpectomy is a treatment option for early-stage breast cancer and that PDT has been used successfully to treat breast cancer recurrences in the chest wall with similar histopathological characteristics to the primary tumours suggests that PDT might replace radiotherapy following lumpectomy in appropriate cases. The idea would be to deliver light to the tumour site with a 1–2 cm margin. By using non-ionising radiation, long-term complications, including the risk of radiation-induced cancer, are avoided. A balloon catheter is used to deliver light to the site to be treated, and this is located using image guidance from ultrasound scans to ensure the treatment does not miss. In contrast to the numerous visits required for radiotherapy, PDT can be given in one simple treatment. The main risk is from infection at the catheter site.

Research is taking place to identify the best drug and light dose combinations. Some trials have shown excellent control of tumours with good recovery of normal tissue, while others have resulted in damage to normal tissue, so it is important that such treatment is given only at centres of excellence at this stage in the development of the procedure.

The limited literature on the use of PDT in the treatment of superficial types of breast cancer such as Paget's disease suggests it might be useful for such cancers.[71]

Side effects

Side effects of PDT can include skin damage and eye damage, if suitable precautions are not taken, and other, usually minor, temporary discomforts, depending on the part of the body treated.

Sunburn and eye damage. As with all kinds of treatment, the side effects of PDT vary from person to person. They also reflect the type of photosensitising drug used and the time between giving the drug and applying the light treatment. Although the drugs used are mostly taken up by cancer cells, they can make normal skin cells, including those of the eyes, highly sensitive to light. People undergoing PDT are advised to protect themselves not only from sunlight but also from bright indoor lighting for a period of time, which can be up to weeks depending on the drug used. Patients may be advised to wear shady hats, and to be well covered and wear gloves and dark glasses if they go outdoors. Sunscreens do not help. It is possible to become severely sunburnt even on a dull winter day or through glass if the sun is strong. Indoors, low-level lighting, maximum 60 W bulb, is advised. Opticians' appointments should be avoided and you should avoid any bright light being shone in your eyes. Your doctor or nurse should advise you on a schedule to expose yourself gradually to normal light when it is safe to do so.

Pain. Treatment with PDT can cause pain in the tumour area, which can be treated with painkillers.

Swelling. This can occur with some drugs. It is usually very temporary and can be treated with steroid drugs to reduce inflammation if necessary.

Depending on the part of the body treated, other side effects can include constipation, which can be helped by a naturally high-fibre diet such as the Plant Programme, or nausea, which can be treated with acupuncture and ginger tea.

Further research
Clinical trials are in hand to maximise the effectiveness and minimise the side effects of PDT. Research is being carried out into different photosensitising agents, which may be green (based on chlorophyll) or red (derived from blood), and on laser versus non-laser light delivered by fibre optics. Your doctor can advise you whether PDT is an appropriate treatment in your situation.

A word of warning and some advice
Because PDT treatment is, in principle, relatively simple, carries little risk to those operating the equipment and is enormously profitable, some private clinics are offering it to patients with advanced breast or ovarian cancer. Unfortunately, they may not be using it a way that will help to treat the cancer. For example,

some patients I have talked to have simply been placed in a whole-body red light field after being given the photosensitising drug. This is Cytoluminescent therapy (CLT), not PDT. It is difficult to understand how the light can reach the tumour in this situation, and I can find no evidence of successful outcomes for people with deep solid tumours such as those of the ovary or deep in the breast. Some private clinics even recommend this treatment instead of chemotherapy. When patients come to see me after CLT (often described wrongly as PDT) it is usually because their symptoms have worsened, in some cases quite dramatically, after being treated in this way. Some of the patients had been doing very well, previously, with their NHS treatment combined with my regime. I have become concerned that the drug that is preferentially absorbed by the cancer if not activated by light may actually stimulate the cancer. I emphasise that I have no evidence for this – it is just my instinct as a scientist. My advice is always to discuss any proposed treatment with your NHS doctor and your oncologist, to confirm that the drugs to be used and the way the light will be administered will be safe and effective.

WHAT WOULD I DO DIFFERENTLY?

I think it might be helpful if I revisit the orthodox medical treatment I received in the light of the recent findings described here. First, it is clear that tumours are best treated by breast-conserving methods (lumpectomy followed by radiotherapy) when they are small, relative to breast size, and isolated. I therefore continue to emphasise breast self-awareness and regular examination, including annual examination by a health professional in women over 40. In my case, I would now choose lumpectomy followed by radiotherapy. I remain unconvinced of the value of annual mammography, even for follow-up after breast cancer. In my case it would have been useless, because tumours were returning at intervals of months, and even weeks. I would still choose ovarian ablation, using radiotherapy, rather than surgery, and in preference to taking Tamoxifen or other selective-oestrogen-receptor modulators (SERMs) or aromatase inhibitors – all which generally have to be taken for a period of several years and can have unfortunate side effects. I would certainly not take Herceptin until there is convincing evidence of improved survival.

There are now many more chemotherapy drugs and regimes available than when I was treated. Their use depends on many factors, including the type and stage of breast cancer, the medical history of the patient, and, in some patients, their state of mind. The oncologist prescribing treatment will consider all of these factors and many others – including their own experience of clinical successes and failures – and I would always follow their recommendations. Overall, I would definitely stay with the NHS in the UK or with doctors who work there.

I emphasise that these would be my personal choices and that you must make your own decisions about treatment options based on the advice given to you by the physicians treating you.

COMPLEMENTARY AND ALTERNATIVE TREATMENTS

The international market for complementary and alternative medicine was worth an estimated $21.2 billion in the United States in 1997, more than half of which was paid directly by patients and £450 million in Britain in 1998, with 90 per cent purchased privately.[72]

Complementary medicine is marginalised in many healthcare systems, but calls for an integrated approach, using both conventional and complementary therapies, are growing louder. Basic courses in various complementary therapies are now available in many medical schools in Britain and the United States, albeit on an optional basis.

Complementary therapies are often seen by patients as more 'natural' and having fewer side effects than conventional treatments. The enthusiasm for them shows people's desire to help themselves, as well as their frustration with the limitations of conventional medicine. The holistic and patient-centred approach of many complementary therapists appeals, as does the sense of empowerment gained from their philosophies of care. One of its great benefits is that users appreciate the greater amount of time devoted to the consultation.[73] Here I shall look only at herbal therapies. Some other complementary therapies, including hypnosis, are considered in Chapter Six.

Herbal therapies

Natural substances have been used in Chinese medicine and Indian Ayurvedic medicine for about 3,500 years, and, as the WHO has pointed out, most of the people on Earth still rely on herbal treatments. Until the nineteenth century, drugs in western Europe, too, came mainly from plants – and botanic gardens were established so that Renaissance medical students could be trained to recognise medicinal plants.

The potential benefits of herbal medicines have been reviewed in an article by Ernst,[74] who suggests that a potential benefit could lie in their high acceptance by patients, their efficacy, their relative safety and their relatively low cost. He nevertheless points out how few clinical trials have been carried out, in view of the very large number – several thousand – of different plants being used for medicinal purposes worldwide. He attributes the relative paucity of such trials to the small size of the sector compared with that of pharmaceuticals. He also points out, however, that records of adverse effects associated with herbal medicine from 55 countries are tiny compared with the adverse effects associated with conventional drugs held on the WHO monitoring centre database for the period 1968–1997.

It is worth remembering that the pharmaceutical industry sources several of its chemotherapeutic drugs from plants, including Pacific yew pine needles, Japanese marine algae and the periwinkle or vinca plant.[75] Taxol, extracted from the bark of the Pacific Yew tree, was first used to treat ovarian cancer with some success in the late 1980s and many other drugs are now based on yew.

Aspirin, which originally was a herbal medicine and one of the first to be commonly accepted by orthodox medicine, has been found to reduce the incidence of several types of cancer.[76] This is attributed to its content of salicylic acid.[77] But remember to keep aspirin-based products – and indeed all medicines – away from children.[78]

Astralagus, a traditional Chinese herbal medicine used for 2,000 years or so for the treatment of cancer, has recently been studied extensively in the West. There are reports that cancer patients receiving Astralagus have twice the survival rate of those receiving placebos. Some herbalists in the West routinely provide chemotherapy and radiotherapy patients with Astralagus, and apart from boosting the immune system (which is damaged by such treatments) it is also claimed to stop the spread of cancer cells. The EU is apparently planning to ban it on the pretext that, although it is a herb, it has not been on sale or in use in Europe for 30 years or more.[79] What a waste of time! Such products are easily available over the internet. Vincristine, an alkaloid from the *Vinca rosea* plant, is also thought to be effective against some cancers.

It is generally accepted that herbs can have a palliative effect, and it has been suggested that their action on hormone function is particularly helpful in cases of hormone-dependent cancers such as breast cancer and ovarian cancer. The herbs used to treat breast cancer include blue flag root, burdock root, comfrey root, Echinacea, mistletoe and red clover. Herbs considered effective in the treatment of ovarian cancer include Agnus Castus, red clover, Thuja and liquorice.[80]

Never self-medicate with herbs. If you are going to use any herbal treatment, inform your doctor and ideally ensure that your treatment is supervised by a suitably qualified doctor, for example from the British Society for Integrated Medicine. Check that your therapist has an MB ChB or equivalent basic medical qualification, or that they belong to the National Institute of Medical Herbalists or the British Herbal Medicine Association (or equivalent bodies outside the UK).

I am aware that herbs can come from unreputable sources. A few years ago, an importer in California brought in a Chinese herb mix, which he named PC-SPES. Word-of-mouth reports said that it relieved pain and symptoms of those with prostate cancer, especially advanced cancer. Researchers recently found, however, that apart from the eight natural herbal ingredients, the mix also contained DES (the synthetic oestrogen used in hormone treatment), indomethacin (an anti-inflammatory drug) and warfarin (an anticoagulant). Apparently, pre-1999, the Chinese had been adding the three compounds to the formula before shipment, and latterly just the warfarin. Doctors had been using PC-SPES with great success but noticed side effects like breast enlargement (typical of taking DES). When some people had blood clots and bleeding problems, investigations started. One wonders why they can't ask the Chinese to provide pure PC-SPES and test whether it works without the addition of Western drugs.

Eye of newt and toe of frog?

There is good reason to think that herbal therapies might be helpful for cancer, not least because several chemotherapy treatments are derived from them, but for many other alternative treatments there is little evidence that they improve outcomes and in some cases such as shark-fin extract their production can involve cruelty. As a scientist, I fail to follow the logic that goes something like this: sharks don't suffer much from cancer, they are cartlilagenous fish therefore if we eat their cartilage it will help treat cancer. I suspect that the real reason sharks don't get cancer is similar to the reason that gorillas in the wild do not get much cancer: because they eat the food they have evolved to eat in environments relatively free from man-made chemicals.

I am also concerned about the use of pancreatic enzymes from young livestock to treat cancer. This dates back to the theory that malignant cancers are false placentas, as first proposed by Scottish embryologist John Beard in 1902. The placenta stops growing on day 56 of human pregnancies, at the same time the pancreas starts to function in the foetus. Beard surmised that the same substances that stopped the growth of the placenta would stop cancer cells growing. He extracted juices from young animals and injected them into cancers and reported that they shrank in animals and humans, but his findings were never duplicated. It has recently been suggested that this is because other experimenters used enzymes that had lost their effectiveness. The ideas are being re-examined by Dr Gonzalez in the USA, according to the theory that cancer reflects the pancreas's inability to produce trypsin, in the same way that diabetes reflects its failure to produce insulin. The enzymes concerned in the enzyme theory of cancer, trypsin and its precursor chymtrypsin, still cannot be synthesised and must be extracted from young livestock. I understand that these enzymes digest protein in the intestines, but I fail to see how such large molecules could enter the bloodstream and tissues and kill cancer cells. I would prefer to eat pineapple, which contains the protein-digesting substance bromelain, on which the first biological washing powders were based, or papaya, which contains the protein-digesting enzyme papain. I am also concerned that pancreatic enzyme might contain growth factors, although I can find no analysis of it, and that some of it is prescribed in a lactose (milk sugar) base.

I also have serious concerns about the use of high concentrations of vitamin C. This treatment derives from the findings of Linus Pauling, winner of the Nobel prize for chemistry, when he developed prostate cancer. He learned that male gorillas in the wild did not suffer from the disease and wisely looked at their diet. Being a chemist, it seems he was looking for the chemical that was protecting the gorillas and calculated that they were having more than 10 times as much vitamin C as there is in a typical Western diet – but he missed the main point that the gorillas were living on a vegan diet packed with fresh fruit and vegetables (see Chapter Six, Lifestyle Factor 1, or www.cancer-supportinternational.com for further evidence against taking man-made vitamins, minerals and extracts). Likewise, apricot kernels which contain vitamin B17, laetrile, were recommended by those studying the Hunza people in Asia who suffer little cancer or other degenerative disease. Again, the answer is most likely to be their vegan diet. Professor Colin Campbell, perhaps the world's greatest ever nutritional scientist describes laetrile as 'a prime example of a health scam' and records that animal studies have repeatedly shown that it had no effect on tumours.[81] Personally, I can see no sense in the use of coffee enemas or colonic irrigation. If the diet is good, elimination of faeces will remove toxins naturally.

Personally, I would always use conventional medical treatment from the NHS combined with the Plant Programme diet and lifestyle, which is natural and healthy and involves no animal suffering. One of the things that occurs to me is that pharmaceutical companies are always quick to move treatments from alternative to mainstream medicine where they can profit by doing so. For example, they have developed several natural plant alkaloids from yew that are used as powerful chemotherapy agents, such as Taxol. There are only two reasons that they have not done so for the therapies described in this section, all of which are amenable to double-blind randomised clinical trials: either they cannot make a profit from them, and they would damage sales of other more profitable anti-cancer treatments – or the treatments do not work. Given the poor outcomes of trials I suspect the latter.

There are many alternative and complementary treatments, from acupuncture to reiki and reflexology, which can help cancer patients a great deal. Moreover, the best alternative and complementary therapists will give you that most precious thing, their time. Just talking to people like Jan de Vries is, I am sure, healing. If your therapist does not help to comfort and support you in this way find a different therapist! At all costs, avoid frenetic people who do not give you time, cannot explain treatments simply and clearly, and push their own pills and potions that they sell at much higher prices than elsewhere.

A FINAL QUOTE
The biomedical community needs to recognise and advocate approaches to prevent cancer with the same enthusiasm that it currently directs towards treating it.

Peter Greenwald,
Division of Cancer Prevention, National Cancer Institute,
National Institutes of Health, Bethesda, Maryland, USA.[82]

Update to Chapter 2. Stem Cells Behaving Badly

It has been suggested recently that tumours arise from specialised cells called cancer stem cells, which have the properties of normal stem cells, particularly the ability to self-renew and differentiate into multiple cell types. This theory explains the genetic instability of cancer which makes it difficult to treat using conventional medicine alone. There are now considered to be three main stages in the development of cancer: initiation, when a cell becomes pre-cancerous because of damage to DNA, followed by promotion, when the initiated cell develops into a population of pre-cancerous cells, and, thirdly, the progression stage. Two groups of powerful biochemicals – hormones and growth factors – are important in regulating growth and differentiation in normal cells, but disturbance of their activity and expression can promote cancer and help it to proliferate.

The word cancer comes from the Greek word 'karkinos', literally meaning 'crab', a word that was first used to describe the disease by Hippocrates. The name is particularly unfortunate, conjuring up, as it does, visions of a creature that won't let go. We shall learn here more evidence that this image is totally wrong and that cancer cells are just some of our normal cells that are behaving badly.

NEW THEORIES FROM OLD

Many of our tissues contain stem cells that help regeneration if tissue is damaged. For example, the hippocampus in the brain, which is responsible for memory, can shrink in people under chronic stress or suffering from severe depression, but it can regenerate when things improve because it contains a large number of stem cells. Unlike normal cells, these cells have the ability to renew themselves and to change into many other cell types. (It is these properties in embryonic stem cells that are under study by scientists all around the world as a means of trying to regenerate damaged tissue: for example, spinal nervous tissue in people paralysed as a result of a serious accident.)

Until recently, most scientists thought that the cells in a cancer were descended from a common ancestral cell, which, until that point, had been a fairly normal cell in the breast or ovaries, for example, and which at some point in time – probably years before any tumour was detected – initiated a programme of inappropriate reproduction. Recently, other scientists have suggested that tumours arise from more specialised cells called cancer stem cells, which have the properties of normal stem cells, particularly the ability to self-renew and differentiate into multiple cell types. These scientists suggest that a distinct sub-population of such cells persists in tumours; and that it is these that cause the cancer to recur and metastasise.[1] Analysis of the cellular origins of cancers of different organs supports this theory because it indicated that the most likely ancestral cell of all the tumours studied was, in each case, a stem cell required for normal tissue renewal. Opponents of the theory do not deny the existence of cancer stem cells. Rather, they suggest that most cells in a tumour have stem-cell properties. The theory explains the genetic instability of cancer cells – which is why they can quickly become resistant to many types of conventional treatment.

As long ago as the mid-19th century, pathologists noted the similarity between embryonic tissue and cancer, and suggested that tumours arise from embryo-like cells. The idea that adult tissues contain embryonic remnants which generally lie dormant but could be activated to become cancer was formalised in 1874 as 'the embryonic rest theory of cancer'. The idea that cancers arise from tissue stem cells in adults is simply a modern version of a theory first proposed more than 130 years ago!

The cancer-stem-cell theory has particular importance when we consider the role of growth factors in promoting cancer, because the fate of normal stem cells (i.e. what type of cells they will finally turn into: for example, breast or ovarian cells or skin cells) depends on cellular signals, especially those from growth factors. It now seems likely that growth factors control what happens to all stem cells, including cancer stem cells. Indeed, cell-signalling pathways are now thought to be the same in embryonic cells and cancer cells.[2] The role of growth factors thus becomes crucial in the development of cancer as a disease. This is discussed further below.

DAMAGED GENES

All in the genes?

Following the Human Genome Project, we have been encouraged to believe that we are simply a bag of genes in a hermetically sealed bag and that developing a disease can be the result of a faulty gene. This simplistic model totally fails to take account of our interface with our environment – such as exposure to toxic chemicals like those in tobacco smoke, which are known to trigger lung cancer. As we shall see, damage to the DNA, the material that makes up our genes, is critical to the initiation of cancer,[3] but both this damage and the promotion and progression of breast and ovarian cancer are critically linked to factors in our lifestyle and environment. There are various repair mechanisms, and it is only when damage persists that cancer becomes established as a disease.

The progression of cancers from an individual damaged cell, now thought to be a stem cell by some scientists, to a cluster of damaged cells, then to non-aggressive cancer and finally to highly aggressive cancer is generally considered to result from the continued accumulation of mutations. Cells from advanced cancer typically have many genetic changes and chromosome rearrangements, although these are considered to be the result rather than the cause of malignancy. The number of mutations required for the development of cancer varies with the cancer type.

Since the first edition of this book, science has come to understand more about the grow, don't-grow and fix-it genes, which, when they malfunction, generate cancer. The **grow genes, or proto-oncogenes**, code for normal growth proteins in the cells that relay signals to the nucleus (the control centre of the cell), stimulating growth in response to proteins and other substances in the intracellular fluid. The signalling process involves a series of steps which begin at the cell membrane, then involve a host of intermediary proteins in the cell cytoplasm, and end with the activation of factors in the cell nucleus which help to move it through its cycle of growth and replication (Figure 2.1). The abnormal degree of proliferation in cancer-cell populations generally results from over-activity in one or more of these steps.[4] Interestingly, one of the diagrams in Woolf's book, *Pathology, basic and systemic*, a basic text for medical students in the UK in illustrating how cancer cells behave, shows a marked increase in growth factors in the intercellular fluid.

The activation of a proto-oncogene to become an oncogene can occur in several ways: by altering DNA at a particular point on the chromosome, by rearranging chromosomes, by increasing the numbers of normal proto-oncogenes in a cell, or by viral insertion.[5] There are several 'grow' genes which, when damaged, become oncogenes involved in breast and ovarian cancer. One of them, ERBB2, codes for an epidermal-growth-factor-like protein; this oncogene is involved in ovarian and other cancers. Others involved in breast cancer include: FGF3, which codes for fibroblast growth factor; MYC, which codes for a factor involved in activating growth-promotion in the cell nucleus and is also involved in ovarian and colon cancer; and ROS1, which codes for insulin-receptor-like proteins in the cell membrane. The location of proto-oncogenes at particular sites on particular chromosomes is now well documented as a result of the Human Genome Project.

In normal cells, the **don't-grow, or tumour-suppressor, genes** suppress the uncontrolled proliferation of cancer cells, but they may fail to do so if they are altered or mutated. BRCA-1 and BRCA-2 are important examples of tumour-suppressor genes that, when mutated, increase the risk of breast and ovarian cancers. Since the first edition of this book, much more has become known about the behaviour of the BRCA genes. More than 2,000 papers have been published in peer-reviewed journals on the BRCA-1 gene alone. From this work, scientists have learnt that this gene in its normal, unmutated form, helps to guard DNA against damage from free radicals, radiation and chemicals. The BRCA-1 protein seems to act like a plumber, fixing breaks in the genome as they occur. The BRCA-1 protein physically binds to damaged DNA and then recruits other molecules to assemble the equivalent of a DNA repair kit. Scientists have further demonstrated that the absence of the BRCA-1 protein does not directly cause cancer but makes cells more susceptible to changes that can lead to cancer.[6,7,8] It has been suggested that the BRCA-1 protein works via the extracellular fluid, from where it interacts with surrounding cells to keep them cancer-free.[9]

More than 100 alterations have been identified in each of the two BRCA genes in families with hereditary breast cancer. There is also evidence of a link to ethnicity. In particular, three alterations of the genes, initially identified in Ashkenazi Jewish

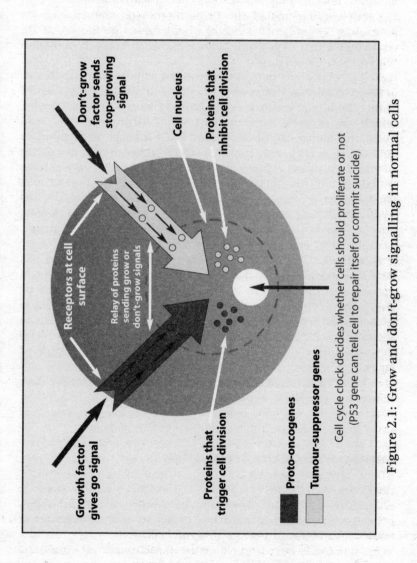

Figure 2.1: Grow and don't-grow signalling in normal cells

families, were later found in an unusually high percentage of the general Jewish population.[10,11] The researchers found that women carrying one of the three alterations studied had, on average, a 56 per cent chance of breast cancer by the age of 70, compared with a 13 per cent chance in the general US population without the altered gene.

The p53 gene, although often grouped with tumour-suppressor genes, actually operates within the cell nucleus, or control centre, by inducing repair or apoptosis. Damage to the p53 gene, which can produce a protein capable of halting the whole cell cycle and hence cell division until DNA damage is repaired or cell-suicide is triggered, continues to be regarded as a key factor in human cancers. More than half of all human cancers have mutations in the p53 gene and hence no functioning p53 (messenger) protein. It has been suggested that a virus called SV40, which knocks out the p53 gene, was a contaminant in polio vaccines administered in the USA and possibly other countries between 1955 and 1963.[12]

New gene therapies that use high concentrations of the p53 gene are becoming available. These carry the gene in a virus and are injected directly into solid tumours, often accompanied by chemotherapy. The side effects from this therapy are claimed to be minimal. These treatments have been tried in America to treat advanced breast cancer and in China to treat several different types of cancer with, it is claimed, a high degree of success. The drug used in China, marketed as Gendicine, was developed by Chinese scientists and is much less expensive than many of the latest drug treatments available in the West. Unfortunately, not all cancers have defective p53 genes, and even in those that do the treatment sometimes fails.

FROM DNA DAMAGE TO DISEASE

There are now considered to be three main stages in the development of cancer (Figure 2.2). The *initiation* stage is characterised by the conversion of a normal cell to a pre-cancerous condition in response to agents that damage DNA. Some cancers are caused by inherited cells which have already been damaged, but in most cases the damage is caused by something in our lifestyle or environment.

The initiation stage is followed by the *promotion* stage, in which the initiated cell is transformed into a population of pre-

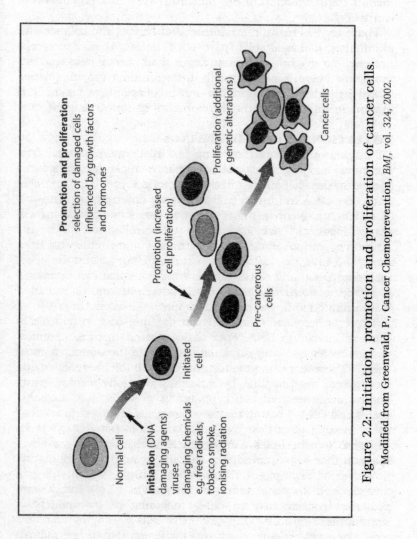

Figure 2.2: Initiation, promotion and proliferation of cancer cells.
Modified from Greenwald, P., Cancer Chemoprevention, *BMJ*, vol. 324, 2002.

The labels within the figure read:

Normal cell

Initiation (DNA damaging agents) viruses damaging chemicals e.g. free radicals, tobacco smoke, ionising radiation

Initiated cell

Promotion and proliferation selection of damaged cells influenced by growth factors and hormones

Promotion (increased cell proliferation)

Pre-cancerous cells

Proliferation (additional genetic alterations)

Cancer cells

cancerous cells as a result of further DNA damage and cell proliferation. Thirdly, there is the *progression* stage, involving the further transformation of pre-cancerous cells to a population of cancer cells.[13]

The body has many mechanisms and checks and balances for eliminating damaged cells (page 58). The fact that cancer cells not only survive but proliferate faster than normal cells suggests that some agent is preferentially fostering their growth relative to normal cells. The promotion and progression stages are thus extremely important in the development of cancer as a disease.

INITIATION OR BAD BEGINNINGS

Of the various factors that damage DNA, environmental contaminants and chemicals such as tobacco smoke are considered further in the chapter on Lifestyle Factors. Viruses, too, are able to change DNA in human cells, by many different mechanisms. They can act to convert normal 'grow' genes into cancer-growth genes (oncogenes), which stimulate uncontrolled cell growth and division by various means. Ionising radiation, including that from medical X-rays, can change the nature of chemicals in the body, including DNA, and cause genetic mutations that can be passed to offspring. Some of the principal sources of ionising radiation were mentioned in the previous chapter, 'Keeping Abreast'.

There is increasing emphasis on the role of free radicals in causing damage to DNA. Free radicals are defined as chemical species that possess an unpaired electron in the outer (valence) shell.[14] This means, in practice, that they are highly reactive and have a very short half-life, because they generally react with any nearby available molecules, including proteins, fats, carbohydrates and DNA. They attack the nearest stable molecule to 'steal' their missing electrons. The attacked molecule that loses its electron then becomes a free radical itself, beginning a chain reaction that, once started, can cascade, resulting in cell disruption. A good example of a free radical is Cu^{2+}, which will grab any electron it can, in order to become Cu^+. Free radicals are produced continuously in cells, including as by-products of normal metabolism.[15]

The best-known defence against the generation of free radicals and the damage that they cause is the activity of antioxidants. These are discussed further in Chapter Five, where we examine the role of diet in the prevention of cancer.

It is worth re-emphasising that, of the tens of thousands of genes in the normal cell, the only genes that are altered in cancer cells are those that control growth, differentiation and proliferation. What we are looking for, therefore, are factors that preferentially promote the growth of cancer cells, with their damaged genes, so that we can eliminate such factors from our lives.

PROMOTION AND PROGRESSION OF CANCER, OR SURVIVAL OF THE UNFIT

Many scientists now think that it is the promotion stage that is crucial to whether cancer develops as a disease or not. I have previously likened the promotion stage in the development of cancer to providing oxygen to a spark, while Professor T. Colin Campbell likens it to watering and fertilising (initiated) cancer seeds.

Since reliable cancer registers began to be kept in the 1950s and 1960s, the age-standardised incidence of hormone-dependent cancers (breast, ovarian, endometrial (lining of the womb), prostate and testicular) have increased in most industrialised countries, over and above that which can be attributed to the introduction of screening.

There is much compelling evidence of links between hormones and the progression of hormone-dependent cancers. For example, some breast cancers may regress following hormone-deprivation therapy, including removal or ablation of the ovaries, or as a result of the use of anti-oestrogens[16] and aromatase inhibitors[17] in post-menopausal women. Conversely, there is evidence that administration of steroid hormones increases the growth of breast tumours.[18,19] Although several classes of steroid have been shown to influence the growth of breast-cancer cells under experimental conditions,[20] oestrogen seems to be the most important (pages 106–110). As discussed in Chapter One, many drug treatments for breast cancer are aimed at reducing tumour levels of oestrogen.[21] The main benefits of such therapy are for oestrogen-receptor-positive cancers.

More recent work has identified the importance of growth factors such as IGF-I and EGF in promoting breast and prostate cancer. One of the methods by which Tamoxifen is thought to work is by preventing IGF-I becoming attached to its receptor, while Herceptin is aimed at preventing the over-expression of the EGF receptor protein.

The evidence that the two groups of biochemically powerful chemicals, hormones and growth factors, promote and cause breast and ovarian cancer to proliferate is considered further below (*see* pp. 315–325).

CHEMICAL MESSENGERS

As discussed above, hormones are secreted in special endocrine glands which contain a rich network of blood capillaries through which the hormones are released into the bloodstream. They circulate in the blood, usually in tiny amounts, until they interact with the target cell by way of highly specific receptors, located either on the cell surface or within the cell cytoplasm. This docking activates a series of intracellular reactions, including gene activation. By this means, hormones and growth factors enable the organism to exert control over a host of metabolic functions and to alter these functions in response to changes in conditions. The sex hormone oestrogen, for example, is involved in the onset of puberty and menopause, ovulation, menstruation, pregnancy, birth and milk production.

Hormones can be divided into two classes, peptides (proteins), which interact with receptors on cell membranes, and steroids (fatty or fat soluble substances), which also interact with receptors but within the cell cytoplasm, through which they can directly affect the proteins released from a large number of target genes.

There is increasing concern now about man-made chemicals which can disrupt our hormone system, in some cases because of their hormone-like behaviour. The most important for breast cancer and perhaps ovarian cancer are thought to be oestrogenic substances (xeno-oestrogens, meaning stranger oestrogens). They include pharmaceutical products such as the female contraceptive pill and hormone replacement therapy as well as some pesticides, plasticisers, fragrances, detergents and chemicals derived from them as a result of their breakdown in the body or the environment.

The second class of chemical messengers – growth factors – also interact with cells by way of specific receptors and are also strongly implicated in the promotion of breast and prostate cancer.[22] They are generally less well understood – even by some medical professionals.

The discovery of growth factors dates back to the early 1950s, when the Italian biochemist and 1986 Nobel laureate, Rita

Levi-Montalcini, was working with tissue cultures of peripheral nerve cells. She found that, while the cultures would maintain themselves in a medium containing the right combination of nutrients, they did not grow much. However, when they were supplied with an extract derived from mouse salivary glands, they grew dramatically, extending towards the highest concentration of the extract. The substance was finally purified and characterised as a low-molecular-weight protein with chemical properties similar to that of insulin, which was called nerve-growth factor (NGF). NGF is now known to be just one of a large number of such small protein growth factors, derived from a variety of tissues and generally named according to the tissue from which they have been purified rather than that at which they act. They include Brain-Derived Neurotrophic Factor (BDNF),[23] as well as IGF-I and IGF-II. The authoritative textbook, *Biochemistry* by Donald and Judith Voet,[24] states that EGF is a hormonally active polypeptide that stimulates cell proliferation.

There is no doubt that an enormous amount of scientific effort continues to be spent on researching growth factors such as IGF-I and IGF-II to prevent them stimulating the growth and proliferation of breast (and other) cancer cells. There are now major text books aimed at cancer scientists and doctors such as the reference book entitled *Growth Factors and Their Receptors in Cancer Metastasis*,[25] which aims to provide state-of-the-art knowledge of the role of growth factors and their receptors in cancer metastasis. The importance of growth factors in promoting breast cancer is no longer in dispute.

In a review of more than 300 publications on the role of insulin-like growth factors in cancer progression, Professor Yu of Yale University and his colleague Professor Rohan stated that the IGFs play a pivotal role in regulating cell proliferation, differentiation and apoptosis.[26] Their binding proteins can inhibit or enhance the actions of the IGFs. They reported that the evidence consistently shows that IGFs exert strong mitogenic effects on cancer cells and prevent their apoptosis. They also act together with other growth factors and steroid hormones in promoting cancer growth. According to Yu and Rohan, high circulating levels of growth factors and low levels of one of the binding proteins are associated with increased risk of several common cancers, including those of the breast, prostate, colorectum and lung.

Levels of IGFs and their binding proteins show little variation with gender, but vary substantially with age. Serum IGF-I and IGF-II levels increase until puberty. IGF-I levels then decline with age, while IGF-II levels remain stable.[27] This evidence suggests that the IGFs instruct cells to proliferate markedly during puberty, but of course such instructions are inappropriate later in life. Such a model would explain how risk of breast and prostate cancer increases with increasing age in those consuming diets high in IGFs.

Many doctors seem to assume that the problem arises from abnormal over-production of growth factors such as the IGFs[28] or their receptors in the body; they do not seem to be aware that dietary factors, especially the consumption of certain types of animal produce, can increase circulating levels of the hormones and growth factors that have receptors in breast and prostate tissue. Yu and Rohan, following their recent comprehensive literature review of the actions of IGF-I and all the evidence incriminating elevated circulating levels of this growth factor with excess risks of breast, prostate and other cancers, emphasise 'the feasibility and validity of implementing dietary interventions to reduce IGF levels with the goal of preventing cancer'.[29] They find that nutritional status is critical to circulating levels of IGFs and that studies of normal adults demonstrate that, as protein levels in the diet increase, so do those of circulating IGF-I. A 50 per cent reduction in calorie intake or a 30 per cent reduction in protein intake significantly reduces levels of circulating IGF-I. Professor Epstein of Illinois University praises the work of Yu and Rohan in showing that circulating levels of IGF-I increase the risk of breast, prostate and other cancers; but he is critical of their apparent lack of awareness of the significance of milk – especially milk that is treated with rBGH – as a source of IGF-I.[30]

We have always used euphemisms for cancer: it is now 'neoplasms', but in my younger days it was 'growths' – and what a clue that was!

Additional information on the role of diet, including limiting exposure to foods with high levels of hormones and/or growth factors likely to promote breast- or prostate-cancer cells, is considered in the update to Chapters Four and Five, together with factors protective against the diseases from studies into the chemoprevention of cancer. Reducing risks from exposure to hormone-disrupting chemicals is considered further in the update to Chapter Six on lifestyle factors.

CHAPTER 2 IN A NUTSHELL

- The word cancer, meaning 'crab', is particularly unfortunate, conjuring up, as it does, visions of a creature that won't let go. This image is totally wrong; cancer cells are just some of our normal cells that are behaving badly.

- Following the Human Genome Project, we have been encouraged to believe that we are simply a bag of genes in a hermetically sealed bag and that developing a disease can be the result of a faulty gene in a cell. The overwhelming majority of cases of breast and ovarian cancer, however, are critically linked to factors in our lifestyle and environment.

- There are now considered to be three main stages in the development of cancer. The *initiation* stage is characterised by the conversion of a normal stem cell to a pre-cancerous condition in response to agents such as chemicals that damage the DNA in our genes. In the *promotion* stage, the initiated cell is transformed into a population of pre-cancerous cells. In the third stage, the *progression* stage, these cells are transformed into a population of cancer cells.

- The body has many mechanisms and checks and balances for eliminating damaged cells The fact that cancer cells not only survive but proliferate faster than normal cells suggests that some agent is preferentially fostering their growth relative to normal cells. The promotion and progression stages are thus extremely important. Many scientists now think that it is the promotion stage that is crucial to whether cancer develops as a disease or not. I have previously likened this stage of cancer to a spark (an initiated cancer cell) in an atmosphere of oxygen.

- There is much compelling evidence of links between hormones and the promotion and proliferation of hormone-dependent cancers such as breast cancer and ovarian cancer.

- Although several classes of steroid have been shown to influence the growth of breast-cancer, oestrogen seems to be the most important. More recently, particular growth factors, such as IGF-I and EGF, have been shown to be important in promoting breast cancer.

- High circulating levels of growth factors such as IGF-I are associated with increased risk of cancer – not only breast cancer but several other common cancers too, including those of the prostate and lung, and colorectal cancer.
- Scientists have recently suggested that tumours arise from specialised cells called cancer stem cells. These cells have the properties of normal stem cells, particularly the ability to self-renew and to differentiate into different cell types. This theory explains the genetic instability of cancer cells – and why they can quickly become resistant to many types of conventional treatment.
- The cancer-stem-cell theory means that the role of growth factors in promoting cancer is extremely important, because the fate of normal stem cells (i.e. what type of cells they will finally turn into: for example, breast or ovarian cells, or skin cells) depends on cellular signals, especially those from growth factors.
- It thus seems likely that it is steroid hormones such as oestrogen and growth factors such as IGF-I that provide 'the oxygen' in which initiated breast cancer and probably ovarian cancer cells are promoted and can proliferate faster than normal cells, thus giving rise to cancer as a disease.
- In Chapters Four, Five and Six of this book we give you the latest information from the scientific literature on how to reduce your levels of oestrogen, other steroid hormones and growth factors to safe levels – levels which will not help cancer to develop and spread in the body.

Update to Chapter 3. Of Strawberries, Lemons and Risk

This chapter compares recent information on the incidence, death rates and survival for breast and ovarian cancer between low-risk oriental and high-risk Western countries. Such comparisons, together with migration studies, continue to support the evidence that breast cancer, and ovarian cancer, too, are closely associated with the Western diet and lifestyle. Despite this association, the conventional medical advice for breast cancer continues to be based on the same old risk factors such as age, gender, age of onset of puberty and menopause, and alcohol consumption; these, and the conventional risk factors for ovarian cancer, are reviewed in the light of recent scientific studies. Unfortunately, most epidemiological studies continue to be carried out within countries rather than between countries, although the latter comparison shows much more significant differences.

THE THIRD STRAWBERRY RULES

In the first edition of this book I used the idea of a slot machine and its combination of strawberries and lemons to communicate the idea that breast cancer is what scientists call a multifactorial disease. I explained that, while there is little that we can do about some of the risk factors – or strawberries – such as our genes, eliminating some controllable risks, and changing at least one strawberry to a lemon, can prevent breast cancer. Indeed, even when we have breast or ovarian cancer, we can put the disease into remission by eliminating one of the strawberries – as I have done for the last 14 years. I went on to try to identify the strawberries or risks we can control, and this led me to compare rates of breast cancer in China with those in the West. What, if anything, has changed in the rates of breast cancer between the West and oriental countries over the past seven years, and what do the data on ovarian cancer say?

BREAST CANCER

Incidence rates

The crude background rate for breast cancer in China remains at about 1 in 100,000 women.[1]

The latest age-standardised rates (ASR) of the incidence of breast cancer in females in China and other oriental countries, with their distinctive diets and lifestyles, are compared with the equivalent rates in a range of Western countries in Table 3.1.* The countries presented are all countries I have worked in, and so I have been able to discuss the data with local doctors. Some doctors in China, for example, hardly remembered treating a case of breast cancer in their entire careers (though this is changing now, as discussed below). I have also selected the countries where data are available for migrant communities (e.g. Chinese or Japanese migrants to America or Australia). These studies show that within a generation or so such communities have acquired the same rates of breast cancer as their host populations – indicating the importance of lifestyle rather than genes as the key factor: the strawberry to be eliminated.

Table 3.1: Age-standardised rates of incidence of breast cancer per 100,000 females for the years 2000 and 2002

	2000	2002
China	16.4	18.7
China Hong Kong	34.4	no longer available
Japan	31.4	32.7
Thailand	15.9	16.6
South Korea	12.5	20.8
New Zealand	82.6	91.9
Australia	82.7	83.2
Canada	81.8	84.3
UK	74.9	87.2
USA	91.4	101.1
Iceland	—	90.0

Data from WHO International Agency for Research on Cancer (IARC)[2]

---

* It is not possible to compare this updated table directly with the earlier version on page 75, because the groupings and methods of age standardisation have been changed by the WHO IARC. Also data for Hong Kong are now included with those of mainland China.

Rising incidence rates of breast cancer

The incidence of breast cancer has been increasing in Western countries for many years. In Britain the age-standardised incidence had increased from 74 per 100,000 women in 1975 to 120 in 2003, a rise of more than 80 per cent in just under 30 years.

Comparison of the most recent data (2002) with those for 2000 (Table 3.1) shows an increase in oriental countries, as they become increasingly westernised, as well as in Western industrialised countries. Rates of breast cancer have increased most dramatically however in the latter, especially in New Zealand, the UK and USA.

The data still clearly show that the incidence rates are much higher in Western countries than in oriental countries. Even Cancer Research UK now includes a sentence that states that breast cancer incidence rates are highest in the developed world and lowest in Africa and Asia, although this is not discussed further.

In the USA, breast cancer is now the most frequently diagnosed cancer in women (more than 30 per cent of all cancers diagnosed there), accounting for 175,000 new cases; it has been estimated that there would be 212,920 new cases in women in 2006. A woman's lifetime risk of developing breast cancer in the USA is now estimated at 1 in 8, moving towards 1 in 7. There were 1,720 new cases of male breast cancer in 2006, and 460 deaths.[3]

In the UK the lifetime risk of breast cancer has risen from 1 in 10 women when I wrote the first edition of this book in 2000 to 1 in 9 women by 2003. The greatest rate of increase in incidence has been in women approaching menopause.[4]

Why is this happening to us?

The continued rise in the incidence of breast cancer cannot be genetic. Genes do not change as quickly as that. Moreover, since the data are adjusted for age the increased rate does not indicate an aging population. Neither can it be attributed to improved screening. In the UK, for example, the trend of increasing incidence predates mass screening and continues today almost 20 years after it was first introduced. The recent rise has been attributed to our increasing wealth and high (material) standard of living by some sources, but countries such as Japan and South Korea have had similar or greater wealth and living standards for decades. The evidence continues to indicate strongly that, as with many cancers, it is an environmental or lifestyle factor which is promoting the diseases in the West and that that factor is now increasingly important in oriental countries. Anyone who has visited or worked in Japan or Korea will know that they live in similar houses, have similar family sizes, dress in similar clothes, wear similar make-up, drive similar cars and watch similar televisions to those of us who live in the West. The only thing that until recently was obviously different was their diet, which was based on rice, soya and vegetables rather than meat and dairy.

Of the oriental countries, the greatest increase in breast-cancer incidence has been in South Korea (Table 3.1). The last time I was there, in 2002, I had to plead for my meal (which consisted of an American-style slab of grilled beef that was raw on the inside and burnt on the outside, followed by cheesecake smothered with cream and ice cream) to be changed to a traditional Korean meal with lots of vegetables and rice. There was much more Western food around generally, and I could not help noticing how young Korean women who used to have neat elegant figures seemed to be taking on a more blousy Western look. (The same is increasingly true of China.) The rising breast cancer incidence rate in Korea most likely reflects the increasing westernisation of their diet.

Still 'Rich Woman's Disease'?

The disease still justifies its Chinese nickname of 'Rich Woman's disease'. The most rapid increase in countries such as Korea is in the richer urban areas that are the most westernised, rather than in poorer, rural areas.

In Europe, the highest incidence rates are in the richest countries in the north and west especially the Netherlands, Denmark, Belgium, France and Sweden, with lower rates in the south and east.

Incidence continues to vary within countries, with the highest socio-economic groups having the highest breast-cancer rates. In the UK, the incidence is 115 per 100,000 women in the highest socio-economic group and 97.3 in the most deprived group. There continues to be a well-defined north–south gradient in England, from low risk in the north to high risk in the south,[5] but now only in older, post-menopausal women. The rates among younger women in northern England who have embraced a similar lifestyle to those in the south are now similarly high.[6]

Migration studies

Migration studies such as those published by Kolonel into cancer incidence in different ethnic populations of first- and second-generation migrants to Hawaii[7] add considerable weight to the evidence of earlier migration studies (*see* pp. 76–77) that most cancers are environmentally determined. Professor Kolonel's research is now focusing on the interaction of diet with genetic susceptibility in determining cancer risk because the potential for understanding cancer through studies of ethnic and migrant populations has, he states, never been greater.[8]

Death rates and survival

The death rate (Figure 3.1) still shows the same two distinct groupings: (1) Western industrialised countries, such as Germany, the UK and the USA, with high mortality rates, and (2) oriental countries, such as Thailand and China, with low rates. The death rate in Japan is rising, however, while that in some Western countries, including the USA and UK, is falling.

In the USA, there were 43,300 deaths from breast cancer in 1999.[9] This was predicted to fall further to 40,970 women by 2006.[10] Breast-cancer death rates in the UK have also fallen markedly in recent years, with a decrease of 31 per cent since 1989. In the UK, breast cancer was the most common cause of death from cancer in women until 1999, when it was overtaken by lung cancer, which, although less common, is more deadly. The decline in death rates from breast cancer has been variously attributed to the introduction of screening, increasing specialisation of care and improved drugs and treatments.

It is important to understand that survival rates for cancer cannot be regarded as 'cure' rates. They represent the number of years that the disease is in remission, and in this respect the situation has improved dramatically. The five-year survival rate for breast cancer improved from 52 per cent for women diagnosed in England and Wales before 1975 to 80 per cent in those diagnosed after 2001. The estimated 20-year survival rate has also improved, from 44 per cent in the early 1990s to 64 per cent today.

Figure 3.1: Breast-cancer mortality (annual, per 100,000), age-standardised rates (Worldwide), 1987 to 2002, by country

Data from WHO/IARC Worldwide Cancer Mortality Statistics.[11]

Because the incidence of breast cancer continues to rise and survival rates have improved, many women are alive having had the disease. The most recent estimate suggests that around 172,000 women are alive in the UK having had breast cancer.

DIFFERENT KINDS OF RISK FACTORS: THE STRAWBERRIES TO TAKE OUT

A risk factor is something that increases your chance of suffering from cancer. Different cancers have different risk factors. For example, smoking is well known to be a risk factor for cancers of the lung, mouth, larynx, bladder and kidney.

However, having a risk factor, or even several risk factors, does not mean that you will automatically develop cancer. Some women who have one or more breast-cancer risk factors, such as a mutated BRCA-1 or BRCA-2 gene, never develop the disease, while many women with breast cancer have none of the conventional risk factors.

There are three main kinds of risk factors. Some, like age or race, clearly cannot be changed. Some risk factors operating through the environment, like man-made chemicals, can be dealt with only at the population level – and new legislation to control the use of harmful chemicals known as REACH (Registration, Evaluation and Authorisation of Chemicals) is to be introduced in the European Union in July 2007. The third type is related to personal diet and lifestyle choices and can be changed. These are known as avoidable risks and eliminating them can help to prevent breast and ovarian cancer and, in combination with conventional medicine, treat the disease. In lung cancer, one of the avoidable risks to eliminate is smoking; in breast cancer, ovarian cancer and colorectal cancer, the avoidable risks are mainly dietary and lifestyle factors; this important information is only poorly reflected by the websites of cancer charities.

Conventional risk factors: some strawberries among the old chestnuts?

According to Cancer Research UK, the UK's leading cancer charity, the risk factors for breast cancer are age, reproductive history, early menarche (onset of periods) and late menopause, hormone exposure, body weight, physical activity, alcohol, diet, height, ionising radiation, socio-economic status, mammographic density, benign breast disease and personal or family history of breast cancer. Let us look at this unhelpful jumble of biological and lifestyle factors and symptoms in a bit more detail to identify which are controllable risk factors – the strawberries that can be eliminated.

Age. Yes, breast-cancer risk does increase with age in the West.[12] Breast cancer is the commonest cause of cancer death in women over 65 years of age,[13] increasing in incidence up to 80 years of age before levelling off between 80 and 85 years of age.[14]

In oriental countries where people maintain their traditional lifestyle this is not the case. I predict that there will be a rise in breast cancer in oriental countries, reflecting the Westernisation of their diet, but that it will occur in younger women who are generally the first to change from their traditional diets.

Family history of breast cancer. Breast-cancer risk is higher among women whose close blood relatives have the disease. Blood relatives can be from either the mother's or father's side of the family.

Reproductive history. According to Cancer Research UK, 'Women in developed countries are at increased risk of breast cancer compared with women from less developed countries.' Much of this variation can be explained, they claim, 'by the fact that women in developed countries have fewer children and a limited duration of breast feeding'. I disagree! Japan was one of the first countries to legalise abortion and has had a Western-type demography for decades now, without our rates of breast cancer, while Catholic Ireland with, until recently, very large families has always had a closely similar breast-cancer rate to that of the UK. China has had a one-child policy now for about thirty years, and this has not caused a change in breast-cancer rates there. Why has Cancer Research UK not carried out proper research into this supposed risk factor, using the data available from cancer registries and population data before putting out such disturbing information?

Breastfeeding. Many studies have shown that breast feeding lowers breast-cancer risk.

Age of menarche and menopause. Early age of menarche is a risk factor, with the relative risk of premenopausal breast cancer being reduced by an estimated 7 per cent for every year that menarche is delayed after 12 years of age. Late menopause is also a risk factor with an approximate 3 per cent increase for each year menopause is delayed. This is true, but Cancer

Research UK appears to be unaware of, or to have ignored, the evidence that clearly shows that early menarche and late menopause are related to diet: Chinese women generally start their periods five years later and start their menopause five years earlier than those eating a Western diet.[15]

Hormones. It has been suggested that the use of oral contraceptives slightly increases the risk of breast cancer, but the evidence is not consistent (*see* p. 395). There is stronger evidence that the use of hormone replacement therapy increases the risk of breast cancer (*see* p. 396). There is also said to be evidence of higher risk in post-menopausal women with higher levels of sex hormones. Again, Cancer Research UK makes no mention of the role of diet in maintaining high levels of hormones (*see* Updates to Chapters Four and Six).

Obesity. Overweight and obesity are said to moderately increase the risk of post-menopausal breast cancer, accounting for about 8 per cent of breast-cancer cases in the UK. Cancer Research UK mentions that it is a modifiable risk factor – although amazingly they do not mention diet! They also mention that a few hours of vigorous exercise a week reduces risk by up to 40 per cent. According to the American Cancer Society, having more fat tissue can increase your oestrogen levels and increase your likelihood of developing breast cancer. Until recently, obesity was extremely rare in oriental countries.

Smoking and drinking. Alcohol may be associated with about 4 per cent of breast-cancer cases in developed countries, but, according to Cancer Research UK, there is no direct link with smoking – but see Chapter Six, Lifestyle Factor 5 where I refer to studies that show an increased risk from smoking. According to the American Cancer Society, women who consume one alcoholic drink a day have a very small increase in risk, and those who have two to five drinks daily have about 1.5 times the risk of women who drink no alcohol.

Ionising radiation. Ionising radiation, according to Cancer Research UK, is responsible for a small number of breast cancers. I agree and wonder if hospitals keep records of the cumulative doses from mammograms, X-rays, CT scans, radiotherapy and other procedures that they use on patients. It is my impression that many do not. The most recent evidence of a link between exposure to ionising radiation and breast cancer has come from areas of Belarus and Ukraine contaminated by the explosion of the nuclear reactor at Chernobyl in 1986. Women in the most contaminated areas were found to be two to three times more likely to develop breast cancer than women in less contaminated areas. Excess cases began to appear 10 years after the incident, with a higher risk among women who were younger at the time of the explosion.[16]

Diet. Cancer Research UK gives just one paragraph on diet, and concludes that fat, particularly animal fat, may cause a small increase in breast-cancer risk but probably does not play as large a role as once thought. Why do they make no connection with their own obesity factor? And why do they ignore all the scientific references by eminent non-aligned scientists, quoted in this and other books?

Mammographic breast density, reflecting the relative amounts of fat and other tissue in breasts is said to be an important risk factor, women with denser breasts having 2–6 times the risk of breast cancer. Again, there is no mention of diet, despite the fact that impeccable research from internationally renowned universities has demonstrated that women on a traditional Chinese diet have sixty per cent less of the high-risk, high-density breast tissue![17]

There are some avoidable risk factors in the Cancer Research UK list, but the most important one, diet, which underlies many of the others, is hardly mentioned.

The American Cancer Society[18] gives some other risk factors (and is especially helpful in relation to male breast cancer: see below). Some of the additional risk factors they list are as follows:

Gender. Simply being a woman is the main risk factor for developing breast cancer. Men can develop breast cancer, but the disease is about 100 times more common among women than men.

Genetics. About 10 per cent of breast-cancer cases are hereditary, as a result of a mutated gene.

Personal history of breast cancer. A woman who has had cancer in one breast has a 3- to 4-fold increased risk of developing a new cancer in the other breast or in another part of the same breast. This is different from a recurrence of the first cancer.

Previous breast biopsy. Women whose earlier breast biopsies detected proliferative breast disease without atypia or usual hyperplasia have a slightly higher risk of breast cancer (1.5 to 2 times greater than other women). Having a previous biopsy as a result of atypical hyperplasia increases a woman's breast cancer risk by 4 to 5 times. Having a biopsy specimen diagnosed as fibrocystic changes without proliferative breast disease does not affect breast-cancer risk.

Previous breast irradiation. Women who as children or young adults have had radiation therapy to the chest area as treatment for another cancer (such as Hodgkin's disease or non-Hodgkin's lymphoma) have a significantly increased risk for breast cancer. There are no data on the repeated use of mammography.

Race. White women are slightly more likely than African-American women to develop breast cancer. African-American women, however, are more likely to die of this cancer because their cancers are often diagnosed later and at an advanced stage, when they are harder to treat and cure. There is also some question about whether African-American women have more aggressive tumours. Asian, Hispanic, and Native American women have a lower risk of developing breast cancer. (Remember that these findings are for women living in the USA.)

Environmental pollution. A great deal of research has been reported, and more is being done, to understand environmental influences on breast-cancer risk.

Physical inactivity. Recent studies show that strenuous exercise in youth might provide life-long protection against breast cancer, and that even moderate to strenuous physical activity as an adult can lower breast-cancer risk.

Medication. Recent work shows that women who took the drug diethylstilbestrol during pregnancy are at significantly increased risk of developing breast cancer. The drug is a powerful non-steroidal oestrogen and was used to prevent miscarriage and complications in pregnancy for almost thirty years from the 1940s.[19]

The risk factors for male breast cancer
The known risk factors for male breast cancer[20] are as follows:

Aging. Aging is an important risk factor for the development of male breast cancer. Men with breast cancer average about 65 years of age at the time of their diagnosis.

Family history of breast cancer. Breast-cancer risk is increased if other members of the family (blood relatives) have had breast cancer.

Klinefelter's syndrome. This is a congenital condition that affects about 1 in 1000 men. Men with this condition have an extra X chromosome. Compared with other men, they have lower levels of androgens (male hormones) and more oestrogens (female hormones). For this reason, they often develop gynaecomastia (benign male breast growth) and have an increased risk of male breast cancer.

Radiation exposure. A man whose chest area has been exposed to radiation (usually for treatment of a cancer inside the chest, such as Hodgkin's or non-Hodgkin's lymphoma) has an increased risk of developing breast cancer.

Liver disease. The liver plays an important role in sex-hormone metabolism by producing binding proteins that carry the hormones in the blood. These binding proteins affect the hormones' activity. Men with severe liver disease such as cirrhosis have relatively low levels of androgen activity and higher oestrogen levels. Therefore, they may have an increased risk of developing gynaecomastia and breast cancer.

Oestrogen treatment. Oestrogen-related drugs are sometimes used in hormonal therapy of men with prostate cancer. This treatment may slightly increase their breast-cancer risk. Men taking high doses of oestrogens as part of a sex change procedure have a much higher breast-cancer risk.

Physical inactivity and obesity. Obesity is probably a risk factor for male breast cancer. The reason is that fat cells convert male hormone (androgens) into female hormones.

OVARIAN CANCER

The incidence of ovarian cancer is much lower than that of breast cancer, but the proportion of ovarian-cancer sufferers who die from the disease is greater, probably because it is often not diagnosed until it has reached an advanced stage.

Incidence

The crude background rate for ovarian cancer in China is about 1 in 100,000 women.[21] The age-standardised rate of 3.2 women in 100,000 may be compared with rates more than 2 to 6 times higher in Western countries (Table 3.2). Like breast-cancer rates, the highest ovarian-cancer rates are in North America and Europe and the lowest rates in much of Africa and Asia. The

Table 3.2: Age-standardised rates of incidence of ovarian cancer per 100,000 females for the year 2002

	2002
China	3.2
Japan	6.4
Thailand	5.6
South Korea	5.7
New Zealand	12.4
Australia	8.9
Canada	11.6
UK	13.4
USA	10.6
Iceland	17.0

Data from WHO International Agency for Research on Cancer (IARC).[22]

lowest rates in Europe are in the south, in Greece, Portugal and Cyprus, while the highest rates are in northern and eastern countries such as Denmark and Lithuania.

Rising trends

As with breast cancer, the incidence of ovarian cancer has been rising in most Western countries. There were 15 cases per 100,000 women in the UK in 1975 and 18 in 2003, an increase of more than 20 per cent. In contrast, the incidence of ovarian cancer declined slightly in the USA between 1985 and 2002. In both the USA and the UK, the disease killed more women than any other cancer of the reproductive tract.

Migration studies

There are fewer migration studies for ovarian cancer than breast cancer, and the results are conflicting.

Death rates and survival

The death rate for ovarian cancer was 10.4 per 100,000 women in 2004 in the UK, where mortality rates have been almost unchanged since the early 1970s. Reduced mortality in younger women has been offset by increased mortality in older women.

The five-year survival rate has increased from 23 per cent for women diagnosed in the early 1970s to almost 30 per cent in women diagnosed in the early 1990s (41 per cent in Scotland). The ten-year survival rate has also increased slightly. In the USA, the five-year survival rate is now 45 per cent. The most important factor in survival is the stage at which ovarian cancer is diagnosed, the greatest improvements being in those with early-stage disease.

Conventional risk factors
The risk factors considered by Cancer Research UK include: a small number of pregnancies, infertility and infertility treatment, contraception and hormone replacement therapy, and sexually transmitted infections.

According to Cancer Research UK, there is a dose response between a lower number of pregnancies and increased risk, although the research for this appears to have been carried out entirely in the USA. They also suggest that there is some evidence that breast feeding has a protective effect. The same arguments apply against such supposed risks as in the case of breast cancer.

Infertility is thought to be linked to increased risk of ovarian cancer, but it is difficult to distinguish the effects of infertility treatment from those of infertility itself.

Hormones. There is evidence that oral contraceptives are protective against ovarian cancer, even in those who have long since discontinued their use. Having fallopian tubes tied and hysterectomy operations also appear to reduce risk. Hormone replacement therapy may increase the risk of ovarian cancer by as much as 20 per cent.

Obesity. Firm evidence on obesity and ovarian cancer risk is lacking, and evidence of links with infectious agents such as Chlamydia is also poor.

There are even fewer avoidable risks given than for breast cancer, and not a hint of the role of diet.

The importance of diet in breast-cancer and ovarian-cancer risk is considered briefly below and discussed further in Chapters Four and Five.

DIFFERENT DIETS
I continue to believe that the distinctive difference in rates of breast and ovarian cancer between Western and oriental coun-

tries relates to diet. The difference between the Chinese and American diets was thoroughly investigated and documented in 1994 by Campbell and Junshi.[23] The advantages of the Chinese diet include the following:

- It is low in fat, which causes oestrogen to be released in women's bodies. Only 14 per cent of calories in the average Chinese diet were from fat, compared with almost 36 per cent in America.
- It is high in fibre, which helps to eliminate excess oestrogen from the body. Animal protein was found to make up only 1 per cent of an average Chinese diet, compared with 11 per cent of the average American diet. Vegetables are the main source of protein in China, giving an average fibre intake of 34 g per day, compared with the average US fibre intake of only 10–12 g per day.
- It is high in phyto-oestrogens, which are protective against breast cancer. Vegetables rich in phyto-oestrogens, such as soya, are the main source of protein in China. A recent study carried out in Singapore by a group of world-leading epidemiologists showed a clear association between high soya intake and a reduced risk of breast cancer.[24]
- Traditionally, Chinese people did not eat dairy produce, whereas in the West this can account for up to 40 per cent of the diet.[25]
- The exposure to animal steroid hormones from a traditional Chinese diet is much lower than from a Western diet. According to the China study, lifetime exposure to oestrogen is 2.5 to 3.0 times higher in those on an animal-based Western diet than in those on a traditional Chinese diet. This translates to fewer reproductive years for Chinese women, with later menarche and earlier menopause.

Interestingly, the study by Campbell and Junshi showed that the Chinese took in more calories than Americans but were much less obese, strongly suggesting that it is the type of food and not the calorie intake that is important.

Unfortunately, the traditional oriental diet is being replaced by the typical Western diet, high in dairy and junk food, leading to an obvious increase in obesity in urban areas. According to Chinese colleagues, just as in the West, dairy is being marketed as being essential for strong bones – an idea widely refuted by informed doctors and scientists.[26]

Figure 3.3: Relationship between breast-cancer incidence for the year 2000 (age standardised rates, worldwide) and the ratio of vegetable protein to animal protein in the diet

Cancer data from WHO/IARC.[27] Diet data from Frassetto and others (2000).[28]

Figure 3.3 shows the proportion of vegetable to animal protein in the diet of 33 countries (compiled from FAO food fact sheets) plotted against breast-cancer incidence. There is a clear relationship between diets with a high proportion of vegetable to animal protein and low breast-cancer risk. The critical change to relatively low risk occurs when the ratio of vegetable to animal protein is about 1.7:1. Put more simply, the data suggest that you can decrease your risk of breast cancer by eating approximately twice as much vegetable as animal protein. **Note that this refers only to protein, and I continue to recommend eating masses of vegetables and fruits as well**.

Nevertheless, despite the mounting evidence of the links between the Western diet and breast and ovarian cancer, conventional medicine continues to promulgate the same old risk factors as outlined above.

Much of the information on convention risk factors may be relevant *within* a single country, such as the USA or the UK, but it completely ignores all the epidemiological evidence of the much lower rates in China and other oriental countries, evidence which strongly implicates the Western diet and lifestyle as the main causative factor.

One of the problems, it seems to me, is that researchers tend to look at their own populations. Using Figure 3.1 as an example, they are frequently looking at minor perturbations in the lines at the top of the graph (i.e. Western countries), while ignoring the much more significant differences between different countries. These differences between Western and oriental countries have been clear and sustained ever since reliable standardised cancer registers were first kept. I remain convinced that the difference in diet and lifestyle, especially to exposure to hormones and growth factors in food and drink and to hormone-mimicking chemicals in food, drink and the environment, are at the root of the problem of the increasing incidence of breast, ovarian and other reproductive cancers in the West.

CHAPTER 3 IN A NUTSHELL

- While there is little that we can do about some factors, such as our genes, eliminating some controllable risks can help to prevent breast and ovarian cancer in the same way that giving up smoking reduces the risk of lung cancer.
- Even when we have breast or ovarian cancer, we can put the disease into remission by eliminating avoidable risk factors – as I have done for the last 14 years.
- The incidence of breast cancer has been increasing in Western countries for many years. In Britain the age-standardised incidence of breast cancer had increased from 74 in 1975 to 120 per 100,000 women by 2003, a rise of more than 80 per cent in thirty years! The lifetime risk of breast cancer has leapt from 1 in 10 women when I wrote the first edition of this book in 2000 to 1 in 9 women by 2003.
- The dramatic rise in the incidence of breast cancer cannot be genetic. Genes do not change that quickly. Moreover, since the data are adjusted for age, the increased rate does not indicate an aging population. Nor can the dramatic rise in breast-cancer incidence throughout the West be attributed to improved screening.
- The data still clearly show that the incidence rates of breast cancer are much higher in Western countries than in oriental countries. Many oriental countries, such as Japan and South Korea, have been densely populated and highly industrialised and urbanised for decades, yet their rates of

breast and ovarian cancer have remained much lower than in the West.

- Migration studies into cancer incidence in different ethnic populations in Hawaii add considerable weight to the evidence of earlier migration studies that most cancers are environmentally determined.

- The death rate from breast cancer still shows the same two quite distinct groupings: of Western industrialised countries, such as Canada, the UK and the USA, with high mortality rates and oriental countries, such as Thailand and Japan, with low rates.

- The death rate from breast cancer in most Western countries, including the USA and UK, is falling. The five-year survival rate improved from 52 per cent for women diagnosed in England and Wales before 1975 to 80 per cent in those diagnosed after 2001. The estimated 20-year survival rate has also improved, from 44 per cent in the early 1990s to 64 per cent today.

- The incidence of ovarian cancer is much lower than that of breast cancer, but the proportion of ovarian cancer sufferers who die is greater, probably because the disease is often not diagnosed until it has reached an advanced stage.

- Like breast cancer, the highest rates of ovarian cancer are in North America and Europe with the lowest rates in much of Africa and South Asia. The age-standardised rate in China is 2–6 times lower than in most Western countries.

- The incidence of ovarian cancer, like that of breast cancer, has been rising in most Western countries. There were 15 cases per 100,000 women in the UK in 1975 and 18 by 2003, an increase of more than 20 per cent. In both the USA and UK the disease kills more women than any other cancer of the reproductive tract.

- The death rate for ovarian cancer in the UK was 10.4 per 100,000 women in 2004. Mortality rates have been almost unchanged since the early 1970s.

- The evidence continues to indicate strongly that, as with many cancers, it is environmental or lifestyle factors that are promoting the diseases in the West and that those factors are now increasingly important in oriental countries.

- People in Japan and Korea live in similar houses and have similar family sizes, and in Japan this has been the case for decades. They dress in similar clothes, wear similar make-up, drive similar cars and watch similar televisions to those of us who live in the West. The only thing that until recently was obviously different was their diet, which was based on rice, soya and vegetables rather than meat and dairy.

• UK Cancer charity websites fail to identify avoidable risk factors clearly and do not acknowledge the overwhelming importance of diet on risk factors such as menarche or menopause – or even obesity.

Update to Chapter 4. Milk Is a Four-Letter Word

In this chapter I explain much of the compelling scientific evidence that has accumulated over the years, even since I wrote Your Life in Your Hands *in 2000, suggesting that breast cancer is associated with the Western diet and its high proportion of dairy produce. Milk contains hormones, such as prolactin and oestrogen, and growth factors, such as IGF-I and EGF, substances which, according to leading international experts, promote breast cancer, ovarian cancer and other types of cancer. The chapter also explains new evidence why giving up dairy is unlikely to cause any health problems, but, on the contrary, is likely to cut your risk of suffering not only from cancer but from many other diseases as well.*

As I indicated in Chapter Three, it was my experience of working in China that first led me to realise that diet was the key factor in promoting breast cancer. The comment by Chinese colleagues about breast cancer being a 'rich woman's disease', which they associated with women who ate Hong Kong (i.e. Western) food, such as ice-cream, milk chocolate and yoghurt, was an important clue. Much recent evidence supports this link. For example, the association between consumption of soya and low risk of breast cancer has been confirmed by scientists from impeccable internationally famous epidemiological centres.[1]

As I have explained, I was one of those who had bought into the image, pushed by the industry, that dairy produce, especially yoghurt, was essential for good health, but this image is just that – a carefully crafted marketing image. The lowing cows roaming lush green pastures used to advertise dairy are a far cry from modern industrialised dairy production systems.

Drinking the milk of another species is a fairly recent practice, dating back only about 6,000 years in Europe and central Asia.[2] This practice was not followed until recently by most of the rest of the world. Seventy per cent of people in the world, more than 90 per cent of the populations of some Asian countries, remain lactose (milk-sugar) intolerant. Most human populations, other than Caucasians, become lactose intolerant after weaning, when the child's body stops producing lactase, the enzyme needed to metabolise lactose. This is a clear signal from nature that, as the

Chinese used to say, 'milk is for babies'. Recent work by an Anglo-German team has shown that Europeans became tolerant to lactose, after dairying began, as a result of genetic changes. They remained lactose intolerant until 5,000 years ago.[3] Five thousand years of milk drinking has masked some of the most obvious ill effects of dairy consumption in Western countries. There is still an enormous variation in the consumption of dairy products. People in most Western countries consume more than 250 kg a year, compared with at most a few kg in oriental countries, such as China, Vietnam and Thailand, and many African countries.[4]

Another clue that milk drinking by adults is unnatural is that no other mammal drinks the milk of another species. Wildlife programmes show animals eating the flesh of other species, and their eggs, and vegetation, but I have yet to see an example of an adult mammal suckling an adult mammal of another species for food.

A recent concern about cows' milk has been its low levels of essential polyunsaturated acids compared with human milk. This is thought to reflect nature putting a higher priority on increased body size in cows and on the development of the brain in humans.[5] Attempts have been made to increase the nutritional value of cows' milk for humans by feeding cattle on fish meal and soya[6] and flaxseed.[7]

Anything naturally good in dairy produce comes from plants or the action on them of microbes in the gut. Surely it is better to eat salads and vegetables, which are not unlike the grasses that cows are supposed to eat in the first place – after all, they are the real source of the immensely strong bones of animals designed to be totally vegan, such as cows and hippopotamuses. It has even been suggested recently that the highly promoted conjugated linoleic acids that occur in dairy fat have a pro-carcinogenic effect.[8]

One best-selling supposedly anti-cancer diet recommends consuming meat and dairy produce to protect against cancer, and another book still available in the UK continues to recommend yoghurt as part of an (anti-breast-) cancer diet. A book by an NHS dietician proposes consuming low-fat dairy to protect against breast cancer. Even ICON, the magazine of the charity, CAN-CERactive, now carries articles suggesting that probiotics – the new marketing name for yoghurt – protect against cancer. This is advice I shall strongly refute, basing my argument on gold-standard scientific publications.

THE CHANGING QUANTITY AND QUALITY OF DAIRY

Many scientists believe that the amount of dairy produce in our diet is now far too high because its role in preventing osteoporosis has been overstated, while its role in cancer has been understated.[9] It has been calculated that the average weekly consumption of dairy by people in the UK is now about the same as the petrol consumption of our cars – approximately 5 litres a week per person! The quality of dairy produce has also changed greatly. The Royal Society, Britain's most authoritative scientific organisation, has suggested that routes of human exposure to oestrogen that changed in the latter half of the twentieth century included increased consumption of dairy produce.[10] They pointed out that dairy practices have changed since World War II, in that pregnant cows continue to be milked, increasing the oestrogen content of the milk. Indeed, in today's large-scale intensive dairy farms cows are pregnant and milked for most of the year.[11] During pregnancy the cow's ovaries secrete high levels of progesterone and the placenta secretes high levels of oestrogen – and the hormone levels in milk from both Holstein and Jersey cows have been shown to have increased markedly.[12]

Milk products now supply between 60 and 80 per cent of female sex steroids such as oestrogen and progesterone in the diet, the remaining 20 to 40 per cent being derived from other animal products such as meat. Significant concentrations of the male hormone testosterone also occur in cheese, milk and milk products,[13] and androgen precursors also occur in dairy.[14] Particular concern has been expressed about the oestrogen content of cow's milk by Ganmaa and Sato,[15] whose study into cancer incidence and food intakes in 40 countries showed an increase in hormone-dependent cancers with increasing cheese and milk consumption. Moreover, selective breeding and high-protein feed to replace grass has increased the average milk yield per cow from nine litres (16 pints) a day to a staggering 22 litres (39 pints) a day,[16] greatly increasing levels of growth factors in the milk.

INCREASING FIGURES

The United States Department of Agriculture has estimated that the average American's diet comprises more than 40 per cent dairy produce, more than double most official guidelines – which distinguished nutritional scientists think are already set too high.[17] The American diet is certainly not a healthy one.

It is estimated that a staggering 60 per cent of Americans are now overweight enough to begin experiencing health problems as a result. About 25 per cent of all Americans under 19 are overweight or obese, a figure that has doubled in 30 years.[18]

A book called *Fat Land: How Americans Became the Fattest People in the World*[19] has been described as a well-written report on the obese American, and how they got that way. And the question was asked 'if America is out in front, can the United Kingdom be far behind'?[20] Some of the latest data from the UK Food Standards Agency (FSA) answer this question. In 2004 the FSA reported that the number of obese men in the UK had risen from 8 per cent in 1987 to 25 per cent; in women the number had increased from 12 per cent to 20 per cent. The influence of vested interests, including the dairy industry, in giving misinformation to consumers is discussed further in Chapter Seven.

MILK – WHAT A COCKTAIL!

Let us now look at a list of the incredibly powerful biochemicals that are contained in milk. Why are they there?

Mammals developed fairly recently in the history of the Earth (they have existed for only about 200 million years, out of the 4,500 million years of the age of the Earth) and are the most evolved and intelligent creatures on the planet. Their high degree of development is achieved by a long period of gestation in the womb, where they are fed a complex cocktail of chemicals, including hormones and growth factors, which bring about cell growth, differentiation and proliferation, including the migration of embryonic stem cells to different parts of the developing foetus. Following birth, infant mammals are suckled (ideally in humans for about one and a half years) because milk carries similar chemical messengers to maintain growth and differentiation. The transport medium for the chemical messengers – plasma – simply changes from red blood to white milk, known as 'white blood' in some cultures.

Milk from every mammal contains hormones, growth factors and other powerful biochemicals. The reason why all mammals, other than humans, stop drinking milk at a certain age is because by then they produce all the hormones, and growth factors they need. The production, secretion and levels of these substances are regulated through a complex, delicately balanced system of interaction. The concern is that by absorbing extra quantities of highly bioactive substances from cows' milk, goats' milk and/or the meat of animals used for dairy production there could be undesirable growth and differentiation of tissues in the human body, leading to cancer.

In fact cows' milk has been shown to contain over 35 different hormones and 11 growth factors![21] Indeed, growth factors for laboratory research studies are normally obtained from milk or cheese whey.[22]

Some of the growth factors, hormones and peptides in milk include the following[23] [my bold]:

- bombesine (a neuropeptide).[24] Milk contains both bombesine and GRP (bombesine-like peptide).[25] Bombesine levels in milk are three times higher than in blood,[26] and GRP and bombesine have been implicated in breast cancer[27] and prostate cancer.[28]
- GRP (Gastrin-releasing peptide).[29]
- substance P (a neurotransmitter),[30] which increases vascular permeability[31] and stimulates[32] histamine secretion, causing allergic reactions.
- CGRP (calcitonin-gene-related peptide, also a neurotransmitter).[33]
- **IGF-I and IGF-II[34] (insulin-like growth factors)**. IGF-I and IGF-II are quite resistant to decomposition by enzymes.[35] They promote both breast,[36] and prostate cancer.[37] See also the work of He[38] and Perks and Holly.[39]
- **EGF (Epidermal growth factor)**.[40] Like IGF, EGF is quite resistant to decomposition by enzymes.[41] EGF enhances breast cancer[42] and prostate cancer,[43] and was the first growth factor to be shown to be absorbed by the blood through the gut wall.[44] It is to be strongly avoided by those with tumours over-expressing the HER-2 protein. EGF has been implicated in androgen-independent prostate cancer.[45]
- NGF (Nerve growth factor).[46]
- **Oestrogen**. There is particular concern about the oestrogen content of cows' milk (see above).
- **Prolactin**. To be able to breastfeed, the female body is better equipped to cope with temporarily increased prolactin

production. Males are not, and prolactin-producing tumours in men are therefore larger, more active and resistant to treatment.[47] Prolactin enhances breast cancer[48] and prostate cancer.[49]

- PRP (Prolactin-releasing peptide).[50]
- **LHRH** (or: GnRH, stimulates secretion of LH and FSH).[51]
- **progesterone**.[52]
- peptide YY.[53]
- peptide histidine methionine.[54]
- neuropeptide Y (stimulating appetite).[55]
- TRH (stimulating TSH secretion).[56] TRH stimulates prolactin[57] and growth hormone (GH) secretion,[58] through T3.[59]
- TSH (stimulating T3 and T4 secretion).[60]
- T3 (Triiodothyronine).[61] T3 increases the number of oestrogen receptors, increasing oestrogen-influence.[62]
- GHRF (Growth-hormone-releasing factor).[63] GHRF stimulates GH and hence **IGF-I and IGF-II** secretion.[64]
- ACTH (regulating cortisol secretion).[65]
- neurotensine.[66]
- cortisol.[67]
- insulin (regulating blood-glucose level).[68]
- beta-endorphine (opioid peptide).[69]

Since many of the powerful chemicals contained in milk are known to have an important role in the development of young mammals, including cell division, and milk is designed for this purpose, it is worth asking the question: what happens if the chemicals which are intended by nature to stimulate cell growth in newly born animals such as cows and goats send similar signals to adult tissue in humans? Much recent scientific evidence reviewed below supports the link between dairy consumption and breast and ovarian cancer and other hormone-dependent cancers.

Many of the growth factors, hormones and other biochemicals contained in dairy milk are implicated in the production and development of cancers, including ovarian and testicular cancer.[70] It has been suggested that different growth factors increase cancer-risk of different tissues. Excessive LHRH, which is concentrated in milk, stimulates secretion of LH and/or FSH, which, in turn, have been implicated in ovarian,[71] prostate[72] and testicular cancer.[73] It has also been suggested that different growth factors promote types of cancer not associated with the reproductive system. There is evidence for the role of milk in promoting lung cancer. For example, in Japan, in 1996 people consumed more than three times as many cigarettes as in Norway,[74] but in Norway lung-cancer mortality in men was higher.[75] Also, in countries such as Russia, UK, France, Canada, USA and Australia fewer cigarettes are smoked,[76] but lung-cancer mortality in men is higher than in Japan.[77] In all these countries more milk, containing lung-cancer-promoting substances, is consumed,[78] again suggesting that dairy contains substances that select for and promote damaged or initiated cancer cells.

IGF-I AND BREAST CANCER

Let us look at the role of IGF-I, for which evidence of its role in breast and other cancers continues to mount.

Why should this substance cause problems such as breast cancer?

In humans, free or circulating IGF-I levels decline with age, consistent with their role in growth. IGF-I levels are higher in teenage girls than boys, and the difference extends into adulthood. Levels are elevated in pregnant women. Although IGF-I is essential for growth, its levels do not correlate closely with growth rates – supporting other evidence that some IGF-I is of dietary origin. It was suggested some years ago by distinguished biochemists that IGF-I levels may reflect nutritional status.[79]

The levels of IGF-I in the blood are highest during the years of puberty, which is, of course, a time of rapid growth. Indeed, at the onset of puberty, IGF-I sends signals to breast and prostate cells to begin dividing so that the breasts and prostate will grow in adolescent boys and girls.

Both insulin and the IGFs cause cells to increase in size. Insulin has a simple short-term action of cleaning excess nutrients from the circulation and storing them in cells. In contrast, the IGFs are involved in cell proliferation and differentiation, and a complex set of factors has evolved to ensure that IGF activity occurs only when conditions are optimal for growth. In 1995 researchers at the US National Institute of Health reported that IGF-I plays a central role in the progression of many cancers. According to Hans R. Larsen, the evidence of a strong link between cancer risk and a high level of IGF-I is indisputable.[80]

Pollack[81] has suggested that the relation of IGF physiology to carcinogenesis will become relevant in cancer-risk assessment and chemoprevention, although he continues to emphasise the potential value of drugs that target the IGF-I receptor and indicates that several candidate pharmaceuticals are being proposed for clinical trials. Lonning also recommends that future therapeutic strategies in treating breast cancer should consider total blockade of the IGF-I receptor.[82] Yee states that there are abundant data from human, animal and laboratory studies supporting a role for the IGFs in cancer and that interactions with their receptors have been shown to stimulate cancer proliferation, prevent cell suicide and enhance metastasis. Again, their research centres on targeting the IGF-I receptor.[83] Pollack raises particular concern about the use of IGF-I and GH in anti-ageing preparations for humans.[84]

Yet another recent study from 1998 confirms that increased IGF-I levels in blood are associated with large relative risks for common cancers including breast cancer and ovarian cancer.[85] Other studies have also linked high circulating levels of bioavailable or bioactive IGF-I with an increased risk of developing[86] cancers. A study carried out by the University of Texas, for example, showed that high circulating levels of IGF-I increased the risk of lung cancer,[87] and a study carried out by Harvard Medical School showed that high circulating levels increased the risk of colorectal cancer.[88] IGF-I has also been linked to an increased risk of childhood cancers, melanoma and pancreatic cancer.[89] Indeed, Campbell and Campbell suggest that IGF-I should be used as a predictor of certain cancers, including breast cancer, in much the same way as cholesterol is used to identify those at risk of heart disease.[90]

Increasingly the evidence suggests that the association between IGF-I and cancer incidence complies with many of the accepted criteria for causality:[91] the association is strong and specific, it demonstrates the correct temporal sequence, it is dose responsive, it has biological plausibility, and it has coherence with other documented associations. According to Holly and others, the last remaining criterion of causality to be satisfied would then depend on interventions, showing that reducing circulating IGF-I levels reduces cancer incidence.[92] They go on to suggest that the fact that circulating IGF-I concentrations are strongly dependent on nutrition raises the prospect of being able to reduce cancer risk by less aggressive interventions. Investigation of nutritional interventions aimed at reducing serum IGF-I concentrations would be warranted if such reductions were confirmed to reduce the risk of cancer.

In summary, the scientific literature strongly supports the link between high circulating IGF-I levels and several types of cancer (including breast cancer). Let us look more closely at what this has to do with consuming dairy produce.

The link between IGF-I and dairy

There is no doubt that the established medical view now is that growth factors promote cancers directly, but much of conventional medicine assumes that growth factors such as IGF-I are made in the body. It would also be true to say that we manufacture our own cholesterol, but cholesterol-related disease (e.g. heart disease) is caused by consuming *extra* amounts of the substance from dairy and other animal products. There is increasingly strong evidence that the same applies to IGF-I.

IGF-I is exactly the same chemical whether it is in the milk of goats, sheep, cows, humans or other mammalian species. Levels of IGF-I are naturally higher in cows' milk (and in that of sheep and goats) than human milk, because these animals grow more rapidly. As pointed out by John Robbins in his book *A Diet for a New America*,[93] while a human normally takes 180 days to double its birth weight, a cow takes only 47 days and a goat even less – just 19 days – so such milk is likely to be particularly bad for us because it will contain more growth factors than human milk. The fact that dairy products are rich in growth factors is illustrated by the normal practice of isolating growth factors for research studies from milk or cheese whey.[94]

The dairy industry tries to argue that IGF-I has no effect on the human body because it is destroyed during digestion and does not cross the gut-blood barrier. Independent studies, however, show that substances contained in milk closely similar to IGF-I are not destroyed by the digestive system because of the protective effect of casein (the principal protein in milk).[95] The 1999 report of the EU Scientific Committee states 'there is clear evidence that orally ingested IGF-I reaches the receptor sites in the gut in its biologically active form.'[96] Moreover, research published by the Cancer Epidemiology Unit at Oxford University[97] has shown that serum IGF-I was 9 per cent lower in vegan men than in meat eaters (also thought to consume dairy produce) and milk-consuming vegetarians. Also, the number of twins born in populations is thought to reflect IGF-I status and the twinning rate in vegans is one fifth of that of vegetarians and omnivores. Moreover the twinning rate in the UK, where recombinant bovine growth hormone (rBGH) is banned and hence IGF-I in milk is lower, increased by 16 per cent between 1992 and 2001. This may be compared with a massive increase of 32 per cent in the USA where rBGH is used.[98] Moreover, recent studies have confirmed that serum IGF-I levels in European women increase significantly with increasing consumption of dairy. Levels also increase with increasing intake of animal protein from meat, poultry, fish and eggs, but these relationships were not statistically significant. There was no relationship with vegetable protein from pulses or cereals, and the more vegetables consumed the lower the serum IGF-I levels.[99]

Milk secretions of mammals contain special forms of IGF-I which are ten times more potent than normal IGF-I. In normal cows' milk, 3 per cent of the IGF-I is reported to be in this form.[100] Interestingly, one study reported a 10 per cent increase in circulating IGF-I levels in people consuming low-fat milk.[101]

Gunnell and others, from a consortium of British universities including Bristol and Cambridge, examined the association of diet with the IGFs in healthy middle-aged men.[102] They found that raised levels of IGF-I, relative to the binding protein that prevents it locking onto receptors, were associated with higher intakes of milk, dairy products, calcium, carbohydrate and polyunsaturated fats, while lower levels were correlated with high vegetable consumption, particularly tomatoes. They found no evidence of an association with red meat. Their findings that vegetable intake was weakly related to lower bioavailable/bioactive IGF-I is consistent with the observation that vegetable-rich diets protect against breast, prostate and colorectal cancer;[103] their findings were not affected by socioeconomic status or other lifestyle factors such as smoking. These associations, with the exception of carbohydrates, support all the factors I proposed as limiting levels of circulating IGF-I in the first edition of this book. Unfortunately, Gunnell and his co-workers looked at carbohydrates as a whole; I advise against refined carbohydrates but not against others, based on scientific evidence that refined white bread increases circulating IGF-I levels whereas whole-grain cereals contain chemopreventative chemicals active against breast cancer (*see* further in Food Factor 6, Chapter Five). Other studies had previously reported reduced levels of IGF-I in those on vegan diets.[104]

Thus, scientific investigations by leading scientists in some of the world's most prestigious universities and research centres show that consuming dairy products increases circulating levels of IGF-I,[105] and this in turn increases the risk of breast cancer,[106] ovarian cancer,[107] prostate cancer,[108] and other cancers. There are a few studies that purport to show the opposite, but, as discussed in the update to Chapter Seven, their validity has been questioned.

Time trends of IGF-I in milk

Following the development of fixed farming communities, Western man has consumed milk and this has always contained some growth factors such as IGF-I. Breast cancers have also existed in Western populations for a long time. The oldest written description of cancer, in fact of eight cases of breast cancer, dates back to 1600 BC and was recorded on an Egyptian papyrus. Throughout the Middle Ages there are many references to cancer generally, and it was noted by early explorers, traders and missionaries that cancer rates were rare in native communities but increased as a result of changing to a modern (i.e. Western) lifestyle.[109]

Modern dairy practices, such as the use of genetically modified hormones in North America and elsewhere, have dramatically increased the levels of IGF-I in milk. One of the most important effects of rBGH, as far as breast and prostate cancer studies are concerned, is that it increases the amounts of IGF-I and IGF-II in milk. Also, the long-term treatment of cows with the hormone implant oestradiol as a growth promoter increases secretion of IGF-I.[110]

Over the years, the dairy industry in most Western countries has chosen to increase the average milk yield by feeding the cows on protein concentrate rather than grass and selectively breeding from cattle which are higher milk producers. This has resulted in the selection of cows such as the Holstein which have higher levels of naturally occurring BGH, so that even before the era of rBGH, levels of IGF-I in milk were increasing. The practice of milking cows when they are pregnant has also increased IGF-I levels in milk, as well as steroid hormones.[111]

EGF

Epidermal growth factor (EGF), which is also a mitogen (promoting cell division), also occurs in milk. It is well established that it stimulates the proliferation of epidermal and epithelial tissues generally and that it crosses the intestinal wall and enters the bloodstream.[112] EGF is implicated in promoting several types of cancer, including HER-2-receptor-positive breast cancer and some types of lung cancer.

GROWTH FACTORS AND TESTOSTERONE AND OESTROGEN

It has been suggested[113] that two possible mechanisms that might explain the strong associations between circulating IGF-I levels and cancer incidence are: (1) IGF-I could be affecting steroid levels and/or amplifying sex steroid actions in the prostate and breast; or (2) IGF-I levels could be having a direct effect on the development of cancer in these tissues. The strength of the associations between IGF-I and breast and prostate cancer suggests that they are unlikely to be due to IGF-I acting merely as a surrogate of steroid status. An alternative explanation might be that IGF-I determines steroid levels or actions, enhancing the production of gonadal steroids from the ovary.[114] The proliferative effects of steroids on the breast can also be made worse by IGF-I.[115] Increased circulating levels of IGF-I could therefore enhance and add to the effects of steroids on the breast. A combination of such potential interacting mechanisms involving IGF-I effects on steroids is a plausible explanation of the associations of oestrogen with breast cancer.[116] Put more simply, the evidence suggests that high circulating levels of IGF-I stimulate the body to produce levels of oestrogen or testosterone more appropriate for teenagers than post-menopausal women or post-andropausal men.

OESTROGEN AND PROGESTERONE

As discussed above the main dietary source of oestrogen and progesterone is dairy, the rest being from other animal products in the diet such as meat. There is overwhelming evidence that oestrogen levels are a critical determinant of breast-cancer risk.[117]

Oestrogen and progesterone have been shown to participate directly in the cancer process.[118]

In the China study, lifetime exposure to dietary oestrogen was shown to be at least 2.5 to 3.0 times higher among Western women than in rural Chinese women, while progesterone levels were also increased with higher levels of prolactin between 55 and 64 years of age.[119] The high oestrogen levels were shown to be associated with early menarche (start of periods) and late menopause. In American girls the age of menarche is 11 years but in rural China it was 17 years old! Menopause began at approximately 55 years and 50 years in America and rural China respectively. Since early menarche and late menopause are two of the main risk factors for breast cancer that we are supposedly unable to change,[120] it is worth asking why we have not been told of this crucially important information by government or breast-cancer charities. According to Campbell and Campbell, it should be shouted from the rooftops![121] 'The sad truth is that most women simply are not aware of the evidence. If this information were properly reported by responsible and credible public health agencies I suspect that many more young women might be taking very real, very effective steps to avoid this awful disease'. I have recounted how I asked the hospital dietician to recommend an oestrogen-free diet and how she appeared not to know what I was talking about. Unfortunately, it would appear that such ignorance of what science has to say about dairy consumption and other animal food and breast cancer remains widespread. This is discussed further in Chapter Seven.

OVARIAN CANCER AND DAIRY

A possible relationship between ovarian cancer and dairy consumption was first proposed in 1989.[122] This study suggested that lactose might be the dietary risk factor. More recently, women who consumed the most lactose in dairy were shown to have twice the risk of developing ovarian cancer as women who consumed the least, and again a lactose component (galactose) was suggested as the risk factor.[123] A study conducted by the famous Karolinska Institute showed that women consuming four or more servings of dairy a day had a risk of ovarian cancer double that of non-dairy consumers. Milk was the product most strongly correlated.[124] The results of three prospective studies also showed a strong association between total dairy intake, low-fat milk and lactose, and the risk of ovarian cancer.[125] Another study into food consumption in different countries in relation to ovarian cancer risk showed that high-dairy-consuming nations such as Iceland had the highest rates of ovarian cancer while countries such as China and Korea, where little dairy is consumed, had extremely low rates. Again, the main finding was that there was a strong link between consuming dairy and ovarian cancer risk. Milk was most strongly correlated, followed by cheese.[126]

Testosterone is thought to be one of the main hormones implicated in ovarian cancer, and dairy produce is one of the main dietary sources.[127]

HORMONES, GROWTH FACTORS AND CANCER AS A DISEASE

As indicated in Chapter Two, DNA can be damaged by many factors, although the body is well equipped to repair or eliminate damaged cells. The problem of cancer developing into a disease is more likely to reflect the influence of factors favouring the growth of damaged, relative to normal, cells over the longer term. Absorbing growth factors and hormones through the diet will preferentially favour such damaged cells – those least able to deal with growth factors – and hence promote cancer. Eventually, tumours can start producing more growth factors, stimulating their own reproduction, but probably only in very advanced cases. Even so, some natural substances can help to block their activity (see Chapter Five).

All these findings provide increasingly compelling evidence that dairy consumption is one of the key factors contributing to breast cancer, ovarian cancer, prostate cancer and many other types of cancer – though all of the other dietary factors in Chapter Five are important too.

I RECOMMEND

I continue to recommend that all women who wish to prevent or treat breast cancer and ovarian cancer and men who wish to avoid breast cancer, prostate cancer or testicular cancer should **totally eliminate all forms of dairy produce from cows, goats or any animal source from their diet and make the other dietary and lifestyle changes recommended in Chapters Five and Six**. Those with active cancer should also cut down their intake of all foods of animal origin as much as possible until their cancer is in remission.

SOME OTHER PROBLEMS WITH MILK AND HEALTH

There are many other diseases which are helped by avoiding dairy, as detailed in *Eating for Better Health*.[128] Some of these are described below, and many of the beneficial effects of a dairy-free diet have been confirmed over and over again by communications from people who have followed the dietary and lifestyle factors outlined in this book.

An increasing amount of scientific evidence shows that dairy milk is not the wonder food the dairy industry would have us believe. Indeed, scientists are now linking cows'-milk consumption to a wide range of human diseases. Milk is one of the commonest causes of food allergies. It is the single commonest cause of allergy in infants,[129] and cow's milk protein (CMP) has frequently been implicated in causing eczema, asthma and migraine. It has been suggested that some of the thousands of cases of cot death that occur in the USA every year might be caused by cows' milk allergy.[130] Respiratory problems, canker sores, skin conditions, and other subtle and not-so-subtle allergies can all be caused by dairy products. Over 70 per cent of the world's adult population are unable to digest the milk sugar, lactose, suggesting that this is the normal condition for adults, not some sort of deficiency.[131] The symptoms, which include abdominal pain, flatulence and diarrhoea, are relieved by taking the enzyme that breaks down lactose, called lactase. Lactose intolerance would seem to be nature's early warning system!

According to the website of the US Food and Drug Administration (FDA),[132] a food allergy, or hypersensitivity, is an abnormal response to a food triggered by the immune system. Many people often have gas, bloating or other unpleasant reactions to something they eat, but this is not a true allergic response. Such a reaction is called 'food intolerance'. Lactose (milk sugar) intolerance is very common, especially among non-Caucasians. This is of particular concern since it is used as the matrix or filler for many orthodox and herbal tablets. The FDA continues:

> The food protein fragments responsible for an allergic reaction are not broken down by cooking or by stomach acids or enzymes that digest food. These proteins can cross the gastrointestinal lining, travel through the bloodstream and cause allergic reactions throughout the body.

The timing and location of an allergic reaction to food is affected by digestion. For example, an allergic person may first experience a severe itching of the tongue or 'tingling lips'. Vomiting, cramps or diarrhoea may follow. Later, as allergens enter the bloodstream and travel throughout the body, they can cause a drop in blood pressure or eczema, or asthma when they reach the lungs. The onset of these symptoms may vary from a few minutes to an hour or two after the food is eaten.

Over 170 foods have been documented in the scientific literature as causing allergic reactions.[133] Most sufferers are affected by the so-called 'big eight': milk, eggs, soya, wheat, peanuts, shellfish, fruits and tree nuts, which between them account for the great majority of food allergies.[134] Cows' milk is known to be a risk factor for many allergic conditions such as asthma and eczema.[135] The most common foods linked to eczema are cows' milk and eggs.

Pending legislation on allergens in manufactured foods, the UK Institute of Food Science & Technology makes the following recommendations for label warnings (to take the example of dairy): 'where calcium caseinate is the MSA (major serious allergen) concerned, the warning should read "Contains MILK PROTEIN". It would be helpful to the purchaser to add to this category of warning the words "to which some people may be allergic"'.[136]

Let me quote from an article in the *Sunday Times*[137] on the role of milk in allergies.

Hippocrates, the father of medicine, swore by milk-exclusion diets for curing all sorts: enfeebled babies, diarrhoea, skin complaints, wheezing, painful joints ... As Hippocrates suspected, the white stuff [milk] is the commonest cause of childhood allergies. Standard medical advice is that such allergies usually desist by the age of three. But in a recent Finnish study, two thirds of a group of 56 infants diagnosed with cows'-milk allergy were still allergic and highly symptomatic at the age of 10. Other studies show that many children are milk allergic but don't know it. Reactions include runny noses, wheezing, coughing, ear infections, rashes and stomach upsets. When milk is withdrawn from their diet, symptoms improve or clear altogether, and reintroducing it leads to relapse in the majority. The chief culprits appear to be lactose and bovine protein.

Diabetes

Recent studies strongly support earlier studies indicating a link between early and adolescent exposure to cows' milk and type-1 diabetes.[138] According to Campbell,[139] the ability of CMP to initiate type I diabetes is now well documented, with many recent studies strongly confirming the danger of cow's milk especially for genetically susceptible children.

Dirty milk and infectious illnesses

Since I wrote the first edition of this book, in which I documented the problem of the contamination of milk by *Mycobacterium paratuberculosis* (MAP), it has made headlines in prestigious newspapers in Britain. For example, an article in the *Sunday Times* discussed links between (MAP) and Britain's 80,000 cases of Crohn's disease.[140] Recent new molecular studies support a causal link between MAP and Crohn's disease.[141] Moreover, up to 7 per cent of samples of pasteurised milk in the UK have been found to contain MAP, increasing at times to 25 per cent.[142] The UK FSA has responded by introducing a strategy to reduce the risk of consuming dairy, but this does not consider other routes of exposure. It has been suggested that drinking water or inhaling particles contaminated by cows' faeces was responsible for a cluster of cases of Crohn's disease on watersheds around Cardiff.[143]

The *Sunday Times* article goes on to describe serious outbreaks of food poisoning also involving pasteurised milk which, in one case, affected sixty people, killing one child and requiring a second child to have a kidney transplant. Hugh Pennington, Professor of Microbiology at Aberdeen University, who traced the outbreak to milk contaminated by manure-related *E. coli* 0157 bacteria, is quoted as saying 'There have been enough problems with milk in recent years to show there is an issue here. Most of the time farmers will get away with dirty milk, but when things go wrong it can be disastrous.' As with Crohn's disease, there is evidence that exposure to *E. coli* is increasingly from cows and sheep via the environment, as a result of contact with animal faeces or water contaminated with faeces.[144]

Drinking milk contaminated with bovine tuberculosis can cause infected glands in children's necks. Bovine tuberculosis now affects more than 700 herds annually in the UK, following the fiasco of the Krebs trial into the extent that badgers are responsible for spreading the disease. There is a simple answer to the problem: remove all the cows and save the health and wealth of the nation. Keep the badgers instead, as there appears to be no evidence of transmission of tuberculosis from badgers to humans.

Most food-poisoning cases in the UK are caused by consuming contaminated meat or dairy products.[145] The dairy industry contributes to the spread of many other nasty infectious illnesses such as brucellosis, leptospirosis (Weil's disease) and cryptosporidium (a malaria-like parasite resistant to normal water disinfection processes, which is now affecting even some of our major groundwater sources), not to mention BSE and new-variant CJD.

Unfortunately, many harmful man-made chemicals which the body cannot distinguish from natural substances also become concentrated in milk. See further in Chapter Six, Lifestyle Factor 6.

Osteoporosis and dairy

Dairy is strongly and wrongly promoted as protecting against osteoporosis. Indeed, the most commonly asked questions from those recommended to adopt a dairy-free diet are 'Won't I get osteoporosis?' or 'Won't my osteoporosis get worse if I stop eating dairy products?' or 'Where do I get my calcium from?' The marketing of dairy produce as an essential source of calcium has been so strong that even some medical professionals, who should know better, insist that eliminating dairy produce from the diet will lead to calcium deficiency and hence increase the risk of osteoporosis. The scientific evidence shows that this is the opposite of the truth. For many people, cheese is likely to be part of the cause, not the cure, of osteoporosis. The widely available scientific evidence on the real causes of osteoporosis, presented in *Understanding, Preventing and Overcoming Osteoporosis*,[146] appears to have made little impact on conventional thinking. We were unable to find a single website from an orthodox medical source, national or international agency or charity that does not recommend dairy as a source of calcium and protection against osteoporosis. Our book presents evidence from the peer-reviewed scientific literature which strongly and convincingly refutes this.

I shall quote here from John Robbins' best-selling book *Diet for a New America*:[147]

> The [US] National Dairy Council has spent tens of millions of dollars to make us think that osteoporosis can be prevented by drinking more milk and eating more dairy products. **But the only research that even begins to suggest that the consumption of dairy products might be helpful has been paid for by the National Dairy Council itself.**

Hegsted's work published in 1986 showed a clear link between excessive amounts of calcium consumed as dairy produce in the diet and increased osteoporosis.[148] He showed that excessively high intakes of calcium consumed over a long time impair the body's ability to control the activity of the activated form of vitamin D, calcitrol. This in turn controls calcium absorption from food, how much is laid down in bones and how much is excreted. According to Campbell,[149] ruining the body's calcium regulatory mechanism in this way is a recipe for osteoporosis in menopausal and post-menopausal women.

The WHO advises that osteoporosis is not a disease of calcium deficiency and Campbell in *The China Study* gives the same advice that I have given: that staying physically active, keeping salt to a minimum and eating plant foods while avoiding animal produce especially dairy is the best way to prevent osteoporosis.

Other problems

There have been several studies recently that link dairy to a wide range of other illness and conditions. In 2005 a paper published in the *Journal of the American Academy of Dermatology* linked teenage acne directly to the consumption of dairy.[150] Moreover, dairy produce such as cheese, butter and whole-milk products supply so much saturated fat that they are now officially classified as junk foods in the UK (*see* Chapter Five). No dairy products contain any fibre at all. It is therefore perhaps not surprising that recent research has confirmed the link between the consumption of cows' milk and constipation.[151] For the same reasons, vegans have healthier levels of cholesterol, LDL and HDL in their blood than vegetarians who consume dairy products[152] and are therefore at significantly lower risk of cardiovascular disease. Recent research also shows that milk intake is associated with increased risk of developing Parkinson's disease. There was a 2.3-fold excess of Parkinson's disease in those consuming more than 16 oz of dairy a day compared to non-milk drinkers.[153]

Let me finish with a statement from a review of an earlier edition of this book, posted on the Amazon.com website by a physician in the USA: 'In my practice I see so many patients with acid reflux disease, asthma, frequent migraine headaches, feeling tired all the time. As soon as we stop the milk and related products their improvement is remarkable. I think it does not make sense that millions of our citizens take medications for the above-mentioned disorders and do not follow a common sense approach by discontinuing milk products and giving themselves a chance to feel better naturally. I switch all my patients from milk to soy on their first visit and in one week they feel the difference.'

For further information on the problems of dairy foods you may wish to update yourself regularly using the website of the AntiDairy Coalition, http://www.antidairycoalition.com.

CHAPTER 4 IN A NUTSHELL

- There is no scientific evidence that we need to consume milk after weaning – indeed, we are the only species that intentionally does so.
- Drinking the milk of another species is a fairly recent practice, dating back only about 6,000 years in Europe and central Asia, a practice not followed until recently by most of the rest of the world.
- Seventy per cent of people in the world, more than 90 per cent of the populations of some Asian countries, remain intolerant to lactose (milk sugar).
- There is still an enormous variation in the consumption of dairy products. People in most Western countries consume more than 250 kg a year, compared with at most a few kg in oriental countries, such as China, Vietnam and Thailand, and many African countries, where rates of breast and ovarian cancer are among the lowest in the world.

- Milk from every mammal contains hormones, growth factors and other powerful biochemicals.
- Cow's milk has been shown to contain over 35 different hormones and 11 growth factors, including IGF-I and EGF which are implicated in promoting cancer. Casein, the main milk protein, has been shown to protect such substances contained in milk from being broken down during digestion and much evidence now shows that circulating levels of growth factors such as IGF-I are higher in those that consume dairy.
- The concern is that by absorbing extra quantities of such highly bioactive substances from milk and/or the meat of animals used for dairy production on a daily basis there could be undesirable growth and differentiation of tissues in the human body, leading to cancer. Increased circulating levels of IGF-I have been shown to increase the risk of breast cancer, prostate cancer, and many other types of cancer, including colorectal cancer. Evidence also suggests that high circulating levels of IGF-I stimulate the body to produce levels of oestrogen or testosterone more appropriate for teenagers than post-menopausal women or post-andropausal men.
- The main dietary source of oestrogen, progesterone and prolactin is dairy produce and there is also overwhelming evidence that oestrogen levels are a critical determinant of breast-cancer risk. Lifetime exposure to dietary oestrogen was shown to be at least 2.5 to 3.0 times higher among Western women than in rural Chinese women, while progesterone levels were also increased with higher levels of prolactin in women between 55 and 64 years of age. This is associated with early onset of puberty and late menopause, two of the main risk factors for breast cancer.
- Studies carried out in 1987 that suggested a strong link between consumption of dairy and ovarian-cancer risk have been confirmed by recent studies.
- Absorbing growth factors and hormones through the diet preferentially favours initiated cancer cells, which have damaged grow and don't-grow genes – those least able to deal with growth factors – and hence promotes cancer.
- Many of the growth factors, hormones and other biochemicals contained in dairy milk are implicated not only in the

development of breast cancer and ovarian cancer but also testicular cancer and prostate cancer as well as non-reproductive cancers such as colorectal cancer.

- Many scientists believe that the amount of dairy produce in our diet is now far too high and that its quality has changed greatly.

- In today's large-scale intensive dairy farms, cows are pregnant and milked for most of the year. During pregnancy, the cow's ovaries secrete high levels of progesterone and the placenta high levels of oestrogen, with the result that hormone levels in milk have increased markedly.

- Moreover, intensive dairying has increased the average milk yield per cow from nine litres (16 pints) a day to a staggering 22 litres (39 pints) a day, also greatly increasing levels of IGF-I in dairy produce.

- Consuming dairy products is implicated in many other diseases, including allergies, auto-immune diseases, diabetes, osteoporosis and Parkinson's disease.

Update to Chapter 5. The Food Factors

Let your food be your medicine and your medicine be your food.

Hippocrates

In the first edition of this book I described seven food factors to help you to prevent and overcome breast cancer. In this edition there are ten food factors to help prevent and treat both breast cancer and ovarian cancer.

THE POTENTIAL OF PREVENTION

Let me begin by stating the potential for cancer prevention generally, as presented in the major report *Food, Nutrition and the Prevention of Cancer: a Global Perspective*, published by the World Cancer Research Fund and the American Institute for Cancer Research.[1] The report reviewed more than 4,500 research studies and involved more than 120 scientists, including from the WHO, the FAO and the US National Cancer Institute. Their conclusions were as follows:

- Eating right, plus staying physically active and maintaining a healthy weight, can cut cancer risk by 30 to 40 per cent.
- Recommended dietary choices, coupled with not smoking, have the potential to reduce cancer risk by 60 to 70 per cent.
- As many as 375,000 cases of cancer, at current cancer rates, could be prevented each year in the USA through healthy dietary choices.
- A simple change, such as eating the recommended five servings of fruits and vegetables each day, could by itself reduce cancer rates more than 20 per cent.

All this agrees closely with the advice of the American-based Physicians Committee for Responsible Medicine[2] of distinguished nutritional and medical scientists such as T. Colin Campbell and John McDougall in the USA, and of nutritionists such as Patrick Holford in the UK. It also agrees with the science-based recommendations on diet and lifestyle in this and my other books.[3] Quite simply, a healthy diet is based on pulses, whole-grain cereals, nuts, seeds, fruit and vegetables, and other foods of plant origin.

The evidence that a diet with lots of fruit and vegetables is preventive against cancer continues to increase. One review of more than 250 studies found that the data overwhelmingly support an inverse association between consumption of fruit and vegetables and cancer risk.[4]

Research in this field is currently focused on identifying biomarkers, such as DNA damage, rather than overt cancer, to allow less expensive trials of shorter duration to be carried out. An example of a useful biomarker for diet is the level of carotenoids in a person's blood as a measure of their fruit and vegetable intake.[5] Even the Beef USA factsheet,[6] aimed at promoting beef and dairy as sources of conjugated linoleic acid (CLA) as anti-carcinogens, states, 'Of the vast number of naturally occurring substances, demonstrated to have anti-carcinogenic activity, all but a very few are of plant origin.'[7] Another source states that CLA is the *only* known antioxidant/anti-carcinogen associated with animal foods.[8]

The numerous components in vegetables and fruit thought to contribute to the reduced risk of cancer include dietary fibre, vitamins, minerals and various phytochemicals (i.e. plant chemicals) including those that act as antioxidants. Phyto-oestrogens have a role in hormone-dependent cancers such as breast cancer and ovarian cancer. Many fruits and vegetables from beetroot to pomegranates and from mandarin oranges to watercress are now being marketed as superfoods! In contrast, animal foods lack any fibre and contain saturated fat, cholesterol and, of course, animal protein, as well as hormones and growth factors, all of which are associated with increased risk of cancer.[9]

Table 5.1 shows the relationship between phytochemicals in plant foods and their suggested modes of action.

It has been known for at least the last 20 years that breast cancer and ovarian cancer have a significant dietary basis. In the case of breast cancer there is overwhelming evidence of the role of oestrogen in increasing risk[10] and a 17 per cent increase in oestrogen levels has been shown to dramatically increase rates of the disease.[11] As discussed in the update to Chapter Four, the most significant source of oestrogen in this diet is dairy produce, the remainder being derived from other animal produce such as meat. All of the evidence supports the case for a change to a predominantly plant-based diet to prevent breast cancer and ovarian cancer and other types of cancer, as proposed in this book and elaborated in *The Plant Programme*.

Table 5.1: Food sources of phytochemicals and proposed mechanisms of action

Phytochemical	Food	Proposed mechanism(s) of action
Allicin Diallyl sulfide S-allyl-L-cysteine	Garlic Onions	Inhibits enzymes that activate cancer-causing chemicals (carcinogens) Stimulates enzymes that detoxify carcinogens
Catechins	Tea (green)	Antioxidant
Ellagic acid	Grapes Strawberries	Antioxidant
Flavonoids: Citrus – Diosmin and Hesperidin Noncitrus – Genistein and Daidzein (Phyto-oestrogens)	Grapefruit juice Orange juice Apples Grapes (red) Soya	Decreases levels of biochemicals that influence cell growth and proliferation Antioxidant Blocks oestrogen and androgen hormones from binding to their receptors (retarding cell proliferation)
Indoles	Cabbage Turnips	Increases conversion of oestrogens to inactive forms Stimulates enzymes that increase carcinogen detoxification
Isothiocyanates	Cruciferous vegetables	Inhibits enzymes that activate carcinogens Stimulates enzymes that detoxify carcinogens

Table 5.1: *Continued*

Phytochemical	Food	Proposed mechanism(s) of action
Lignans	Flaxseed and grains	Prevents oestrogen and prostaglandin hormones from binding to their receptors (retarding cell proliferation)
Lutein and Zeaxanthin	Kale Okra Romaine lettuce Spinach	Antioxidant
Lycopene	Tomatoes Watermelon	Antioxidant
Monoterpenes: Limonene	Lemon peel Orange peel	Decreases cell proliferation by decreasing activity of ornithine decarboxylase (ODC), an enzyme that helps trigger cancer Decreases activity of growth-promoting proteins Prevents expression of oncogenes Stimulates enzymes that detoxify carcinogens
Phenols	Berries Grapes Mustard Tea Turmeric Sesame seeds	Antioxidant Inhibits formation of carcinogens such as nitrosamines Stimulates enzymes that detoxify carcinogens

Table 5.1: *Continued*

Phytochemical	Food	Proposed mechanism(s) of action
Phytate	Grains Nuts Seeds Soya beans	Inhibits cell proliferation and the spread of cancer cells (metastasis)
Polyphenols	Artichokes	Antioxidant Stimulates enzymes that detoxify carcinogens
Protease Inhibitors	Dried beans Lentils Soya beans	Antioxidant Inhibits transformation of normal cells into cancerous ones Inhibits expression of certain genes and cellular processes that promote cancer
Sulforaphane	Broccoli	Stimulates enzymes that detoxify carcinogens

Adapted from the MD Anderson Practice Guidelines on Nutrition and Cancer Risk Reduction.[97]

DIET AS TREATMENT

When I wrote the first edition of this book, some conventional doctors agreed that the available evidence suggested that the risk of women developing breast cancer or ovarian cancer could be reduced by changing to a regime like the Plant Programme. They maintained, however, that once cancer had developed, changing diet would not help to treat the cancer or prolong survival, and that to do so could be detrimental.[12] This view is not evidence-based. There is only one small study into diet and cancer survival, and that shows improvement in early prostate cancer following dietary change (see below). Other studies have been started in the US, where it is now recognised that more scientific evidence on the role of dietary changes in cancer survival is needed (*see* further in Chapter Seven).

I disagree strongly with the advice of doctors who argue, without any scientific evidence, that changing diets has no influence on outcomes in cancer treatment. This is contrary to the reports I receive from breast-cancer and ovarian-cancer sufferers and my experience of working with people with these diseases, even at an advanced stage. The conventional medical view fails to understand that removing the factors that favour the promotion of cancer will help treatment. Moreover, evidence is accumulating that dietary changes can help to treat cancer. T. Colin Campbell in his book *The China Study*[13] reports animal experiments published in some of the most prestigious scientific journals in which diets rich (more than 20 per cent) in protein (specifically the cows' milk protein, casein), promoted several types of cancer after initiation, but the disease regressed dramatically when the dietary intake of animal protein was reduced to less than 5 per cent. Campbell states in his book 'Like flipping a light switch on and off we could control cancer promotion merely by changing levels of protein, regardless of initial carcinogen exposure.' A study of the effects of changes in diet and lifestyle has been carried out on men with early prostate cancer who were not undergoing conventional surgery, chemotherapy or radiotherapy at the Preventive Medicine Institute in California. This showed clearly that those who changed to a diet like the Plant Programme, consisting mainly of fruit, vegetables, whole-grain cereals and legumes, supplemented with soya, had a 10 per cent lower PSA level than the control group and the level of cancer inhibitors in their blood was eight times higher than that of patients keeping to a typical Western diet.[14]

Nevertheless, I emphasise that the Plant Programme is meant to complement, not replace, conventional medical treatment.

JUNK SCIENCE AND SOUND SCIENCE

No intelligent doctor should object to any of the scientifically based recommendations of the Plant Programme. It includes a diet packed with healthy, natural, nutritious food. So why is it that when you mention using diet to complement your treatment for cancer there can be such a negative,[15] or at best a lukewarm, response from many doctors?

I think there are several reasons for this. First, some people follow diets that are so strict and extreme that they become undernourished at a time when they need all their strength. In extreme cases they may even have been persuaded to use diet instead of conventional medicine to treat their cancer – advice I strongly disagree with. Frequently, cancer patients have been recommended by their alternative practitioner to follow a diet that eliminates all wheat products, potatoes, tomatoes, peppers and other vegetables belonging to the deadly nightshade family and all fruit on the grounds that it contains sugar; increasingly they are told not to have soya products. None of this has any scientific basis. The same practitioners that recommend such diets frequently sell their own synthetic chemical versions of vitamins and minerals and a range of wacky extracts often at exorbitant prices (see further in Chapter Six, Lifestyle Factor 1). Such an approach is likely to be unhelpful and even make matters worse, and the advice to cut down on vegetables such as tomatoes and fruit demonstrates their total ignorance of the peer-reviewed scientific literature.

There is also much confusing advice in anti-cancer diet books and magazines. One such book suggests avoiding parsnips, broad beans, pumpkins, honey, watermelon, pineapple, couscous and muesli (all excellent foods as part of an anti-cancer diet) because they are said to promote cancer by stimulating insulin production. This is nonsense! The problem is insulin-like growth factors, not insulin!

Some books claim that yoghurt is protective, while others group soya, rice and vegetable milks with goat's milk. One recently published book even claims that low-fat dairy is protective against breast cancer and states that those who say anything to the contrary do not understand science. Her evidence appears to be based mainly on one flawed study funded by the UK dairy industry (*see* Update to Chapter Seven). The person making these bold statements however is not a research scientist, she is an NHS dietician who appears not to have much of a grasp of science. There must be serious concern for anyone taking her advice.

All this is junk science and it causes serious problems in using diet to prevent and treat cancer. First, it eliminates cancer-protective foods from the diet: for example, tomatoes which contain lycopene, shown in many studies to be anti-cancer. Secondly, it diverts attention from the real culprit foods such as dairy products that internationally renowned nutritional scientists and doctors agree promote cancer. Thirdly, it causes confusion, which is used by producers of cancer-promoting foods to keep pushing their dangerous produce (*see* further in the Update to Chapter Seven).

The Plant Programme is based on sound science from the peer-reviewed scientific literature and it follows the principles of diets that have been studied by teams of internationally renowned scientists from universities that are centres of excellence such as Oxford in the UK and Cornell in the USA.[16] Such diets have been found to prevent not only breast cancer and ovarian cancer and the other 'cancers of affluence' such as colorectal cancer and pancreatic cancer but also a host of other diseases. These include type 1 and type 2 diabetes, cardiovascular disease and strokes, osteoporosis, food poisoning, kidney disease, and a whole range of auto-immune diseases including hyperthyroidism and multiple sclerosis as outlined in *Eating For Better Health*.[17]

BACKGROUND TO THE DIET

The food factors that follow are based on the principles of the Chinese diet. The recipes in *The Plant Programme* and *Eating for Better Health* are designed to accompany the food factors, with recipes adapted to suit Western tastes. All the recipes contain high levels of foods known to be protective against breast cancer and ovarian cancer and other types of cancer and to contain no foods known to promote these diseases. The recipes are delicious – and are also practical and easy to make for busy people.

Before discussing the food factors further, I want to tell you a little more about the Chinese diet. This has evolved over thousands of years of observation and practical experience and has been thoroughly documented and referenced. It is not a new fad diet based on the latest single-issue biochemical theory, but has evolved over more than 5,000 years as a sustainable system of nutrition and agriculture by one of the most biologically successful people on Earth.

In Japan, where the traditional diet is similar to that of China, a healthy diet is believed to be based on eating at least thirty different ingredients a day. Compare this with the diet of the average American, for whom 40 per cent of all they consume is dairy.

THE CHINESE WAY

In some parts of China, less than 3 per cent of the population under 65 years of age die from any form of cancer, breast cancer is rare and ovarian cancer is almost unknown. Although cancers such as stomach cancer are more prevalent in China,[18] they are attributed to chronic infections rather than diet.

The Chinese diet has been handed down from generation to generation using the pictogram system of writing, which was developed early in their history. Chinese writing has evolved progressively into the sophisticated system in use today (an educated person in China is expected to know at least 10,000 different pictograms) and, like the diet that is recommended here, continued to evolve.

Legend in China describes how Emperor Shen Nung, revered as the founder of Chinese agriculture, set out in 3494 BC to discover the healing properties of plants. Each day he would taste various plants to determine their properties – poisoning himself several times in the process, so that he also had to find many antidotes. This story of Emperor Shen Nung may well be a metaphor for the trial and error method of the discovery of the properties of plants, but there is little doubt that Chinese agriculture and medicine are derived from knowledge accumulated over the last 5,000 years. It is worth recalling that China had reached a considerable level of sophistication while the British Isles were emerging from the Stone Age.

To those used to modern Western science and medicine, some concepts basic to the Chinese approach to diet, such as balancing yin and yang foods, may sound strange, but the observations provide excellent responses to nutritional and environmental problems and have sustained the Chinese population for thousands of years. The Chinese diet has been shown to be one of the healthiest diets in the world.[19]

It is this kind of well-tried, observation-based traditional diet, particularly from China and other parts of South East Asia that is the basis of the food factors described here.

FOOD FACTOR 1: FROM DAIRY TO SOYA

Soya consumption has been shown to be inversely related to breast cancer risk.[20] As discussed on pages 128–129, it contains a wealth of anti-cancer agents and helps to prevent the spread of cancer generally.

Since the publication of the first edition of this book in 2000, there have been many attacks on soya (frequently on untraceable and unattributable websites), even suggesting that soya causes cancer. Such is the scare campaign that some men even express concern to me that eating the phyto-oestrogens in soya will feminise them. Many of the questions put to me express concern about these issues. So what are the facts? First we need to learn about the different types of oestrogens that we are exposed to.

Phyto(plant)-hormones, xeno(stranger)-hormones and animal hormones – the good, the bad and the deadly

There is a consensus among mainstream scientists that phyto(plant)-hormones are protective against hormone-dependent cancer, and this is discussed further below.

It is worth noting here that there are two groups of hormones to which we are exposed that can increase cancer risk: animal hormones such as oestrogen and progesterone, and man-made chemical hormone mimics known as xeno(stranger)-hormones. The former are overwhelmingly from dairy in our diet (*see* Chapter Four), while the latter are from pesticides, plastics and detergents in consumer products and contaminants in the environment (*see* further in Chapter Six, Lifestyle Factor 6).

It is also worth noting that, in experiment after experiment, casein (cows' milk protein) has been shown to promote cancer whereas soya protein has no such effect. In *The China Study*, Campbell describes the powerful effects of casein on cancer promotion and then states 'So the next logical question was whether plant protein tested in the same way has the same effect on cancer promotion as casein. The answer is an astonishing "NO"' (the capitals are his). Neither soya nor wheat protein were found to promote cancer, even at the highest levels of intake. In fact, the phyto-oestrogens in soya are particularly helpful in all cases of hormone-dependent cancers, such as breast cancer and ovarian cancer, because they block receptor sites for hormones and growth factors in the cell or on the cell surface.

Recently there have been attempts to relaunch yoghurt as a probiotic, with no mention of dairy, but this is the type of dairy that has been known to be a particular problem since Cramer's work, published 20 years ago in 1987. Also, remember that low-fat organic yoghurt was the only type of dairy I was consuming when I had repeated recurrences of cancer in 1993. Within six weeks of eliminating it from my diet, my cancer disappeared and has not returned 14 years later.

Anti-soya propaganda

The soya bean, just like all other beans and peas, is packed with phyto-oestrogens; and I do not know of any non-aligned scientists who believe that beans, especially soya beans, and peas in a diet such as the Plant Programme cause health problems. Moreover, despite exhaustive studies, there is no evidence that soya feminises males.[21] Certainly a lack of male potency and reproductive capacity does not appear to have been a problem in China or other oriental countries over the fifty centuries or so that they have used soya. Rather the reverse.

Gynaecomastia (man-boobs) is an increasingly important problem in the West. According to a recent article in The Times, 4,000 men had their man-boobs removed by plastic surgery in 2003 in the UK alone. There is even a dedicated website here, Man-breasts.co.uk. In all my years of working in China and other oriental countries I did not see a single man with boobs there although it is hard to avoid seeing men with them in the UK or US. Unfortunately they are becoming more apparent in China as they follow the Western diet. Man-boobs are far more likely to reflect intake of animal oestrogens, or xeno-oestrogens, than eating soya.

The argument that soya is carcinogenic centres on the fact that it contains phyto-oestrogens – but the fact is that most vegetables naturally contain phyto-oestrogens or substances that are converted to phyto-oestrogens in the gut. Such foods include berries such as strawberries, cranberries and bilberries, whole-grain cereals, seeds and spices, peanuts, cabbage, hops, tea and, of course, peas and beans (the legume family, to which soya belongs).[22] In general, phyto-oestrogens are found in the seeds, stems, roots or flowers of plants, serving as natural fungicides and acting as part of the plant's defence mechanism against micro-organisms.[23]

Phyto-oestrogens are chemically and structurally similar to the mammalian oestrogen, oestradiol, and have oestrogenic properties. However, their oestrogenic activity is much less than that of human oestrogens (their oestrogenic activity ranges from 1/500 to 1/1,000 of that of oestradiol), and they have been found to be protective against prostate cancer and other hormone-dependent cancers.[24] All the experiments on soya-bean phyto-oestrogens (isoflavones such as genistein) continue to indicate that such chemicals help prevent the growth of hormone-related cancers such as breast cancer and ovarian cancer by a variety of mechanisms.[25]

Much of the evidence used to attack soya is from animal experiments which appear deliberately designed to demonstrate some adverse effect of eating soya. For example in some experiments ridiculously large amounts of raw soya were fed to experimental animals. Marilyn Glenville[26] poses one of the key questions in relation to such 'research': 'Who eats raw soya anyway?'

In other experiments, laboratory animals are fed extracts of soya processed in aluminium vessels, which, it has been claimed, causes Alzheimer's disease, in such a way that the soya absorbs aluminium. Such soya isolates can turn up in soya 'meat' or 'cheese' products and as flavour enhancers in soups and sauces and other processed foods such as cakes, bread and biscuits. They are not present in the traditional whole-soya products such as natto, tempeh or bean curd (tofu) recommended in the Plant Programme. The 'scientists' behind the scare stories also seem unaware that the association of Alzheimer's disease and aluminium has long been discounted in favour of a link with a protein called beta amyloid which forms plaques in the brain. Most respected non-aligned scientists think that the plaques are formed as a result of eating a diet too high in animal protein such as dairy and meat.[27]

It would make sense that the anti-soya campaign is led by vested interest groups such as the dairy industry. Marilyn Glenville in her book *The New Natural Alternatives to HRT*,[28] which recommends soya to treat menopausal symptoms, states 'the good publicity for soya tends to alarm another section of industry, the pharmaceutical giants who stand to lose a lot of money if alternatives to HRT are found. The dairy industry, which would lose out if the population shifts to soya instead of milk and other dairy produce, is also affected.'

Of course, the dairy industry have tried to fight back, and as their propaganda about the need for dairy calcium to prevent osteoporosis increasingly founders,[29] they have latched on to the presence of substances called CLAs in dairy products and the meat of ruminant animals such as cows and sheep, which they claim to be preventive against cancer. CLAs are natural derivatives of the essential fatty acid, linoleic acid, which is found in vegetable seeds and the oils produced from them, such as soya. Interestingly, the dairy industry is trying to increase the amount of CLA in milk by adding extracted whole soya-bean and linseed oils to a corn-alfalfa diet.[30] As queried in an article in the *Sunday Times*,[31] how much artery-clogging saturated fat would we have to consume (as dairy) to have enough CLAs to be protected against cancer?

One final question
If soya is so bad for health why is so much used to feed dairy cows and why is it being used to improve the nutritional quality of cow's milk?

The Japanese rule
At this point I would like to re-emphasise that simply adding soya to a typical dairy-rich Western diet will *not* decrease breast-cancer or ovarian-cancer risk. It is absolutely essential to eliminate ALL animal dairy produce, including 'hidden dairy' such as casein whey and lactose. Other vegetable milks, creams and yoghurts, besides soya, are all OK, including coconut, rice, oat and pea milks, but I recommend only organically produced GM-free products.

I also emphasise that I am not advocating that people live on an entirely soya-based diet, and I continue to recommend the Japanese principle, on which *The Plant Programme* cookbook is based, of eating at least thirty different food substances every day. I also agree with the advice of the American Cancer Society that eating a balanced diet should include five or more servings a day of fruit and vegetables (though I think it should be much more – see Food Factor 2), along with foods from a variety of other plant sources, such as cereals, legumes, seeds and nuts; this is more effective than consuming one particular food in large amounts.[32]

Just one word of warning about soya: along with many other vegetables such as turnips, broccoli and brussel sprouts, it contains substances called goitrogens which can cause the thyroid to be underactive, so ensure that you take your kelp tablets (*see* p. 200) to counteract the effects of goitrogens on the thyroid, and be especially careful if you have hypothyroidism. There is further information on goitrogenic foods and thyroid disease in *Eating for Better Health*.

FOOD FACTOR 2: VITAL VEGETABLES AND FREQUENT FRUIT

Vegetables and fruit are the energy foods we evolved to eat. They are packed with healthy antioxidants, vitamins and minerals, fibre, live enzymes and other good-for-health phytochemicals – which help to fight cancer. There is no dispute about their health benefits among mainstream scientists.

The US National Cancer Institute has launched a publicity campaign to boost fruit and vegetable consumption from the 'bare minimum' of five servings a day to nine servings a day. Only 4 per cent of men in the US consume nine servings. More than a third of the population eat only one or two servings, and 4 per cent eat less than that.[33] The official recommendation of five portions a day, especially when each portion can comprise a glass of (commercial) fruit juice and a tablespoon of dried fruit,[34] was always completely inadequate.

Based on this new information and many other findings described below, the second food factor is to increase the amount of vegetables and fruit you consume. The evidence that an abundant intake of vegetables and fruit can play an important role in reducing cancer incidence is becoming overwhelming.[35] The only people who recommend elimination of either fruit or vegetables from the diet now are fringe practitioners ignorant of the scientific literature.

Anti-cancer chemicals

The list of anti-cancer chemicals identified in vegetables and fruit just keeps on growing (Table 5.1). Indeed an increasing number of chemotherapy agents are purified plant alkaloids.

In addition to the phyto-oestrogens discussed above, plant-derived foods contain thousands of other phytochemicals, many of which have been investigated in laboratory and clinical studies to determine their effects on cancer risk and their mechanisms of action.[36] The Division of Cancer Prevention of the US National Cancer Institute is currently sponsoring more than 65 chemoprevention trials, many of them concerned with food substances in relation to particular cancers. They include, for example, three trials of lycopene in preventing prostate cancer.[37] Salvesterol, which is concentrated in fruits such as tangerines, has been found to inhibit the enzyme CYP IBI which occurs in cancer cells but not normal cells, and this substance as well as bromelain in pineapple and papain in papaya are protease inhibitors which means they can damage cancer proteins.

In general, the outcomes of studies into protective substances in fruit and vegetables highlight the difficulty of identifying single dietary components such as beta-carotene as chemopreventive agents (*see* further discussion in Chapter Six, Lifestyle Factor 1).[38] This may be because substances such as beta-carotene are simply biomarkers for other protective components of vegetables and fruit, or because it may not react in the same way when separated from the chemicals with which it is associated in natural food substances.

Eating your greens and other colours

Recent research has provided new evidence in favour of my rainbow rule of eating as many different coloured vegetables as possible.[39] Include lots of salad vegetables, and make sure they are fresh and ripe. Most vegetables and fruit include such vitamins as beta-carotene (which is the precursor of vitamin A and is especially rich in yellow and orange vegetables such as carrots, saffron, red and yellow peppers, pumpkins and sweet potatoes, and fruit such as peaches, cherries and apricots, including the dried variety). It has long been suggested that beta-carotene protects against several forms of cancer, including by acting as an antioxidant. Other vegetables and fruit also contain other carotenoids such as lycopene, vitamin C (in most fresh or very lightly cooked vegetables and fruit) and vitamin E (in most fresh fruit and vegetables), which counteract the activity of free radicals and stop our tissues being damaged by them. Garlic and Brussels sprouts are also especially rich in antioxidants. The pigment in red vegetables and fruit – lycopene (which is enriched in tomatoes (especially cooked ones), pink grapefruit and red grapeskins) – is also a powerful antioxidant and may have other cancer-preventing properties. Lycopene binds to fats and lipids in the blood stream, protecting against some of the worst aspects of Western diets.

Increased consumption of tomatoes and products containing tomatoes has recently been shown to be associated with lower bioactive IGFs[40] supporting the results of earlier findings reported for Greek men.[41] Other good sources of natural lycopene include strawberries, red grapes, peaches, peppers and carrots. One large helping of freshly made tomato soup or red pepper soup contains masses of lycopene (see the easy-to-follow recipes in *The Plant Programme*). I recommend against tinned or packaged tomato soups, since they frequently contain cream, whey or other dairy products, and many tin cans are lined with a substance which can leach BPA, an endocrine-disrupting chemical (*see* p. 387). If you eat tinned baked beans, be very careful to read the label, because even some brands that claim to be in tomato sauce might be more accurately described as being in a milk or cream source.

Fresh red peppers, as well as being rich in lycopene, are a particularly good source of vitamin C, which strengthens the immune system and neutralises toxins. Other especially good sources of vitamin C include papaya, berries, cherries and all citrus fruits. Salad vegetables, especially watercress, and raw or lightly cooked broccoli are also good sources.

Good sources of folic acid include green leafy vegetables, avocado, beans, carrots, pumpkins, apricots, melons and newly sprouted shoots such as bean sprouts and alfalfa. We should *all* be eating a diet that has adequate quantities of folic acid without having to resort to taking pills (*see* Chapter Six, Lifestyle Factor 1). Drinking lots of juices rich in folic acid helped me to keep my hair during chemotherapy, though this does not work with some of the new chemotherapeutic agents with a different mode of action.

Protective phyto(plant)-oestrogens
Other rich sources of protective phytohormones, in addition to those listed on page 336, are wild yam (or sweet potato) and

fennel, which contain both phyto-oestrogens and phytoproges-terones. Flaxseed has a high content of lignans, which are converted in the digestive tract into substances that help to regulate endocrine function. Much research on flax has been carried out by the US Food and Drug Administration (FDA), the National Cancer Institute and the Canadian Food Protection Branch.[42] The recommendation is to take about one tablespoon a day of flaxseed in your diet for each 100 pounds of body weight (but be prepared to go to the loo more often!). As well as being a good source of phyto-oestrogens, seeds can be good sources of zinc, selenium and vitamin E. Sunflower and sesame seeds, especially when sprouted, can be particularly good sources of zinc, which helps vitamin C work and accelerates healing.

Some really powerful cancer-busters – are you getting enough?

There is increasing evidence that all cruciferous vegetables, as well as garlic, onions, leeks and chives are protective against cancer. They also contain good amounts of fibre, which helps to eliminate toxins, and have been shown to protect against both breast cancer and colorectal cancer.[43] Intake of vegetable fibre has been shown to reduce the risk of ovarian cancer, with a 37 per cent decrease for each additional 10 g a day consumed.[44]

You should have at least two to three raw cloves of fresh garlic a day to prevent and treat cancer and to ward off infectious illnesses when your immune system is impaired from cancer treatment. Many people worry about smelling of garlic but if everyone eats it, no one notices – just as everyone who has dairy products does not notice that they and others smell of sour milk (a much more unpleasant smell to me)! I have a friend who kept telling me that I smelt of garlic. I simply put on a worried face and replied 'Oh dear, if you can smell it that means you are not getting enough!' She doesn't comment any more.

Juices and smoothies

If you're thinking of cheating by drinking bottled or frozen juices instead of freshly made ones, there is simply no point. If you cut an apple, it immediately starts going brown (because it has oxidised), and what you need is the green unoxidised juice.

The same is true for all juices. If you buy commercial juices they will be far more oxidised and chemically far less potent as anti-cancer agents. Also, they may contain some type of preservative or have undergone some type of process to stop them going rotten (just think about it, how else could carrot juice be sold weeks after it is prepared?) so they will be chemically changed. The only exceptions are good frozen juices, not made from concentrates. I have discovered people with colon cancer changing the diet I recommend by eating vegetable pills instead of raw vegetables and their juices – a complete waste of time!

Smoothies have become very popular as a way of having fruit. They are delicious – but make your own with banana not dairy yoghurt as a thickener. I buy them only if they are in glass containers or are freshly made at a juice bar.

Soups, salads and stir fries

In addition to juices, I continue to have masses of fresh salads and vegetables including in soups and stir fries. Stir fries are delicious and a good way of persuading young people to eat vegetables, but try to avoid actually frying the food. Lightly sauté vegetables for just a few minutes in olive oil and then pop on a lid so the vegetables cook in their own juices

Let the wind go free

When you begin to follow the Plant Programme you are likely to suffer from 'wind', but don't worry – after a few weeks of the diet recommended here the body will adjust and you will have no further problems. My late mother-in-law, a wonderful Highland Scot with a great sense of humour who became Mayoress in the Borough of Southgate and a Justice of the Peace, knew a little rhyme that might help when you first change to the Plant Programme. It went like this:

Where'er ye be
Let the wind gang (go) free
Except at the kirk (church) or taking tea.

Remember to eat fresh, whole **fruit and vegetables as nature intended, not man-made pills or potions extracted from them.**

Also, remember to be like Chinese people and eat everything when it is as fresh and ripe as possible. This is much healthier than eating dead junk food and trying to make up the difference with synthetic chemicals sold as vitamin and mineral supplements.

Sea vegetables

Sea vegetables are especially valuable sources of nutrients such as calcium, magnesium and iodine. Seaweed also protects against radiation. Alginate, a mucous material extracted from seaweed, is a standard protective agent against radioactivity, so kelp and other seaweeds help reduce the side effects of X-rays and radiotherapy. Agar-agar, which is widely used to replace gelatine in vegan foods, can also be used in your diet as a source of iodine. Other seaweeds which I use include: arame, hiziki, dulse and wakame (which I add to some soups immediately before serving). Nori, which is commonly sold in sheets, can be used to wrap rice balls, sushi and many other foods. A lunch box containing this is available from at least one supplier of ready-to-eat meals – much better for you than grabbing a sandwich or baguette!

One final question

With all this accumulated evidence on the beneficial effects of vegetables and fruit in protecting against cancer and other diseases, why did it take so long for us to be told? (*See* Update to Chapter Seven for further discussion on this point.)

ORGANIC FOOD AND PESTICIDES

The establishment point of view

I'd like to tell you why we must continue to insist on as much high-quality organic food as possible, despite the efforts of organisations such as the Food Standards Agency when it was under the direction of Sir John Krebs to persuade us that there is no difference between organic and conventionally produced food.[45] The evidence of the presence of pesticide residues in conventionally produced food continues to mount, as do the beneficial effects of eating organic food. For example, a study published in 2006 demonstrated that an organic diet provides a dramatic and immediate protective effect against exposure to

organophosphate pesticides commonly used in food production.[46] Moreover, the synthetic nitrogen fertilisers used in
industrial agriculture leach into ground and surface water,
encouraging the spread of bacteria and toxins that may be
linked to some types of cancer.

I think it is particularly important to limit exposure to
harmful chemicals. I believe the food industry contributes
significantly to modern health problems with their widespread
use of chemical fertilisers, pesticides, plant and animal hormones and other veterinary medicines, and genetically modified crops, designed to survive being dowsed with herbicides
that kill other plants. Thus, even eating an apparently healthy
diet can lead to an increasing burden of man-made toxins, many
of which have not been properly assessed for their carcinogenicity, especially in the cocktail we consume.

The establishment view was that not more than 2 per cent of
cancers are attributable to the use of pesticides.[47] There is,
however, mounting evidence that many pesticide formulations
are endocrine-disrupting (see further below and in the Update
to Chapter Six) and are thus likely to increase the risk of
hormone-dependent cancers. Moreover, it has emerged recently that one of the authors of the key 1981 paper on chemical
exposure and cancer, Professor Sir Richard Doll, had a conflict
of interest, inasmuch as since 1979 he had been paid large sums
of money by pesticide manufacturers, which he failed to
declare.[48]

In July 2006 the EU stated 'Long term exposure to pesticides
can lead to serious disturbances to the immune system, sexual
disorders, cancers, sterility, birth defects, damage to the nervous system and genetic damage.'

Pesticides, endocrine disruption and cancer
In 1993 a distinguished American scientist, Theo Colborn,
coined the term endocrine-disrupting chemicals[49] to describe
chemicals that interfere with the functioning of the hormone
system by mimicking or blocking the action of hormones such
as oestrogen or testosterone. Endocrine-disrupting chemicals
are increasingly linked to hormone-dependent cancers such as
breast cancer and ovarian cancer. Recently more than 100
pesticides have been identified as having endocrine-disrupting
properties[50] and these are just the active ingredients. Many

pesticide formulations also contain other chemicals such as nonyl phenol ethoxylate (NPE), designed to achieve good dispersion of the active ingredients over crops. NPE is one of the most notorious endocrine-disrupting chemicals known,[51] and it is now being banned for use on food crops across Europe. One of the things that always occurs to me when this happens is how do all those who kept reassuring us that a substance was safe or that there is no benefit to eating organically produced food manage to keep their jobs when they are proved wrong? Because they are part of the establishment?

A study on women aged 55 or younger in one of Canada's largest fruit- and vegetable-growing regions showed that women who have worked on farms are up to nine times more likely to develop breast cancer than those who have never been employed in agriculture.[52] These findings raise further suspicions that the array of fungicides, herbicides and insecticides used on many farms is a factor in the 'huge increase in the rates of breast cancer' in Canada and may be responsible for at least some cases of breast cancer in the population as a whole.

According to McMichael,[53] there has been a 30-fold increase in global pesticide use and a nine-fold increase in chemical fertiliser use since the 1950s. This has increased food yield, but it has also caused widespread chemical pollution, destruction of wildlife and disturbance of ecosystems. In Western countries, millions of kilograms of pesticides are used each year for agricultural and non-agricultural applications, including forestry, landscaping, gardening, food distribution and home pest control.

Fortunately, in the UK, more than seventy such products, including some that were in use for growing vegetables, have recently been cleared from garden-centre shelves because they have been banned by the EU – but why did it take so long?! After banning DDT in the 1970s, followed by other organochlorines including the drins and many, many other pesticides, it might have been expected that there would have been a speedier reaction to limit our exposure. I am still left with the question: What are we still using today that in the future we shall find evidence to ban?

Avoiding the chemical nightmare
The alternative to the chemical nightmare of industrialised agriculture continues to be to buy organically produced food,

ideally grown to the standards of and policed by the UK Soil Association – their symbol is a circle with the words 'soil association' around the top and 'organic standard' round the bottom, and a sort of curly, triangular design inside the circle. I object to buying so-called organically produced food, produced to no particular standard, which is then expensively flown in to supermarkets from across the world – long-distance air transport causes pollution too.[54] Choosing food that carries symbols such as that of the Soil Association also means you will avoid genetically modified food. A recent report into the environmental performance of supermarkets by the UK National Consumer Council rated Sainsbury's and Waitrose best for organic food and responsible use of pesticides on non-organic produce. If you are unable to obtain good organically produced food at your local supermarket, use a search engine on the internet to identify local suppliers – who will often deliver to your door. If you cannot afford the additional expense of buying organically produced food for all your needs and cannot grow your own, make food that will not be cooked (such as salad vegetables and fruit) your spending priority, since at least some of the damaging chemicals in pesticides break down during cooking and processing.[55] See further in Update to Chapter Six, Lifestyle Factor 3.

A problem with some organically grown food such as peanuts stored in hot, humid conditions, usually in developing countries, is that it may be contaminated with high levels of carcinogenic fungal substances called aflatoxins, which, it is claimed, are killed off by the use of pesticides. If buying peanuts, simply buy them in their shells and discard the shells.

FOOD FACTOR 3: HEALTHY NOT WEALTHY PROTEINS

The first thing to say about protein is that in the West we generally eat far too much of it. Protein is needed only to repair our cells and tissues and it is quite unsuitable for energy generation. It is estimated that only 5 to 6 per cent of our daily calorie intake should be protein, with a maximum intake of about 10 to11 per cent. Many people in the West consume much more, some people having an unhealthy 20 per cent or more, especially those who followed the infamous Atkins diet. Too much animal protein such as cheese makes the body too acid, increasing the risk of a range of diseases from cancer to osteoporosis.

To make matters worse, much of the protein consumed is animal rather than vegetable protein. The Western diet, with its high content of animal protein, is linked to many of the cancers of affluence: prostate cancer, breast cancer, ovarian cancer, colorectal cancer and pancreatic cancer.[56] These diseases all have the highest incidence and mortality in wealthy Western countries and increase as wealth increases in developing countries, as their populations abandon their traditional diets in favour of the Western diet.

Undoubtedly one of the main differences between the Western and traditional oriental diets is the amount of animal protein in the former, while the latter is heavily based on foods of vegetable origin. So, if you wish to prevent breast, ovarian or other types of cancer, don't even think about going on a high-animal-protein diet to help weight loss. I advise people who have active cancer of the breast, ovary or colon to eliminate all animal produce from their diet until they are better, always ensuring that their diet is balanced. For other people, a small amount of animal protein in the diet is fine provided it is balanced by at least twice as much vegetable protein and lots of other vegetables and fruit as well.

It is worth remembering that all vegetable protein provides dietary fibre, whereas no animal protein has any. A good dietary fibre intake has been shown to be important in preventing ovarian cancer, colorectal cancer, diverticulitis, haemorrhoids and varicose veins. The association with colorectal cancer was first proposed by Professor Dennis Burkitt in the 1950s, based on his studies of African diets, and has recently been confirmed by the European Prospective Investigation of Cancer (EPIC) study, which found that those having the diets highest in fibre had a 43 per cent lower risk of developing the disease.

Soya has a complete range of amino acids, and other pulses such as peas and beans, cereals (see below) and nuts are also good sources of protein – without the unhealthy animal fat. All pulses are also very good sources of fibre, including a type that binds and inactivates free radicals in the gut and bloodstream. As discussed above, they are also valuable sources of phyto-oestrogens. Eat at least one good-sized portion a day.[57] Cereals are a good source of vegetable proteins, complementing those in pulses, and are discussed further under Food Factor 6. Another good protein source is nuts: I continue to eat lots.

Now my cancer is gone, I eat one small portion of animal protein (such as an organic egg) a day, although I always keep to a vegan diet for at least one day a week. I eat fish, but no more than once a week and only if it is wild or organically farmed, since this is less likely to contain antibiotic residues and other man-made pollutants. Oily fish such as salmon, herring and mackerel are rich in vitamin D, essential for healthy bones, and omega-3 fatty acids. Vitamins A and D, found in oily fish and in fish oils, may work to reduce the risk of breast cancer by lowering blood levels of IGF-I. I particularly avoid farmed trout, which may have been treated with steroid hormones to produce only female fish. If I eat salmon, I buy that produced to the standards of the Soil Association. This is much paler than most farmed salmon on the market, because it does not contain the artificial colouring agent which makes other farmed salmon so vividly pink; one such agent, canthaxanthin, has been implicated in damaging eyesight. The same additive is used to feed non-organically produced chickens to colour their skins and the yolks of their eggs.[58] Non-organically produced farmed fish can also contain antibiotic residues and toxic chemicals used to control sea lice and to prevent growth of other organisms on the cages in which the fish are kept. In the past, the latter have included tributyl tin, a powerful endocrine-disrupting chemical (see p. 109).

Fish-liver oil is a good source of omega-3 fatty acids and vitamins A and D – but ensure that you buy the ultra-pure varieties which have had harmful chemicals such as PCBs (see p. 220) extracted. I take a teaspoon of Seven Seas cod-liver oil a day, the type which is labelled 'original and ultrapure', which is slightly more expensive.

When I eat meat, I choose organically reared lamb or chicken, or wild game such as rabbit or venison. Game generally has higher levels of nutrients and far lower levels of fat than concentrate-fed animals which have led a sedentary life.

On page 163 I wrote 'If I were an American, I would never eat beef or pork unless it was absolutely guaranteed to be organically produced.' In 2006 research carried out by some of the world's leading epidemiologists at Harvard showed that eating red meat was linked to breast cancer, and it was suggested that this might reflect the hormone residues contained in the meat.[59] Although the use of all such hormones is banned throughout Europe, on a BBC Radio 4 programme, British pig farmers complained that European farmers were allowed to feed their animals on sewage sludge – a practice forbidden in Britain! The message is clear. If you wish to eat pork, bacon or ham, eat organically produced British products, especially from traditional rare breeds such as Gloucester Old Spot and Tamworth pigs. High intake of red or processed meat has also been shown to increase the risk of bowel cancer and stomach cancer.[60]

Populations such as the Eskimos living on a predominantly fish diet have long been known to have less breast cancer than those eating other animal foods.

Fish, chicken and eggs, especially fried eggs, have been shown to be associated with increased risk of fatal ovarian cancer.[61]

One valuable tip for those who like the taste of meat or fish but wish to cut down the amount they eat is based on my husband's experience as a young soldier in Nyasaland (now Malawi) in the 1950s. The African soldiers he was responsible for were very fit and healthy and ate a diet consisting mainly of 'Mzima' or mealy meal made from maize, flavoured with small amounts of 'Ndiwa' which was a sort of stew made from rabbit, chicken or fish with lots of vegetables. At mealtimes the Mzima was just dipped in the Ndiwa so that the overall amount of animal food was low but it flavoured most meals. You can easily copy this idea, for example, by making fish stew or spicy chicken with extra tomato and vegetables, and use the juice to flavour vegetable-based rice or pasta dishes over a few days.

In summary, I try to maximise the amount of vegetable protein and minimise the animal protein in my diet to cut my risk of suffering from any of the cancers of affluence or other chronic degenerative diseases linked to the Western diet. As for eating cheese and yoghurt – I don't even consider it!

FOOD FACTOR 4: OILS AND FATS

It is increasingly recognised that it is not the total fat in the diet that is associated with increased risk of hormone-dependent cancer, including breast cancer and ovarian cancer. What is significant is the amount of saturated fats, most of which are from animal sources (i.e. dairy products and meat) and trans fats.[62] New evidence confirms that high intakes of saturated fat increase the risk of breast cancer: women with the most fat in their diet doubled their risk.[63] Increased consumption of saturated fat is also associated with increased risk of ovarian cancer,[64] as is eating cholesterol from animal foods such as eggs.[65]

It is important to note that breast cancer and ovarian cancer are not the only human diseases that appear to be associated with dietary animal fat intake. High-animal-fat diets have also been correlated with prostate and colon cancer, heart disease and hypertension, and most cancer and heart charities recommend reduction in the amount consumed. Breast-cancer and ovarian-cancer patients and those people wishing to reduce their chances of developing these diseases would be wise to reduce their intake of animal fat to an absolute minimum.[66] Many people do not realise just how much fat there is in our food now. Intensively reared animals have much more saturated fat relative to protein than in the past, when animals could exercise and were fed natural foods. For example, the amount of saturated fat in chickens has increased from 2 per cent thirty years ago to 22 per cent now.[67]

Many people are confused about the type and quantity of oils and fat they should be eating. At a meeting on Cancer Prevention at Bethesda, USA, it was noted that the move towards lower dietary fat had failed to distinguish between unhealthy, saturated fats and healthy fats – and this matters. Apparently, some tomato sauces available in health-food stores have had olive oil removed so they could be labelled 'fat free'.[68] Also, we continue to be persuaded to buy spreads based on (usually altered and processed) polyunsaturated fats.

Yet, the advice against consuming trans fatty acids, which can be formed during the manufacture of margarine and which can be high in many bought cakes and biscuits, remains unchanged. Since January 2006, trans fats have to be listed on products sold in the USA and they have been banned in Denmark. In the UK, action appears to be being left to large retailers. Most spreads now state the amount of trans fatty acids they contain: one organic soya spread my family uses contains only trace quantities. The advice to eat polyunsaturated fats and to use olive oil for cooking remains the same as on pages 170–177.

FOOD FACTOR 5: SEASONING, FLAVOURING AND ADDITIVES

One of the most dramatic differences in our diet now compared with the end of World War II is the increase in fast and convenience foods. There are now more than 320,000 different processed foods and drinks on the market.[69] As well as preservatives to give it a long shelf life, such food frequently contains artificial flavouring and colouring agents. Eric Schlosser in *Fast Food Nation*, his book about the problems caused by the fast-food industry in America, recounts how the strawberry flavour in milkshakes sold by one outlet is prepared from more than 55 different artificial chemicals. Such chemical concoctions are used to give a consistent taste and improve the acceptability of low-cost food.

Overuse of salt and sodium bicarbonate was linked by Gerson to cancer and some researchers say that it promotes certain types of cancer.[70] Other common sources of sodium include monosodium glutamate, the 'extra meaty flavour' in cheap meat products and some soya sauces, and sodium sulphite used as a preservative in many wines. One London clinic actually gives out sodium bicarbonate to alkalise the body instead of adjusting the diet (see further below). Recent research by Djamgoz and his team at Imperial College, London[71] has shown that cancer cells metastasise more readily in the presence of sodium, so it is best to avoid concentrated sources such as salt added to food. After a time your body will cease to crave salt or 'extra meaty flavour'.

Instead, use herbs and spices to flavour food. Many anti-cancer diet books recommend against the use of spices, but Korean and Thai food, and food from Hunnan and Szechuan provinces in China, are very heavily spiced, and the rates of prostate and breast cancer there are exceptionally low. Many of the delicious recipes in *The Plant Programme* and *Eating for Better Health* include spices, since we are aware of the use of many spices as anti-cancer treatments in traditional Indian Ayurvedic and Chinese medicine. Turmeric, for example, one of the main ingredients of curry powder, contains curcumin, which has been shown to have powerful antioxidant and anti-cancer properties, suppressing the proliferation of cancer cells. Curcumin has even been shown to help prevent cancer cells producing their own growth factors, as they do in advanced cases of the disease. In particular, curcumin inhibits the growth of oestrogen-receptor-positive breast cancer.[72]

Celery seed, garlic, onions, ginger and turmeric contain substances which stimulate the activity of an important detoxifying enzyme GST (glutathione-S-transferase), and are useful for making delicious food.[73] Rosemary, sage, oregano and thyme are also strong antioxidants,[74] and rosemary and sage have documented anti-tumour activity.[75] Ginger contains more powerful antioxidants than even vitamin E,[76] and many other herbs and spices contain substances considered to be cancer-preventive agents.[77]

FOOD FACTOR 6: CEREAL FOODS, SNACKS AND TREATS

Eating good food is one of life's great pleasures, and the Plant Programme is not a hair-shirt regime! I eat sorbets and soya ice creams and organic dark dairy-free chocolate for occasional treats.

On the run, I often buy a lunch box full of delicious vegetable sushi from a Korean or Japanese shop for lunch or to snack on.

Whole-grain versus refined

Most cancer-prevention diets include plenty of whole-grain cereal foods such as bread and pasta.[78] Clearly if you are intolerant of or allergic to gluten you may need to avoid food and drink containing wheat, rye or barley, although many people can tolerate some gluten-containing foods better than others (wheat contains the most gluten). Good substitutes include rice and corn, and some new scientific evidence suggests that oats may be safe.[79]

Whole grains contain a wide range of phytochemicals that reduce the risk of cancer.[80] The active phytochemicals are concentrated in the bran and the germ, so that refining wheat causes a 200- to 300-fold loss in valuable phytochemical content.[81] Tumour cells synthesise and accumulate cholesterol faster than normal cells, and one group of chemicals in whole-grain cereals (and fruit and vegetables) suppress tumour growth by limiting cholesterol synthesis.[82] Other anti-cancer substances in whole grains induce the production of the detoxifying enzyme GST.[83]

On the other hand, consuming highly processed bread and cereals that are too easily digested floods the body with sugar, stimulating it to produce high levels of IGF-I.[84] Acne may be an indicator of the over-production of IGF-I as a result of this process. (Several people following my diet have reported that their acne has disappeared, but I think that giving up dairy produce helps this too.)

Try to eat only organic wholemeal brown bread made with stone-ground flour. I continue to eat many other types of organically grown cereals, including porridge and oatcakes, organic whole-grain brown rice and wholemeal brown organic pasta, all widely available in health-food stores and supermarkets.

FOOD FACTOR 7: SWEETENERS

Use raw cane sugar molasses, unrefined honey (preferably wild) or maple syrup as sweeteners. Refined white sugar (called 'pure, white and deadly' by Professor Yudkin) is just empty calories stripped of nutrients; I never eat it. A natural herbal substance called Stevia, which has been used as a sweetener and flavour enhancer in Paraguay for centuries and is also suitable for diabetics, is now available from good health stores.

I avoid any products containing man-made sweeteners such as aspartame,[85] cyclamates, saccharin, or refined sugar. I do so because some of these artificial sweeteners have been linked in laboratory studies to a range of diseases.[86] Artificial sweeteners are frequently found in soft drinks, over-the-counter and prescription drugs, vitamin and herbal supplements, yoghurt, confectionery, some processed cereals, sugar-free chewing-gum, some desserts, some ready-made meals, some milk-shakes, sweeteners, and some instant teas and coffees. So read all labels carefully!

Traditionally, Chinese children have eaten very few sweets. Their treats were pumpkin seeds or dried fruit.

FOOD FACTOR 8: WHAT TO DRINK

Many medical professionals seem to be unaware of the problems associated with the use of recycled treated sewage water as the principal drinking-water supply in urban areas (*see* further under Lifestyle Factor 6 in Update to Chapter Six) – or so it seems to me. For example, I remember a TV interview in which a senior cancer specialist from a famous London hospital accused me of putting cancer patients to unnecessary trouble in advising them to filter and boil their water before drinking it. It emerged that he had no idea that levels of natural and synthetic oestrogens (the latter from the female contraceptive pill and other endocrine-disrupting chemicals) in water from sewage-discharge systems could be so high in the UK that 100 per cent of the male fish downstream of such discharges are feminised.

Some water from extraction wells has also been found to contain an amazing range of pharmaceutical residues – everything from the female contraceptive pill and HRT to Viagra, antidepressants and chemotherapy agents. For these and other reasons, I do not drink water straight from the tap. Nevertheless, I continue to advise against bottled water, since some bottled waters can contain such high levels of radioactivity or nitrates that they would be illegal if they came out of the tap. This is important advice when travelling. For example, the Indian government has ordered a revision of national safety standards for drinking water after the Centre for Science and Environment in New Delhi found pesticide residues in bottled drinking water that were 36 times higher than the maximum limits set by the European Commission.[87]

One recent book about fighting cancer recommends reverse osmosis to clean up tap water, but this generally involves forcing chlorinated water through plastic membranes so I prefer to keep my simple jug filter.

Evidence of the cancer-protecting properties of green tea continue to emerge. Recent studies have confirmed that epi-gallo-catechin-3-gallate has a protective role against several types of epithelial cancers. It has also been suggested that green tea is a stronger antioxidant than vitamin C[88] and helps to neutralise free radicals.

Interestingly, new research has shown that adding cow's milk to tea removes its health benefits. Once again the problem is casein (milk protein), which blocks the beneficial effects of catechins.[89]

I recommend drinking at least six cups a day of organic green tea certified by the Soil Association (and buy Fair Trade, which guarantees a better deal for Third World producers, whenever you can). I also drink herbal teas, mostly peppermint or camomile with honey (many people do not like the taste of pure camomile at first).

Studies linking coffee consumption to cancer are conflicting, but there is a suggestion of a higher incidence of cancer of the ovaries (and pancreas, bladder and kidneys) among coffee drinkers.[90]

Alcohol has been incriminated in breast cancer, but all the studies I have found were carried out on Western women likely to be eating a typical Western diet. Studies are being carried out in Sweden to assess the effects of alcohol on IGF-I and the proteins which can inactivate IGF-binding proteins.[91]

Alcoholic beverages such as red wine can contain hidden animal-produce ingredients which it would be difficult to take account of in such studies. Also, if wine is stored in plastic-lined vats it can contain the endocrine-disrupting chemical bisphenol A (BPA).[92] According to the website of the Vegan Society,[93] many wines on sale have been fined, or cleared, using one of the following: animal blood, bone marrow, chitosan (from the hard parts of insects and crustacea such as shrimps and crabs), albumen (egg white), fish oil, gelatin (obtained by boiling animal tissues such as skin, tendons, ligaments or bones), isinglass (a fish's swim bladder), milk or milk casein (precipitated from milk). Non-animal alternatives used in wines labelled as vegan include limestone, clays and silica gel. But remember that wines labelled as vegetarian may have been fined using casein (milk protein). In the case of beer, isinglass is used especially for real ales. Keg, canned and some bottled beers are usually cleared without the use of animal substances. The production of spirits generally does not involve the use of animal substances (vodka is filtered using birchwood charcoal). The Vegan Society website[94] gives a list of good sources of vegan alcoholic beverages. I continue to drink organically produced cider, perry and beer. I avoid all diet drinks since these are likely to contain man-made sweeteners. Some ciders also contain man-made sweeteners.

I drank very little alcohol before I had cancer and I had none during treatment. I drink some alcohol now.

FOOD FACTOR 9: ACID-ALKALINE BALANCE

The correct balance of foods in our diet influences how acid or alkaline our blood can become, which can in turn affect how our bodies function. Cancer is thought to thrive better in an acid environment. If we eat too much protein, especially animal protein, the body becomes too acid. Interestingly, hard cheese is the most acid-generating food in the Western diet, about three times as acid-generating, weight for weight, as roast beef.

If you are well, you should aim for a diet that is 60 per cent alkali-generating foods and 40 per cent acid-generating foods. If you are ill, you should try to increase your alkali-generating food to about 80 per cent of your diet – but beware! There is a lot of misleading information about which foods generate acidity and alkalinity in the body. For reliable information based on sound scientific research, go to www.janeplant.com, www.cancersupportinternational.com or the charts in my books *Osteoporosis* or *Eating for Better Health*.

FOOD FACTOR 10: SOCIAL EATING

Boredom and loneliness can make matters worse when there is nobody to share our worries with. Buying processed convenience food and eating alone is not good for health. Humans evolved as social animals, hunting, gathering, preparing and eating food in groups; and preparing and eating food with others is a good way to improve your mood and your diet. So, depending on your circumstances, try to learn to make a few simple wholesome meals, ideally preparing them and eating with others. Simple vegetable soups, salads and baked potatoes are easy and provide good wholesome nutrition. Substitute them for sandwiches, burgers, pizzas and other processed food.

THE PLANT PROGRAMME

A report from the Royal College of Physicians asks doctors to pay more attention to nutritional status, something they have neglected in the past and which can cause many health problems and delay recovery. It can also increase health-care costs. Their report calls for nutrition to be tackled seriously and included in undergraduate and post-graduate training of doctors and other health-care staff.[95] Hear! Hear! – and about time too!

In the meantime, *The Plant Programme* gives full details of what to eat and what not to eat for those with breast cancer, ovarian cancer or other types of cancer, and provides dietary regimens for those suffering from active cancer and for those wanting to avoid recurrences of cancers. Living on processed food, as many cancer patients I see have done, is not good for health, so above all learn to cook – starting with the easy-to-follow recipes in *The Plant Programme* or *Eating for Better Health*.

CHAPTER 5 IN A NUTSHELL

- Organisations such as the WHO, the FAO, the US National Cancer Institute and the Physicians Committee for Responsible Medicine,[96] all agree that up to 40 per cent of all cancers could be prevented by diet.
- Evidence is accumulating that dietary changes such as those in the Plant Programme can also help to *treat* cancer, although diet should be used to complement, not replace, conventional medical treatment.
- Vegetables and fruit are the energy foods we evolved to eat. Numerous components in vegetables and fruit, including dietary fibre, vitamins, minerals, live enzymes and various phytochemicals (i.e. plant chemicals), including those that act as anti-oxidants, contribute to a reduced risk of cancer. In contrast, animal foods lack fibre and contain saturated fat, cholesterol and animal protein as well as hormones such as oestrogen and growth factors, all of which are associated with increased risk of cancer. There is no dispute about the health benefits of fruit and vegetables among mainstream scientists.
- The Plant Programme is based on sound science from the peer-reviewed scientific literature, and it follows the principles of diets that have been studied by teams of internationally renowned scientists. Such diets have been found to prevent not only breast cancer and ovarian cancer but other cancers such as colorectal cancer and pancreatic cancer as well as a host of other diseases.
- Many anti-cancer diets are based on junk science. Advice to eliminate all fruit and vegetables such as potatoes and tomatoes from the diet demonstrates total ignorance of the peer-reviewed scientific literature and diverts attention from the real culprit foods.
- One of the first and most essential things you can do to reduce your risk of breast cancer and ovarian cancer is to remove **ALL** dairy products (whether from cows, sheep, goats or any other animals) from your diet. You can replace them with soya, oat, rice or any other vegetable substitutes. The important thing is to ditch the dairy.
- Forget the anti-soya propaganda. It is not based on good science. In experiment after experiment, casein (cows' milk protein) has been shown to promote cancer, whereas

soya protein has no such effect. Dairy milk contains *dangerous* growth factors *and* animal hormones such as oestrogen while soya, just like other peas and beans, contains *protective* phyto-oestrogens.

- Some men express concern that eating the phyto-oestrogens in soya will feminise them. In all my years of working in China and other oriental countries I did not see a single person with man-boobs (gynaecomastia), although it is hard to avoid seeing men with them in the UK or USA. It is far more likely that man-boobs reflect intake of animal oestrogens from eating animal produce or xeno-oestrogens from the environment than eating soya.

- The evidence of the presence of pesticide residues in conventionally produced food continues to mount, as do the beneficial effects of eating organic food, but it should be produced to the standards of and policed by organisations such as the Soil Association.

- It is estimated that only 5 to 6 per cent of our daily calorie intake should be protein, with a maximum intake of about 10 to 11 per cent. The protein intake should consist predominantly of vegetable protein, with a smaller proportion of animal protein. The typical Western diet contains too much animal protein, in the form of meat or cheese. Instead of dairy and an excess of other animal protein, eat plenty of organic whole-grain cereal foods and other seeds, pulses and nuts as a source of protein.

- The risk of breast and ovarian cancer has been linked to high dietary animal-fat intake. Substitute vegetable oils. Extra-virgin cold-pressed oils are excellent for salad dressings, and use extra-virgin olive oil for cooking too.

- Use herbs and spices to flavour food and cut down or cut out salt and other sources of sodium.

- Use raw cane sugar, molasses, unrefined honey (preferably wild) or maple syrup as sweeteners, rather than refined white sugar or artificial sweeteners.

- Drink freshly made vegetable and fruit juices from organic produce, lots of green tea and some herbal teas made with filtered tap water.

- The correct balance of foods in our diet influences how acid or alkaline our bodies can become, which can in turn affect how our bodies function. Cancer is thought to thrive better in an acid environment. If we eat too much protein, especially animal protein, our body becomes too acid. There is a lot of misleading information about which foods generate acidity and alkalinity in the body. For reliable information based on sound scientific research, go to www.janeplant.com, www.cancersupportinternational.com or the charts in *Osteoporosis* or *Eating for Better Health*.

- Buying processed convenience food and eating alone is not good for health. Humans evolved as social animals, and preparing and eating healthy nutritious meals with others is a good way to improve your diet, your health and your mood.

Update to Chapter 6. Ten Lifestyle Factors

On pages 198–231, five lifestyle factors were presented to help you cut your risk of suffering from breast cancer. Here new evidence that has emerged since the first edition was published is considered. In addition, there are five new lifestyle factors as well as information to help prevent and treat ovarian cancer.

LIFESTYLE FACTOR 1: VITAMINS, MINERALS, SUPPLEMENTS AND FOOD FORTIFICATION

Most vitamins (A, B complex and folic acid, C, D, E and K) and several minerals, including selenium, zinc and iodine, are considered to protect against cancer, partly because of their antioxidant properties. Zinc, for example, helps to maintain epithelial and tissue integrity and acts as an antioxidant.[1] After iron, zinc is the next most important trace nutrient needed by our bodies,[2] and it is an active participant in maximising the effect of several other antioxidants.[3] It is involved in more than 200 enzymes in the human body and is essential for healing, so it is important to have adequate zinc to help recover from surgery, radiotherapy and chemotherapy.

Zinc is involved in cell division, and in the way IGF-I is controlled. Researchers at the University of Illinois, USA have shown that a complex interactive set of factors are required to ensure that IGF-I activity occurs only when conditions are right for cell growth, and they describe a discrete role for trace nutrients – especially zinc – in regulating IGF-I activity.[4] They have suggested that one of zinc's functions is to help to inactivate IGF-I. Good sources of zinc include crabs, snails and oysters (especially Atlantic oysters) or, if you are a vegan, sesame seeds (best as tahini – a delicious spread made from sesame seed), pumpkin seeds, sunflower seeds or wheat germ.

A study published in the *Journal of the American Medical Association* claims that nearly all adult Americans have dietary deficiencies in one or more vitamins and should be taking multivitamin supplements.[5] In the UK it has been suggested that in the last half of the 20th century intakes of vitamin A, iron, iodine, magnesium and potassium were lower than recommended.[6] There is little doubt that levels of essential minerals such as copper, zinc and iodine have fallen in soils and the crops grown on them, while levels of toxic elements such as cadmium have increased as a result of modern intensive agriculture.[7]

Let us look in a bit more detail at why we might have developed deficiencies and what we can do to overcome them without taking man-made vitamin and mineral pills, using the example of the chemical element iodine. It was suggested as long ago as 1976 that geographical differences in the rates of breast, endometrial and ovarian cancer reflect iodine status, in that low iodine status leads to too much oestrogen and increased cancer risk.[8] Iodine is called a conservative element because it prefers to stay in water. This means that it is most highly concentrated in the oceans and the main dietary source of iodine is seafood. A hundred years ago fish waste and seaweed were used as fertiliser, but these have now been mostly replaced by inorganic fertilisers, especially rock phosphate, which generally has low iodine content but high levels of the toxic element cadmium. The Soil Association are careful to limit the amounts of cadmium and other toxic substances allowed in rock-phosphate fertiliser for food production, and they ban the use of sewage sludge, which can also have high levels of cadmium and other heavy metals. Another reason to eat organic!

To ensure that I have enough iodine I take kelp tablets. All seaweed has high concentrations of iodine and other nutrients, but it can also concentrate pollutants. I therefore try to buy kelp from Iceland, which has a low population, uses only natural geothermal energy, and is further away from most pollutant sources than any other supplier of seaweed I know of. Taking kelp in my diet has improved my skin enormously. If I run out of tablets for any length of time my skin becomes rough, initially around my elbows and knees and the roughness gradually extends over progressively larger areas until I take kelp again, when the roughness retreats.

An extra bonus is that iodine is good for the brain.[9]

Vitamin and mineral pills and cancer

Taking foods such as kelp which have high concentrations of nutrients is helpful, but there can be many problems as a result of taking man-made vitamins and minerals for cancer patients. One of the first experimental and observational studies to show that taking vitamin pills does not help prevent or treat cancer involved beta-carotene. In a study beginning in 1985, beta-carotene was included in two large long-term chemo-prevention trials sponsored by the National Cancer Institute in the USA. Previous epidemiological studies had suggested that diets high in beta-carotene (e.g. from carrots) reduced lung cancer incidence. In the trial studies, daily doses of beta-carotene in combination with either vitamin E or vitamin A were administered for several years to tens of thousands of people thought to be at high risk of developing lung cancer. What happened? The rate of lung cancer in those taking the pills increased in both trials![10]

A recent Canadian study also showed that women who took large doses of vitamins and minerals during conventional treatment for breast cancer were more likely to relapse and die than women who did not.[11] The five-year survival rate for patients prescribed vitamin C, beta-carotene, niacin (vitamin B3), zinc, selenium and coenzyme Q10 was 72 per cent, compared with 81 per cent for the control group. Over a ten-year period, those who took large doses of vitamins and minerals were 10 per cent more likely to die. The investigators were surprised with the results, because they were expecting that the patients prescribed vitamin and mineral supplements would have a 25–30 per cent increase in survival rates.

In an editorial article in the *BMJ* in July 2002,[12] consideration of the value of daily doses of multivitamin tablets concluded that regular consumption would probably do no good unless your intake is inadequate as a result of poor diet. The article recommends only folic acid for women before and after conception [but if you eat enough green leafy vegetables – or fruits such as melon – this is unnecessary], and perhaps vitamin D in elderly people. Regarding cancer, the article refers to unexpected results that more people receiving supposedly protective supplements died than people receiving placebos.

The vice chair of the panel of US Preventive Services Task Force has also stated that there is insufficient scientific evidence to support the notion that taking vitamin supplements will prevent cancer. She pointed out that people should strive to eat the healthiest diet possible and that nutrients from supplements may not offer the same benefits that they do when consumed as part of a healthy diet.[13]

In the UK, the Food Standards Agency has suggested that many people could be damaging their health by taking vitamin and mineral supplements in doses that are too high. The agency's expert group on vitamins and minerals spent four years looking at the evidence on the potential harmful effects of taking high doses of 34 vitamins and minerals that can be bought over the counter. It found enough evidence to suggest safe upper levels for eight of them and suggested guidance on 23. It also issued statements on three minerals. Two supplements – namely beta-carotene and chromium – were found to have the potential to cause cancer in some people and should be avoided by smokers and those who have been exposed to asbestos. Chromium picolinate supplements may also cause cancer and should be avoided.[14]

Other evidence against taking pills involves zinc. Men who took more than 100 mg a day of zinc supplements were found to have more than twice the risk of advanced prostate cancer. These levels are far above the recommended doses. However, in the USA, a significant number of men take zinc supplements higher than the recommended levels, partly because of their supposed benefit in preventing colds. Again the message is clear: DO NOT take man-made vitamin or mineral supplements. Have them as nature intended – as part of a good diet.[15] A recent paper on the subject[16] concluded 'there is absolutely no benefit from taking these supplements and I would suggest people avoid them.' The study found, for example, that those taking a supplement containing vitamin A were 16 per cent more likely to die than those not taking supplements. The comparable figures for beta-carotene and vitamin E were 7 per cent and 4 per cent respectively.

Oakley has suggested that as many as 350,000 deaths from coronary heart disease could have been prevented over the last decade in the UK if the government had fortified flour with folic acid when the evidence was first published.[17] According to Reynolds, however, fortifying flour with folic acid understates the potential risks to the nervous system. Experimental studies confirm that folates cause convulsions if the blood-brain barrier is circumvented.[18] We should oppose fortification of our food or water, whether by folic acid or fluoride.

Calcium and vitamin D

There is often a lot of pressure on women, especially menopausal women, to take calcium supplements to avoid osteoporosis Let us look in more detail at how taking calcium can adversely affect breast and ovarian cancer.

There is much evidence that vitamin D blocks breast cancer by several mechanisms, including by interfering with the IGF-I signalling pathways, decreasing cancer-cell proliferation[19] and increasing apoptosis.[20] Studies of the effects of vitamin D on IGF-I and its receptor show a similar relationship.[21] Vitamin D has been shown to cut the risk of pancreatic cancer by 86 per cent and it has also been suggested that vitamin D compounds help to normalise telomerase activity (see Chapter Two).[22]

Vitamin D is present in small quantities in our food and it has been proved to reduce the incidence of cancer significantly, but its ability to do this is limited by the effects of excessive calcium (and protein) in the diet.[23] Dairy milk is loaded with calcium and taking large amounts of calcium, whether as supplements or otherwise, lowers blood levels of the type of circulating vitamin D which prevents cancer.[24] Colleen Doyle, director of nutrition and physical activity for the American Cancer Society in Atlanta, explains: 'Calcium, especially when it is taken as a supplement, has the ability to suppress the amount of vitamin D that circulates in the blood.'[25] One cannot help wondering how much cancer is being caused by people taking too much calcium as pills or as dairy.

Vitamin D forms in the skin under the influence of solar ultraviolet light, so that outdoor exercise wearing light clothing in sunny weather usually enables your body to produce all that it needs. Good food sources include oily fish and eggs, so only vegans living in cold climates or the housebound elderly need consider taking supplements. In the latter case I would recommend the ultra-pure versions of fish-liver oils. Always remember that too much vitamin D is toxic. Also that the emerging consensus is that the beneficial effects of vitamin D in protecting against cancer or osteoporosis is blocked by taking too much calcium as dairy or supplements. Calcium is best obtained from green leafy vegetables, whole-grain cereals and pulses.

Selenium supplements

The only synthetic supplement I have taken since my first diagnosis of cancer 20 years ago is selenium. Selenium is important for thyroid function, immune function generally and as an antioxidant, but its status is often marginal to deficient in UK diets. It works best in conjunction with vitamin E, since both are antioxidants and can increase the production of antibodies by up to thirty times,[26] greatly enhancing the immune response. For over 20 years animal studies have shown that tiny amounts of selenium in the diet can suppress several types of cancer, but equivalent data on humans are only just emerging. It has been suggested that selenium has a protective role against breast cancer and ovarian cancer. There is also evidence that low selenium status may be a predictor of ovarian cancer and that it helps to decrease the side effects of chemotherapy in the treatment of ovarian cancer.[27] Although selenium is essential to health, it is required only in minute quantities. Although it is not certain at precisely what level it begins to cause adverse effects, it has been found that doses of 900 micrograms (0.9 mg) per day can make hair and nails fall out and affect the nervous system.[28]

Selenium is best from natural sources. In addition to seeds and garlic, good sources include wholemeal bread, organic eggs, onions, broccoli and tomato, but I do not eat brazil nuts as a source of selenium for the reasons given on page 167.

Whole foods not pills

In general, I prefer to eat whole foods because problems tend to arise when we try to separate food into its constituent parts.

Food such as fruit, vegetables and whole grains contain hundreds of antioxidants (and other phytochemicals) and at least some of them work together (i.e. synergistically).[29] The protective effect of a mineral-vitamin-phytochemical-rich diet is best obtained from the consumption of adequate amounts of fruit, vegetables, legumes and whole-grain produce[30] based on a good, well-balanced diet such as that in the Plant Programme. All this was confirmed by a recent report in New Scientist.[31] Paul Coates, who is responsible for dietary supplements in the US National Institute of Health, is quoted as saying, 'just because a certain compound in food is beneficial it does not mean that a nutraceutical (with the same chemical compound in it) is.' The article goes on to say, 'the advice is simple, stick to foods such as flavanoid rich vegetables and fruit but do not take high dose supplements or fortified foods.' Hence fresh or frozen cranberries are recommended rather than cranberry capsules, green tea rather than green tea extract and fresh fruit is recommended rather than vitamin C pills. This is advice every cancer patient needs to take on board, because it seems that they are often prey to unscrupulous practitioners selling pills and potions at exorbitant prices, cashing in on their distress. Some people who come to see me have bags full of pills. One woman with breast cancer, who had been seeing only alternative practitioners, was given a very bad prognosis initially when persuaded to seek medical help. She had more than twenty preparations in a bag of everything from megadoses of vitamin C to shark's cartilage to laetrile. Some were in a lactose (milk sugar) base and some were coloured with E number substances. We agreed to junk them all and she is now doing much better. Save money by not buying potentially harmful vitamins, minerals supplements and extracts and spend it instead on the best locally grown organic vegetables and fruit you can find.

The food supplements I use

The supplements I use are still available, despite the new EU legislation, because they are simply foods that are naturally enriched in trace nutrients. I continue to take kelp* to avoid iodine deficiency and also brewer's yeast,* which is a good source of many trace elements such as iron, selenium, chromium and zinc and B vitamins. These are important if the body is to synthesise important compounds such as co-enzyme Q10, which is essential to the optimal functioning of all cell types and is also an antioxidant. Note that brewer's yeast will not cause Candida, as some practitioners might try to persuade you. Candida infection reflects overuse of antibiotics, other medications or a diet that is too acid-generating with too much animal protein and white sugar.

I now take balanced omega-3, omega-6 vegetable oils* daily and Seven Seas ultrapure cod-liver oil*, which I store in a cool, dark place. These are all natural, not synthetic, substances. I

---

* Follow the manufacturer's instructions and do not exceed the recommended amount – the quantity of tablets or oil depends on the brand.

always follow manufacturers' instructions. I took tablets containing selenium and vitamins A, C and E when I had active cancer.

If you must take man-made minerals, vitamins, supplements or any pharmaceutical products, make sure that they are not in a lactose matrix and do not contain artificial colouring or flavours.

LIFESTYLE FACTOR 2: FOOD PACKAGING

As discussed on pages 200–201, the fact that most of the hazardous chemicals from packaging are highly fat soluble is of particular concern if you are buying oily foods such as oily fish. My fishmonger now wraps my fish in paper or foil. Try to minimise consumption of water or juices sold in plastic bottles, food purchased in cans, and wines stored in vats[32] lined with plastics, which can contain the endocrine-disrupting substance bisphenol A. Try to eat fresh or frozen food, and drink wines stored in oak. Also try to cut down on plastic bags to carry shopping. I have a battered old shopping trolley for shopping, and for buying a small number of items I do what our mothers used to do – I use a shopping bag. Evidence that phthalates from soft plastics can feminise baby boys thus confirming their oestrogenicity is discussed under Lifestyle Factor 6.

LIFESTYLE FACTOR 3: COOKING

The style of cooking recommended in the Plant Programme ensures that fresh, wholesome ingredients are cooked in the healthiest way possible and served as soon as possible. Here are some additional important rules:

- Never use a microwave cooker, because free radicals are formed in the food (although acrylamide levels may be lower than if you fry foods)
- Never use a pressure cooker, because it destroys vitamins and other important nutrients
- Never dehydrate food between plastic sheets because the food could absorb harmful chemicals from the plastic.
- How you store food is also important. Do not store unripe fruit and vegetables in the fridge or vital vitamins and other important phyto-chemicals will not build up. Melons, citrus fruits and avocados are all best stored at room temperature and eaten ripe.

Meat

The way meat is cooked is important. My mother and all her generation of British women were taught to cook meat thoroughly, and that meant slowly. For all sorts of reasons, including preventing cancer, I will not now eat undercooked meat under any circumstances. Meat is a poor conductor of heat and if it is not cooked properly hormones in it (whether natural or introduced by man, as in the USA) will not be destroyed. Even if it is well-cooked, steroid hormones such as oestrogen may survive. Remember that official figures show that dairy-cow meat contains even more IGF-I than milk, so I avoid cheap processed meat, mince, sausages or burgers made from this type of beef.

I never eat grilled or barbecued steak. Cancer-promoting chemicals (heterocyclic amines (HCA), the most abundant of which is known as PhiP) are likely to be formed in burned meat, while cancer-promoting chemicals including hormones will remain intact in the relatively raw meat inside. Amounts of HCA range from very low in poached, steamed or stewed meat and fish to very high levels in grilled or barbecued meat. PhiP has been linked to breast, prostate and colon cancer.[33] High levels of HCA also occur in pan-fried meat.[34] Other toxic by-products of interaction between sugars, fats and proteins also form when food is cooked at too high a temperature.[35] Recent research carried out at Harvard University confirms that eating red meat is an avoidable risk factor for breast cancer and the EPIC study confirms that it is a risk factor for colorectal cancer.

Seafood

It is important to cook seafood in a way that will preserve essential minerals such as iodine. The distinctive chemistry of iodine means that it is easily lost when processing and cooking food (Chinese people tend to cook fish in sealed containers and use the juices to make soup. This ensures that all the iodine in the fish is consumed.) Baking fish in foil or cooking it in a fish kettle with a well-fitting lid helps to preserve all the nutrients it contains.

Fried Foods

The Gerson diet recommends avoidance of all fried foods, and fried eggs were shown in 1985 to increase the risk of fatal ovarian cancer.[36]

In the last few years there has been concern about the presence of a potentially cancer-causing chemical called acrylamide in fried food, including chips and potato crisps. Swiss researchers have also reported high levels of the substance in ground roast coffee.[37]

The levels of acrylamide in some foods are compared with the US Environmental Protection Agency (EPA) limit for this chemical in water in Table 6.1.

Table 6.1: Levels of acrylamide in foods, in micrograms per serving[121]	
Water, 8oz, EPA limit	0.12
Boiled potatoes, 4oz	<3
Taco shells, 3, 1.1oz	1
French Fries, uncooked, 3oz	5
French Fries, baked, 3oz	28
Breakfast cereals, 1oz	6–7
Tortilla Chips, 1oz	5
Corn Chips, 1oz	11
Potato crisps, 1oz	25
French Fries, 5.6–6.2oz, and potato wedges, 6.2, purchased from fast-food outlets	39–82

Studies to date suggest that a minimum temperature of 120°C is needed to form acrylamide in food, with levels increasing further with increasing temperature. There is a ten-fold difference between normal and overcooked chips.[38]

Previously, concern about acrylamide had centred on occupational exposure (i.e. through the skin, or by inhalation of dust or vapour) during its manufacture and use by industry, and environmental exposure.[39] Acrylamide is used in the manufacture of adhesives, dyes, soil-conditioning agents, products for sewage and waste treatment, chemical grouting, the manufacture of non-iron fabrics, crude oil production, the processing of paper and pulp, and some ores and concrete.[40] Some home appliances and parts of cars and other vehicles are coated with acrylamide resin and other acrylics. Acrylamides are also contained in some cosmetics and soaps, in which they act as thickeners, in dental fixtures, hair-grooming preparations and pre-shave lotions.[41] Until recently, acrylamide was not thought to occur naturally.[42]

All this information tends to suggest that acrylamide might be expected to occur at low levels in the environment from man-made sources in industrialised countries.[43] It is a water-soluble, rather than fat-soluble, substance,[44] with a high water solubility which increases with temperature.[45] Hence, despite the statement by the UK Food Standards Agency[46] that 'frying and baking create high levels of acrylamide in a wide range of food', the levels could partly reflect environmental pollution. When food is fried, the acrylamide will not be dissolved out into the fat and is likely to become more concentrated in the food as water is lost in cooking. On the other hand, where food is boiled, the highly soluble acrylamide is likely to be lost to the cooking water. My advice remains the same as for avoiding other harmful man-made chemicals in food and drink: eat as organically as possible and follow the methods of preparation and cooking set out in *The Plant Programme*. This also includes plenty of fresh fruit and vegetables, which experts recommend to help to counteract the effects of high acrylamide.

Living dangerously

An amazing number of people I see who have cancer do not cook at all. They simply buy pre-prepared meals from super-markets and reheat or microwave them. I have no scientific data to prove my theory, but I think this really is living dangerously. The meals in the Plant Programme are all healthy and nutritious and many are very easy to make. Start with a simple soup, salad or curry.

LIFESTYLE FACTOR 4: DEALING WITH STRESS

The stress of coping with cancer

The word 'cancer' is terrifying to most people, and earlier I described the horror I felt at discovering I had breast cancer. But remember that new medicines have been developed that effectively relieve most of the worst symptoms of cancer, such as pain and nausea – including that caused by treatment. Modern treatments, especially for breast cancer, are effective and are given with an increasingly significant chance of remission.[47]

In an article entitled 'ABC of psychological medicine: Cancer',[48] White and Macleod point out that cancer is the most feared of diseases and causes considerable psychological distress, including depression and anxiety, in patients and their families, and even in health professionals who care for them. A diagnosis of cancer can precipitate feelings similar to bereavement (it is worth noting that a recent study showed that people who profess stronger spiritual beliefs seem to resolve grief more rapidly than people with no spiritual beliefs).[49] Severe and persistent depressive disorder is up to four times more common in cancer patients than in the general population, and occurs in 10–20 per cent of people affected by the disease. Feelings of loss may be a reaction to perceived loss, for example of one's role in family or society, or impending loss of life. Anxiety can manifest itself as apprehension, uncontrollable worry, restlessness, panic attacks, and avoidance of people and of reminders of cancer. Patients may overestimate the risks associated with treatment and the likelihood of a poor outcome. Anxiety may also exacerbate or heighten perceptions of physical symptoms that patients can interpret as cancer symptoms, and post-traumatic-stress symptoms occasionally follow diagnosis or treatment that the patient has found particularly frightening. Certain cancers and treatments are associated with specific fears. For example, patients may develop phobias and conditioned vomiting in relation to treatments such as chemotherapy.[50]

Distress is more likely to occur at specific points in a patient's experience of cancer. These include:[51]

- *Diagnosis*, when doctors should explain that feelings such as shock, anger, disbelief and distress are normal.
- *During treatment*, especially at times when treatment appears to be failing.
- *At the end of treatment*, because of the fear that the cancer might recur.
- *After treatment*, because of fear of recurrence and misinterpretation of symptoms (such as believing that pain associated with a muscle strain represents a recurrence of cancer).
- *Recurrence*. Most patients report recurrence of cancer as more distressing than receiving the initial diagnosis.

The principles of treatment[52] to help such patients involve:

- A clearly identified principal therapist to coordinate care.
- Sympathetic interest and concern.
- Effective symptomatic relief.
- Understanding the patient's concerns and needs.
- Collaborative planning of continuing care.
- Good information and advice.
- Involvement of the patient in treatment decisions.
- Involvement of family and friends.
- Early recognition and treatment of psychological complications.
- Clear arrangements to deal with urgent problems.

As discussed on pages 203–215, the idea that cancer could be cured by positive thinking had always seemed to me to be ill-founded. A recent systematic review of the influence of psychological coping on survival and recurrence in people with cancer[53] supports the view that positive thinking is not the key to fighting cancer. It found that most of the studies that investigated fighting spirit or feelings of helplessness or hopelessness found no significant associations with survival or recurrence. The authors conclude that people with cancer should not feel pressured into adopting particular coping styles.

Another recent study has suggested that women who had one or more severely stressful life experiences in the five years after diagnosis had a lower risk of recurrence than those who did not.[54] The authors of the study conclude that women with breast cancer need not fear that stressful experiences will trigger a recurrence of their disease.

Some people feel guilt that their cancer is some form of punishment. I certainly felt that, but, as I now say in the many lectures I give, cancer is not brought about by a wrathful God. Almost all cancers, and certainly breast and ovarian cancer, have far more rational explanations, as discussed in this book.

Because stress has been implicated as an important factor in cancer generally, people can become worried and hence more stressed by problems, so that a vicious circle is set up. Over the last fourteen years I have faced up to some extremely stressful situations in my family life and at work, and yet my cancer has not returned – because fundamentally it was a problem caused by harmful chemicals from my food and the environment. Now that my diet and lifestyle are sound, I cope much better with stress.

Helping yourself cope

Nevertheless, it is helpful to reduce the stress and distress in your life as much as possible. In situations of acute stress, hormones from the adrenal gland increase the amount of blood sugar available, boost the heart rate and slow down digestive function to equip us for fight or flight. Too much stress for too long, however, can affect the immune system and increase prolactin levels. Other damaging hormones and biochemicals that increase under chronic stress include cortisol, noradrenaline, growth hormones, thyroxin, testosterone and oestrogen.[55]

Several complementary and alternative-medicine treatments have been shown to improve the well-being of patients with cancer. These include: mind-body programmes for stress, including yoga and reiki; acupuncture or acupressure for nausea; tai chi and other gentle exercise techniques to improve strength; therapeutic massage and relaxation techniques to reduce stress; and herbal medicines for depression and anxiety.[56] Certainly, talking therapies such as counselling, cognitive behavioural therapy (CBT) and psychodynamic therapy (PDT) can be very helpful. CBT is becoming increasingly available on the NHS. According to MIND, the mental health charity, cognitive therapy is about learning to think and behave in positive ways. It is a type of behavioural therapy which is helpful in overcoming negative thinking. If you think this would be helpful, ensure that you consult an expert in cognitive therapy, since most GPs have had little training in this field.[57] Psychotherapy may last for several years and is particularly helpful in understanding, and coming to terms with, past events. It is expensive and would normally be available from the NHS only in extreme cases.

Above all, as I emphasised earlier, try to develop loving caring relationships with your family and friends and to let go of negative situations. This is a time to improve the emotional basis of your life.

Dealing with the stress of breast and ovarian cancer

Let us look at some of the particular problems associated with coping with breast and ovarian cancer. Women who have undergone mastectomy or hysterectomy may experience feelings of a loss of femininity and desirability. Men with breast cancer can feel embarrassed, and health professionals need to be particularly sensitive to their needs. It is important to discuss worries with partners, because they are affected as well and they are usually concerned about how to express their love and support during and after treatment. Suggestions that may help them to cope better include involving them as soon as possible in all decisions about treatment, openly communicating feelings, needs, and wants, and seeking the support of others.[58] Some marriages and family relationships break down following the wife and mother suffering from breast cancer, and I know of some such cases personally, but I cannot think of a single case of this happening to someone with ovarian cancer. The vast majority of men are very supportive if their wives have cancer and they usually make it clear that they value them for so many reasons other than physical perfection. Women with ovarian cancer may become emotionally distressed, especially if they have a hysterectomy. Even women who are long past their child-bearing years may become very emotional at the loss of their womb or ovaries. Certainly I sobbed every time I attended to have my ovaries irradiated. This is an entirely natural reaction, but it is sometimes difficult for males to understand. Male surgeons are often perplexed by this reaction.

Working through

I found it helpful to keep working during my treatment because it took my mind off my cancer, and I took the minimum of sick leave; the ability to do this varies and depends on having a supportive environment at work and on your health and stamina. The level of fatigue after cancer treatment is the largest factor in predicting a return to work. Nearly two thirds (64 per cent) of cancer survivors in a study of 235 patients were back at work within 18 months; the duration of sick leave depended on diagnosis, treatment, age, physical complaints and workload.[59] If you need to take time off, do so. This is a time to follow your instincts and do what you feel is right for you.

LIFESTYLE FACTOR 5: SLEEPLESSNESS AND FATIGUE

One of the common problems of cancer sufferers is that of sleeplessness. Almost fourteen years on, I am still affected by this problem. In my case, it was probably made worse by the strong tranquillisers I was prescribed to make me sleep when it was thought that I was terminally ill.[60]

Alternative techniques for helping people to sleep include herbal substances, but I have found these to be ineffective.

Methods I have found to be helpful include the use of acupressure cones, which can be bought from high-street chemists and applied to the acupuncture sleep points on the wrists as shown in the accompanying leaflets. One tip is to buy travel bands instead, since, unlike the cones, they can be re-used many times. They work on the same principle as the cones, but are intended for use on different acupuncture points on the wrists, to prevent nausea. I use them with the studs placed on the sleep pressure points, which saves money and reduces using yet more plastic.

I listen to self-hypnosis tapes, available widely in bookstores and health food shops. I also find it calming to have a bowl of organic porridge with a little soya milk before going to bed (though this may not be suitable for those with a gluten allergy); oats were the traditional treatment for hyperactivity in children and are still used by herbalists to help overcome benzodiazepine and valium addiction, alcoholism and some other types of drug addiction.[61]

If I cannot sleep I listen to the world service of the BBC and comfort myself that I am learning a lot. One or two sleepless nights do not matter, and usually you will make up for any sleep deficit later. Also remember that people who think they have had a sleepless night may have slept quite a lot intermittently. Whatever you do, try not to take sleeping tablets such as benzodiazepines. They can make natural sleep almost impossible and increase your levels of anxiety.

LIFESTYLE FACTOR 6: AVOIDING HARMFUL SUBSTANCES IN YOUR ENVIRONMENT

Despite the information on the website of Cancer Research UK that smoking is not a risk factor for breast cancer (see p. 301), it was strongly recommended on page 217 that smokers should give up smoking on the basis of scientific evidence. It has been shown,[62] for example, that non-smokers not exposed to active or passive smoking have a much lower probability of contracting breast cancer. However, women exposed to passive smoking had a breast-cancer rate which was approximately 80 per cent of that of active smokers.

The carcinogenic effect of cigarette smoke on developing breast tissue has been shown to increase risk of breast cancer. A recent Canadian study showed that the risk of breast cancer was significantly increased in women who had started to smoke within five years of puberty.[63]

Smokers may be helped to quit smoking by using nicotine-enriched chewing gum or patches, since it is the contaminants in the smoke rather the nicotine that are the carcinogens. It is also important to avoid passive smoking. So avoid smoky bars and restaurants, and **if somebody asks 'Do you mind if I smoke?', just say 'Yes'**.

On pages 216–217 I gave several reasons for not smoking or subjecting yourself to passive smoking. Since then I have learned also that cigarettes contain a lot of the heavy metal cadmium, which is a carcinogen.[64] It is also an endocrine-disrupter and is particularly damaging to bones,[65] which need to be specially protected in breast cancer. Other authors have also indicated that there is a positive association between smoking history and IGF-I level.[66]

Since the first edition of this book was published much more has emerged on the harmful effects of man-made chemicals used in pesticides, plastics, detergents and cosmetics and fragrances. There is now mounting concern about endocrine-disrupting chemicals. Below is a list of some of the most important harmful substances and their links to cancer.

CANCER HAZARD: ENDOCRINE-DISRUPTING CHEMICALS (EDCs)

The term 'endocrine disruptor' was first introduced by Theo Colborn.[67] Following Colborn's work, it was realised that a lot of man-made chemicals that are manufactured in large quantities and to which we are exposed in consumer items and through the environment might be implicated in many health problems including cancer. When I first described endocrine-disrupting chemicals in relation to cancer in the first (2000) edition of this book, I was attacked for being alarmist by some doctors, despite the fact that scientists were already aware that 100 per cent of male fish in many of our rivers had been feminised. Since that time there have been many articles about such substances, described as 'gender benders' in the press; and many people writing about cancer have picked up this theme. Because breast and ovarian cancers are considered to be hormone-dependent, avoiding EDCs is particularly important in their prevention and treatment, and I do a full check on exposure on all my patients in the SuPPort Clinic and advise them how to reduce their risks.

EDCs are defined by the UK Environment Agency as 'naturally occurring or synthetic substances that interfere with the functioning of hormone systems resulting in unnatural responses.'[68] They cause problems, including by (1) mimicking the natural hormone and producing a similar response by the cell, (2) binding to cell receptors and preventing a normal response and (3) interfering with the way natural hormones and receptors behave. Perhaps of most concern is the evidence that EDCs or their breakdown products can directly damage DNA to alter the cell cycle, affect repair processes, or interfere with cell-to-cell signalling – all processes implicated in the initiation of cancer.

Concern about this group of chemicals has mushroomed in recent years. The concern reflects: (1) the discovery that a range of widely used man-made chemicals, including substances used in detergents, herbicides, pesticides, plastics, the female contraceptive pill, hormone replacement pills and by-products of other industrial and waste-disposal processes, to which we are exposed daily, can act as EDCs[69] (127 pesticides have recently been suggested to be EDCs[70]); (2) hypothetical links to an increase in disorders of reproductive development and function in the human male and in some species of wildlife;[71] and (3) the striking coincidence between human exposure to these chemicals and the increase in prevalence of a range of hormone-dependent human reproductive cancers (prostate, breast, endometrial, testicular and ovarian). Some of the substances have been used for a considerable length of time in household and personal-care products and even in the manufacture of children's toys and teething rings. One particularly powerful EDC, nonyl phenol ethoxylate (NPE), has been used for at least twenty years in the formulation of many herbicides and insecticides to spray on food crops – although its use has now been banned. Bisphenol A (BPA), an oestrogenic EDC, can leach from the plastics used to line tin cans and even from some types of composite dental fillings.[72] Countries around the world are only now phasing out the use of many of these substances of concern.[73] The European Union is leading the world in managing chemicals, with new legislation for the registration, evaluation and authorisation of chemicals (REACH) being introduced from 2007.

In addition to oestrogen-mimicking substances, EDCs include chemicals that are thought to block oestrogen, mimic or block testosterone and other androgens (male hormones) and possibly also mimic or block thyroid hormones. Most people now have body burdens of EDCs similar to those that cause abnormalities in other vertebrates.[74] Proving a causal link between EDCs and cancer is difficult for many reasons, including the multifactorial nature of the disease and differences in the duration and intensity of exposure. Despite these difficulties, evidence is accumulating from laboratory animal, wildlife and human studies that exposure to EDCs can promote hormone-dependent cancers.[75] Case-control studies, for example, have found that breast-cancer risk is increased in women with high body burdens of organochlorine pesticides.[76] Organochlorines have also been shown in laboratory experiments to alter tumour-suppressor genes, promoting the growth of breast-cancer and ovarian-cancer cells.[77]

One of the most important recent papers showing the effect of EDCs on humans[78] reported that prenatal phthalate exposure of baby boys reduced the volume of their penises, increased the likelihood that they would have undescended testes and reduced the ano-genital distance (AGD) closer to that of females (which is about half that of males). This study confirmed the results of earlier studies on rats. Other studies are confirming these findings. The fact that a new index of feminisation of males – the AGD – is now available provides a powerful new research tool into the effects of EDCs, especially oestrogenic chemicals and anti-oestrogens which are implicated in breast and ovarian cancer.

Recent advances in molecular biology demonstrate that the hormones used by vertebrates all have a similar structure.[79] Because EDCs are related to hormones, an infinitesimal quantity can have a significant effect.[80] Indeed, recent evidence suggests that extremely low doses of EDCs can have effects as damaging as higher doses.[81] Male frogs suffer from conditions such as undescended testes and even hermaphrodism when exposed early in their development to tiny doses (1–2 parts per billion) of a commonly used herbicide called atrazine. Some persistent EDCs can accumulate in the body and be passed from one generation to the next.

Some researchers have suggested that xeno-oestrogens are unlikely to cause harm because we are already exposed to phyto-oestrogens. Humans and their pre-human ancestors have been eating phyto-oestrogens for millions of years, however, whereas most xeno-oestrogens have been around for, at the most, a few decades. Moreover bioaccumulative persistent xeno-oestrogens and other endocrine disrupters accumulate in body tissues to much higher levels than phyto-oestrogens.[82] All of the epidemiological and other research I have read, including papers from the authoritative Royal Society, indicates that phyto-oestrogens are protective while xeno-oestrogens are potentially very harmful.

There are now many sources of information on EDCs. For example, a new database (REDIPED), launched in 2002 by the Department for Environment, Food and Rural Affairs in the UK, provides information on 79 confirmed or suspected EDCs.

SOME OTHER HAZARDOUS ENVIRONMENTAL CHEMICALS

The occurrence of pharmaceuticals in the environment and the extent to which they pose a risk to the environment and humankind has also received considerable attention since the early 1990s. An initial risk assessment for the UK,[83] covering more than sixty compounds thought to account for more than half of the known tonnage of pharmaceutical consumption, suggested that the substances of most concern were paracetamol/acetminophen, aspirin and dextropropoxyphene (pain killers), fluoxetine (antidepressant), oxytetracycline (antibiotic), propranolol (for heart disease and migraine), aminotriptyline (for neuralgia) and thioridazine (for adult schizophrenia).

Recently the United States Geological Survey carried out the first nation-wide reconnaissance of the occurrence of pharmaceuticals, hormones and other organic contaminants in water.[84] The most frequently detected compounds were coprostanol (faecal steroid), cholesterol (plant and animal steroid), N,N-diethyltoluamide (insect repellent), caffeine (stimulant), triclosan (disinfectant), tri(2-chloroethyl) phosphate (fire retardant) and 4-nonylphenol (detergent breakdown product). More than one of the contaminants was commonly detected in samples, and there were as many as 38 in some samples. Little is known about the potential interactive effects that occur from such complex mixtures and their breakdown products and their overall effect on human health and the environment.

Other monitoring programmes in Europe and the Americas have detected pain-killers, cholesterol regulators, antiseptics, chemotherapy agents, antibiotics and hormones in water.[85] One of the problems is that conventional sewage-treatment technologies vary greatly in their ability to remove drug residues and, in some instances, have even been shown to increase the bioactivity of the pharmaceutical residues.[86] Activated carbon filtration, which is used by some states in the USA, continues to be one of the most effective known methods of removing drug and other contaminant residues from drinking water. Please see the section on Food Factor 8 'What to Drink' in Chapter Five, to reduce your risk of taking in harmful substances through your drinking water.

HARMFUL GASEOUS SUBSTANCES

Brominated flame retardants (BFRs), widely used for fire proofing everything from televisions and computers to carpets and curtains, are now known to be persistent, bioaccumulative and toxic – and have been detected in human breast-milk samples![87] Harmful gaseous substances are increasingly of concern in buildings and vehicles. The Hamburg Environment Institute has analysed gaseous emissions from household and office appliances such as computer mice and mobile phones.[88] They have also tested carpets and wallpaper. Their study identified a hundred compounds emitted from the products tested, including carcinogens and EDCs. Volatile organic compounds can reach particularly high levels in new cars.[89] A useful leaflet entitled *Volatile organic compounds (including formaldehyde) in the home* has been posted on the website of the UK Institute for Environment and Health.[90]

HARMFUL SUBSTANCES AND BREAST AND OVARIAN CANCER

Many studies indicate an increased risk of hormone-dependent cancers (such as breast and ovarian cancer) due to exposure to chemicals in the environment, especially EDCs.[91] Timing and dose in relation to the developing female body are likely to be crucial factors. The pesticides most strongly implicated in increasing breast-cancer risk include DDT/DDE, hexachlorobenzene (HCB), lindane, a breakdown product of the insecticide heptachlor and triazine herbicides such as atrazine. Women with high body burdens of the insecticide dieldrin have been shown to have twice the risk of developing breast cancer and to have higher mortality from the disease. A study carried out on women aged 55 or younger in Ontario, in one of Canada's largest fruit and vegetable growing regions, showed that women who have worked on farms are up to nine times more likely to develop breast cancer than those who have never been employed in agriculture.[92] These findings raise further suspicions that the array of fungicides, herbicides and insecticides used on many farms is a factor in the 'huge increase in the rates of breast cancer' in Canada. The article notes that over the past three decades the incidence of breast cancer has risen by about 1 per cent every year.

In the early 1990s a substance 'leaching from plastic tubing' as well as some pesticides were shown to promote the growth of breast cancer cells.[93] Studies have also linked drastic changes in mammary-gland development to exposure to BPA (from epoxy resins, polycarbonate plastic and dental sealants) while PVC has been linked to the development of breast cancer. Occupational exposure to solvents such as benzene, styrene, carbon tetrachloride, and formaldehyde in the electronics industry and fabricated metal, printing and clothing and textile industries has also been shown to increase breast-cancer risk. Some solvents such as ethylene glycol methyl ether (EGME) have been suggested to increase the sensitivity to breast tissue of oestrogen and progesterone.

Other probable links between breast cancer and man-made chemicals have been established with combustion by-products such as dioxin and PAHs, chemicals in sunscreens, phthalates from plastics and electromagnetic fields.

Increased risk of ovarian cancer is associated with employment in the graphics and printing industries, in which many chemicals ranging from solvents, mineral oils, PAHs, inks and pigments are used. Hairdressers and beauticians also appear to be at increased risk.[94] Some evidence links ovarian cancer to exposure to the herbicide atrazine. Recent studies also link ovarian cancer to exposure to ionising radiation, and there are conflicting studies of a link with the use of talc in the genital area.

Chemicals in the environment and ignorance

The Royal Commission on Environmental Pollution's Report 24 'Chemicals in products: safeguarding the environment and human health' states that 'ignorance outweighs knowledge at every stage in our understanding of synthetic chemicals.' Recently, Professor Sir Richard Peto, co-author with Doll of the now notorious 1981 paper that discussed risk from pesticides and other chemicals in the environment, pronounced in an article in the *Independent* that links between chemicals in the environment and breast cancer are 'rubbish'. Mmm . . . what did the Royal Commission say about ignorance and chemicals?

The tiniest amounts

As discussed in Chapter Four, dairy milk contains oestrogen and progesterone. These chemicals are powerful EDCs and can cause severe biological damage, even at very low levels. Natural oestrogens have been classified as known human carcinogens.[95] One illustration of how tiny amounts of EDCs can cause problems was the problem caused by the effects of a chemical called tributyl tin (TBT) on dog whelks on Britain's south coast. The chemical was developed for use in paint to coat the underside of ships to prevent fouling, or the growth of creatures such as barnacles that increase friction and thus slow down ships and boats. The levels of TBT in water were only about five parts in a million million and were barely detectable. Nevertheless, in the 1980s, over a wide area of Britain's south coast where minute traces of the chemical occurred, female dog whelks died when their egg tubes became blocked by their own eggs because they had developed male organs which had overgrown their female organs. It is difficult to comprehend that such an infinitesimal amount of a substance could, in the open sea, have such a profound effect: but it did. Unfortunately, the chemical is still licensed for use in larger ships including those used by the British Navy. Interestingly, TBT's mode of action is thought to be by blocking the conversion of testosterone to oestrogen in organisms because it inhibits aromatase. Aromatase inhibitors are now being widely prescribed for breast cancer, and I have yet to meet an oncologist who has heard of the damage caused by TBT.

Making sense of it all – the practicalities

Here is some more practical advice to cut down your individual exposure to such chemicals and that of society more generally, although it is impossible to do this completely. Indeed, many of the chemicals of concern are distributed across the globe and are even found in the blubber of seals and other creatures at the Polar Regions.

My advice continues to be to have as few man-made chemicals in your life as possible and avoid using perfume, fragrances or perfumed soap, aftershave, deodorant or similar products, especially in the genital or under-arm areas. Use natural crystal deodorants and try to avoid people who use lots of perfume. I never sleep with face cream on, and after removing make-up I remove the make-up remover with cotton wool soaked in hot water.

Try to avoid new products steeped in flame retardants, especially carpets, curtains and upholstery, computers and TVs.

If you do buy such products, ensure that you buy them from a company with an ethical policy on chemicals such as Marks and Spencer, and, particularly when they are new, ensure you are in a well-ventilated environment. Remember that the characteristic smell of a new car reflects the fact that it is emitting nasty chemicals such as plasticisers and brominated flame retardants. Although more than 120 gardening chemicals have been banned since the first edition of this book was published in 2000, it is still necessary to be careful. To avoid irresponsible use of chemicals in the environment, I never buy or give cut flowers. It is much better to give a garden plant. In my garden, Susan's rose, Eileen's buddleia and Georgina's astilbe bloom, reminding me of them every year. Many organophosphates, well known to be damaging to the central nervous system, are now known to be EDCs. Aside from sheep dip and shampoos to kill headlice, many familiar products are based on these substances, including many insecticides, sprays and treatments for lice or fleas on pets, including flea collars. Avoid all such products, and never use aerosol sprays for hair, deodorants, cleaning, gardening or any other purpose because of the increased risk of inhaling man-made chemicals. Evidence has recently emerged of the high levels of EDCs that we can be exposed to in cabin air when flying.

Pesticides are also widely used in some leisure industries. Golf courses, for example, are often kept looking perfect as a result of using large quantities of killer chemicals including herbicides, insecticides and rodenticides to kill moles. Try to persuade those in charge of any facilities you use, from tennis courts to cricket pitches and golf courses, that you would prefer less visual perfection in return for less use of toxic chemicals.

Where you live can also be a factor in increased exposure to harmful substances. Areas affected by pesticide spraying ranging from farms to golf courses, landfill and hazardous-waste sites, and areas downwind of certain industrial activities or hazardous-waste incinerators can all increase exposure. If you are concerned about any such hazards where you live, consult the Environment Agency in England and Wales or its equivalent in other countries.

Finally, remember: whenever you read or hear a new advertisement for a new 'personal care' product, man-made fabric or garden spray, for example, think very carefully whether you really need it. Almost certainly you do not. People who avoid such products are frequently portrayed as odd, especially by those wishing to sell us products that we do not need in order to make money. No one looking at me, spending time with me or visiting my home would think I was a crank. Unless pointed out to them they probably would not notice anything is missing or different. Indeed, people comment on how normal I am (presumably despite being a scientist)!

There is much additional information on hazardous substances at www.cancersupportinternational.com, and this site is constantly updated.

NEW LIFESTYLE FACTOR 7: OBESITY, EXERCISE AND SUNLIGHT

It has been suggested that women who are overweight or lead a sedentary lifestyle are more likely to express increased levels of insulin and growth factors that are associated with an increased risk of cancer.[96] Evidence of a link between breast cancer and ovarian cancer and obesity continues to mount. It is thought that the excess oestrogen produced by obese women increases the chance of developing hormone-dependent cancers. Other cancers for which obesity has been shown to be a risk factor include kidney and oesophageal cancers, while apple-shaped people with a large waist relative to their hips have been shown to be at increased risk of pancreatic cancer.[97]

A number of studies have shown that regular exercise, particularly if it is vigorous, offers some protection against breast cancer by modulating oestrogen. Exercise may also be helpful for women with early-stage breast cancer, by improving physical function and blunting some of the negative effects of treatments.[98] Vitamin D metabolite receptors are found on endocrine and reproductive organs and are known to play a role in inhibiting several types of cancer. The most beneficial form of vitamin D is created in the skin by the action of sunlight, and the amount of sunlight has been shown to decrease ovarian-cancer deaths in 100 of the largest cities in the USA.[99] A recent review of epidemiological studies into the association between cancer and vitamin D, sunlight, ultraviolet radiation and latitude confirmed that vitamin D is protective against several types of cancer including breast cancer and ovarian cancer.[100] Outdoor exercise in daylight may therefore be especially helpful. Try to incorporate exercise into your daily routine. A brisk walk for 30 minutes a day in daylight is good for the body and mind.

NEW LIFESTYLE FACTOR 8: HORMONES, THE FEMALE CONTRACEPTIVE PILL AND HRT

The most convincing evidence that exposure to hormones given to women raises breast-cancer risk relates to the use – in the past – of very high doses of diethylstilboestrol (DES) given to pregnant women.[101] Daughters of these women had an increased incidence of cancer of the vagina and cervix and there was a 35 per cent increase in breast cancer in the mothers themselves. However, it took twenty years before the hazard of DES in breast cancer became apparent, emphasising the long period between exposure and the appearance of the disease. Miller and Sharpe conclude that there is little additional convincing evidence to prove that circulating levels of other pharmaceutical hormones are related to the risk of breast cancer. However, they find that the evidence for links between hormones and the progression of established cancers is much more compelling.

Currently, two types of oral contraceptives (OCs) are available in the United States and many other countries.[102] The most commonly prescribed OC contains two synthetic versions of the natural female hormones (oestrogen and progesterone).

The second type of OC available in the United States is called the minipill and contains only a progestin. The minipill is less effective in preventing pregnancy than the combination pill, so it is prescribed less often.

Because medical research suggests that cancers of the female reproductive organs sometimes depend on naturally occurring sex hormones for their development and growth, medical researchers have focused a great deal of attention on OC users over the past 30 years. This has produced a wealth of data on OC use and the development of certain cancers, although the results are not always consistent. A new study shows that older women who have used OCs are no more likely to develop breast cancer than those who have not, according to the *BMJ*, bolstering a growing body of evidence that no link exists, although the researchers cautioned that the new findings were limited to the age group studied – women aged between 35 and 64.[103]

Most orthodox doctors in Western industrialised countries believe that the decline in oestrogen production at the menopause is one of the major factors in promoting osteoporosis and other conditions in women over the age of 50. The simplistic solution has been to replace the oestrogen with oestrogen replacement therapy (ORT, or ERT in North America where oestrogen is spelt estrogen). It soon became clear that this was associated with increased risk of endometrial cancer, which was attributed to prescribing unopposed oestrogen. This treatment was therefore replaced by tablets containing both oestrogen and progestins (hormone replacement therapy: HRT). Recent trials of one of these products has been abandoned, however, because the preliminary results, in line with the results of earlier studies, showed that the treatment carried an increased risk for breast cancer, coronary heart disease and strokes of 26 per cent, 23 per cent and 38 per cent, respectively.[104]

In a similar study of ORT/ERT, women were also found to be at increased risk of breast cancer which continued for four years after stopping therapy, when risk returned to normal.[105] One recent observational study also found that risk of breast cancer increased with longer duration of HRT use and only returned to the risk of non-users five or more years after use was stopped.[106] Another study suggests that the risk begins to return to normal about six months after women stop taking the hormones.[107]

While observational studies indicate that both groups of HRT users have a higher risk of breast cancer than non-users, the risk appears to be greater among women using combined therapy than in women using oestrogen alone.[108] Recently a big fall in breast cancer cases in the US has been attributed to the decline in use of HRT from about 30 per cent to about 15 per cent of women.[109] After rising steadily for 20 years, new cases of breast cancer fell by 7 per cent in 2003, about 14,000 fewer women affected than in 2002. In the UK there was a slight drop in breast-cancer cases in 2003 in women aged between 50 and 64 years, which is consistent with declining use of HRT – but by 2006 the cases in the UK had increased again to reach a new record high of 1 woman in 9 being affected by breast cancer.

If it is unwise to use HRT, is there anything that can be used instead? We have already mentioned the benefits of a diet rich in phyto-oestrogens. *The Desktop Guide to Complementary and Alternative Medicine: an evidence based approach*[110] indicates that there are no known contra-indications for phyto-oestrogens consumed as part of diet, although there are some for concentrated supplements. The guide concludes that increasing consumption of phyto-oestrogens in the diet has few risks and various potential health benefits.

JR Lee,[111] who, in the first edition of *Natural Progesterone*, was one of the first people to publish warnings that HRT increased the risk of breast cancer, has pointed out that over 5,000 plants contain progesterone-like substances. He suggests that creams derived from plants that are especially rich in these substances, such as wild yam, are more effective than conventional ERT/ ORT and HRT and lack the harmful side effects. He also suggests that restoring proper progesterone levels helps to protect against breast cancer. He cites a prospective study[112] in which pre-menopausal women with low progesterone levels were found to have 5.4 times the risk of developing breast cancer and a ten-fold increase in deaths from all cancers, compared with those with normal progesterone levels. The differences remained true despite differences in other commonly cited risk factors including age at onset of puberty, age at menopause, history of oral contraceptive use, history of benign breast disease and age at birth of first child.

Another relevant factor, according to Lee, is the survival rate after breast-cancer surgery of women with differing progesterone levels, and he refers to improved survival rates when breast-cancer surgery is performed in the second half of the menstrual month, when progesterone levels are highest.[113]

In a 20-year prospective study published in 1996 in the *British Journal of Cancer*, it was shown that women with a higher progesterone level had a significantly better survival rate (65 per cent) at 18 years than those with lower levels of progesterone (35 per cent).[114]

On the other hand, Lee quotes research which suggests that progestins (man-made, patentable pharmaceutical versions of the female hormone, progesterone) do not prevent breast cancer, and indeed seem to be associated with increased risk of the disease. He repeats that progestins are *not* the same as progesterone and that they do not stimulate the tumour-suppressor genes that fight cancer.

Lee notes the findings on the harmful effects of oestrogenic chemicals, including oestrone and oestrodial (produced in the body and also contained in some foods) and expresses concern about the conventional practice of prescribing oestrogen-replacement therapy (ORT) to women without a uterus or HRT using oestrogen with progestins. In his conclusion, he claims that progesterone creams decrease cell proliferation in breast cells by more than 400 per cent. He also claims that several men with prostate cancer were able to reduce their prostate-specific antigen (PSA) level by using a daily dab of progesterone cream, with no progression of their prostate lesions.

Personally, I would not use progesterone cream prepared from the urine of horses or other animals. I have used wild yam cream, which contains some of the herb black cohosh and which I buy from health food shops, in place of hormone replacement therapy for some considerable time with no ill effects. **Before using this yourself, you should discuss it thoroughly with your medical professional, bearing in mind that some breast tumours are progesterone-receptor positive**.

Ovarian cancer

The combined female contraceptive pill has been shown to be protective against ovarian cancer, but there may be an increased risk from the prolonged use of fertility drugs[115] and HRT.

There is some evidence that women who are lesbian are at increased risk of developing ovarian cancer. It has been suggested that this reflects the absence of such protective factors as pregnancy and the use of birth control pills.[116]

NEW LIFESTYLE FACTOR 9: PREGNANCY AFTER BREAST CANCER

Young women diagnosed with breast cancer before completing their families face difficult decisions about future child bearing. Because of the well-established link between oestrogen levels and the growth of breast-cancer cells, many doctors have advised breast-cancer survivors not to become pregnant. Although few studies have been performed, nearly all have found that pregnancy does not increase the risk of recurrence after successful treatment of breast cancer. Indeed one recent study concludes that the results do not support the current medical advice given to women with a diagnosis of breast cancer to wait two years before attempting to conceive unless they are receiving certain treatments or have other systemic disease. For women with localised disease the authors suggest that early conception, six months after completing treatment, is unlikely to reduce survival.[117] Women are advised to discuss their risk of recurrence with their doctors. In some cases, counselling can help women with the complex issues and uncertainties regarding motherhood and breast-cancer survival.[118]

NEW LIFESTYLE FACTOR 10: ABORTION AND BREAST CANCER

There are two different types of abortion, induced abortion, when a woman chooses to end a pregnancy, and spontaneous abortion, which most people refer to as a miscarriage. No link has been found between breast cancer and miscarriage (or stillbirth). In the case of induced abortion, the largest and most reliable study, conducted in Denmark, studied women born there between 1935 and 1978[119] and provided substantial evidence that induced abortion does not affect a woman's risk of developing breast cancer. Two other smaller studies reached similar conclusions. According to the American Cancer Society[120] the scientific evidence does not, at the present time, support a causal association between induced abortion and breast cancer. Any suggestions of a link appear to be from people who oppose abortion on religious or moral grounds.

CHAPTER 6 IN A NUTSHELL

- Scientific evidence shows there can be many problems as a result of taking man-made vitamins and minerals for cancer patients. Instead, use supplements that are naturally enriched in trace nutrients, such as kelp and brewer's yeast, but most importantly have a healthy diet with lots of organic fruit and vegetables. The use of calcium supplements may give rise to particular problems.
- Harmful chemicals can leak from plastic wrappings into food, and then accumulate in our body fat. Try whenever possible to buy food in good old-fashioned brown paper bags.
- Try not to live on fast and convenience food. Learn to cook and prepare healthy nutritious meals such as those in *The Plant Programme* or *Eating for Better Health*.

- It is helpful to reduce stress as much as possible, because scientific evidence indicates that it can have adverse physiological effects. Methods of reducing stress include meditation, relaxation and visualisation. Some cancer patients will benefit from professional help from a counsellor or psychologist.
- Try not to punish yourself. Some people feel that their cancer is some form of punishment but cancer is not brought about by a wrathful God. Almost all cancers and certainly breast cancer and ovarian cancer have far more rational explanations, as discussed in this book.
- The problem of chemicals in consumer products and as contaminants in food, air and water is not helped by the fact that many doctors take little or no interest in such chemicals or their effects. So learn how to cut down your exposure for yourself.
- Evidence of a link between breast cancer and ovarian cancer and obesity continues to mount.
- Outdoor exercise in daylight increases levels of a beneficial form of vitamin D that helps protect against breast cancer and ovarian cancer; other forms of gentle exercise, such as yoga or tai chi, may be helpful in coping with stress.
- There is no consistent evidence of a link between the female contraceptive pill and breast cancer, but its use appears to protect against ovarian cancer. HRT is strongly linked to increased breast-cancer and ovarian-cancer incidence. It is better to have a diet high in phyto-oestrogens to reduce menopausal symptoms. There is some evidence of increased risk of ovarian cancer as a result of prolonged use of fertility treatments.
- Although few studies have been performed, nearly all have found that pregnancy does not increase the risk of recurrence after successful treatment for breast cancer. Women are advised to discuss their risk of recurrence with their doctors. In some cases, counselling can help women with the complex issues and uncertainties regarding motherhood and breast-cancer survival.
- Scientific evidence does not, at the present time, support a causal association between induced abortion and breast-cancer or ovarian-cancer risk.

Update to Chapter 7. Why Our Lives are in Our Own Hands. Ten Simple Guidelines

I am convinced that our lives really are in our own hands. Much of the advice given to us, even from some government sources and charities, cannot be regarded as reliable, because of the overwhelming influence of vested-interest groups such as the food and pharmaceutical industries. We must, therefore, rely on ourselves and our own efforts in safeguarding our health, and try to distinguish objective, unbiased information based on good science from data biased by commercial or political interests. This chapter gives some advice on how to do this and concludes with ten simple guidelines.

As I wrote in the first edition of this book, much of the scientific evidence presented here has been widely known for decades by scientists around the world, so why have we, the public, not been told? Let us look first at dietary factors.

According to T. Colin Campbell,[1] scientists know an enormous amount about the links between nutrition and health, but the real science has been buried beneath a clutter of junk science, fad diets and food-industry propaganda. Many elements of the Western diet, such as the high levels of saturated fats and cholesterol in dairy products and meats, have been known to cause disease for decades. In 1961 the results of the seminal Framingham study in the USA showed clearly that cardiovascular disease did not reflect the heart wearing out, as previously thought; it reflected instead high intakes of animal fats in the diet.[2] These findings have been confirmed time and time again, and it has even been shown that heart disease can be reversed using diet alone.[3] Yet this has never been clearly communicated to the public, who, instead of being helped to change their diet and lifestyle, have been treated with a succession of pills and potions, many with unfortunate side effects and now with dairy-based spreads containing plant extracts!

In presenting the preliminary results of the China study, Campbell and Junshi[4] speculated that pressure from the food-industry lobby had distorted their important message to base diet mainly on fruit, vegetables and cereals and influenced both the media (and hence the public) and also policymakers simply to concentrate on low-fat foods.

According to an article entitled 'Food industry obfuscates healthy eating message'[5] this practice continues to the present day. The article describes how food giants are still going to enormous lengths to obfuscate US government messages on healthy eating. To counteract this problem, one US-based organisation is now sponsoring 'Clean Science in Regulation' to explore how to establish a proper relationship between an independent scientific community and the business community. The centre wants to prevent regulated industries from attacking and discrediting valid scientific information, and to examine bias in the membership of advisory committees and conflicts of interest in the sponsorship of scientific studies. Dr Marion Nestle of the Department of Food and Nutrition Studies, New York University, sums up the situation: 'Food is big business, $1.3 trillion . . . and the food industry will do everything to make sure that no regulatory agency and no nutritionist ever suggests eating less . . . and what [we] should eat less of'.

Recently the food industry in the USA has been accused of generating a 'toxic food environment',[6] dominated as it is by animal products, refined cereals and chemical concoctions that bear little resemblance to natural food.[7] Americans are increasingly sick, despite having the highest per capita spending on health care of any country in the world. An amazing two thirds are overweight and over 15 million have diabetes – and America has some of the highest rates of breast and ovarian cancer in the world.

Let us look in more detail at the role of the food industry in marketing food that is damaging to health, using the dairy industry as an example.

DAIRY IN THE DOCK

As discussed in Chapter Four and *Eating for Better Health*, in addition to the overwhelming evidence that dairy products are implicated in breast and ovarian cancer and osteoporosis, dairy is associated with a very wide range of diseases, including serious infectious illness. Industrialisation of the dairy industry has made matters worse. Cows are kept in large industrialised units, in which they are fed concentrates rather than being allowed to graze naturally, and they continue to be milked when they are pregnant. To quote from the *Sunday Times*, 'In reality, the modern high-yield dairy cow is a pitiful ramshackle embodiment of market-driven exploitation. The new UK model, so help us, is the American Holstein battery cow. A shed-housed fermentation vat on legs, teats dragging on the ground, it's a sight to frighten children.'[8] The article includes a photograph of 'a large-uddered milker, one of the grotesque products of the modern dairy industry'. The article goes on to point out that farmers have not been able to resist the genetic promise (of developing such creatures) – a 2 per cent compound increase in milk yield annually.

In the UK, the industry has been immensely damaging to our economy, including tourism, as a result of BSE, which was mainly a disease of dairy, not beef, cows, the foot-and-mouth crisis of 2001, and more recently bovine tuberculosis. Milk makes up 14 per cent of EU agricultural output and the annual turnover in the dairy-processing sector is about 117 billion euros.[9] Yet it continues to be heavily subsidised under the European Common Agricultural Policy. In fact, the EU's support for dairy farmers amounts to around £11 billion per year, which works out as about £1.40 per day for each cow. Put another way, the average EU cow now receives more than the income of half the world's population.[10] Dairy is big business, with the total value of milk production in the UK estimated at £2.7 billion, 3 times the value of the production of fresh vegetables.[11]

Concerns about marketing cows' milk to replace breast feeding have been around for many years. The late Dr Benjamin Spock, in *Baby and Child Care* (the United States' best selling book, other than the Bible, over the past fifty years), after recommending that no one consume cows' milk and cataloguing a host of ills associated with milk consumption (heart disease, cancer, obesity, antibiotic residue, iron deficiency, asthma, ear infections, skin conditions, stomach aches, bloating and diarrhoea*), concludes: 'In nature, animals do not drink milk after infancy, and that is the normal pattern for

---

* Other scientists link type 1 diabetes to the consumption of cows milk by babies and infants, especially genetically susceptible children.

humans, too . . . Children stay in better calcium balance when their protein comes from plant sources.' Dr Spock recommends human mother's milk for baby humans.

Dr Spock's book has been hugely influential. A great deal of his advice has been followed conscientiously by parents in America and all round the world. Why has his simple advice on milk not been followed equally conscientiously? And why has it taken about fifty years since Dr Spock's book was published for the UK Department of Health to endorse the resolution passed at the World Health Assembly in May 2001 that babies should be exclusively breast fed for the first six months of life?[12]

One of the reasons action has taken so long is perhaps illustrated by the example of the recent prosecution of SMA Nutrition, part of Wyeth, one of the world's biggest manufacturers of infant formula milk. This company was fined and ordered to pay legal costs after being convicted of six separate breaches of illegal advertising direct to consumers. In what is thought to be the first case of its kind, the judge described the company's breaches as 'cynical and deliberate . . .'[13]

The insidious ways that milk has been marketed to us are outlined by Butler.[14] She describes, for example, how school milk has been central to the promotion of dairy, most recently through the School Milk Project (TSMP) funded by the Milk Development Council. Dr Peter Atkins of Durham University has reviewed the motivation behind the introduction of cows' milk in schools early in the twentieth century. He concludes that the nutritional benefits were debatable, possibly even negative where dairy replaced other foods, but the dairy industry did well for itself creating new markets at a time of depression.[15] Free school milk continued until 1971 when Margaret Thatcher withdrew school milk on economic grounds. The emotional argument that followed and the nickname 'Thatcher, Thatcher milk snatcher' is a warning to anyone acting against the interests of the powerful dairy industry lobby.

I have certainly come under strong personal attack for my anti-dairy advice. For example, 'Jane Plant's statements are truly unfortunate. A study describing a single case history, particularly when it is the author's own, is scientifically unacceptable and lacks any objectivity', says Gregory D. Miller, PhD, FACN, vice president of nutrition research for (guess who!) the US National Dairy Council. He continues, 'There is no scientific evidence . . .'[16] Those of us in the UK know how little state-ments beginning 'There is no scientific evidence . . .' mean after the problems with BSE and new variant CJD that we have experienced. What the US National Dairy Council website attacking this book totally fails to mention is that it contains more than 600 references, mostly from the peer-reviewed literature, medical textbooks and websites such as those of the WHO. I have become accustomed to such arm-waving attacks which are deliberately misleading. As an experienced scientist, I am quite prepared to listen to specific facts that are wrong and to change my book accordingly. In the seven years since it was first published I have received no such comments.

As well as attacks on my work, there have been several attempts to buy me off. The latest, amazingly in the presence of my lawyer, was an offer by a probiotics (or yoghurt) company mediated by the head of a well-known cancer charity to persuade me that 'probiotics were not such a bad food after all'. In return for changing my position I would be given funding for my new website. Of course I was not prepared to accept such an offer and we left, indeed we swept out of the meeting immediately.

But back to the attacks, the study most frequently quoted against my books and in favour of the health benefits of dairy products is the Harvard Nurses' Health Study (HNHS), which purported to show the benefits of dairy products.

Dr R. M. Kradjian, Chief of the Breast Surgery Division, Seton Medical Center, California, in his book *Save Yourself from Breast Cancer*,[17] has much to say about the Harvard study in relation to breast cancer. In Appendix 1 of his book, he strongly criticises the methodology of the study, documenting several serious flaws in the scientific methodology. He concludes:

When one carefully dissects this report, it is revealed as a very peculiar piece of work. The problem is that very few physicians, American women, or members of the press seem to have read the article in close detail; nor did more than a handful apparently read the twelve pages of remark-able supplementary material. They were apparently com-forted by the names – Harvard, National Institutes of Health, and the American Cancer Society – and looked no further.

Kradjian himself discourages all use of cows' milk and all other dairy products. He notes that human beings are the only mammals on earth that continue to drink milk after weaning. 'Despite the fact that milk drinking is widespread among Westernised people, it is a truly bizarre habit.' Appendix 2 of his book is entitled 'Research Funding: an incentive for bias'. The first question is 'Who sponsored the Harvard Nurses' breast cancer study? At issue is the funding of university studies and university researchers by interested food-industry groups. Such funding could clearly result in pressure on those investigators to deliver conclusions that are acceptable to the sponsors, should the investigators hope to continue receiving funds from those sponsors.'

Much of the following section of the Appendix describes how he repeatedly contacted the Freedom of Information Office at the (US) National Institute of Health, but was unable to obtain an answer to the simple question 'Is the food industry involved in the funding of the Harvard Nurses' Health Study?' After a year of persistent probing, he had received 'only a verbal acknowledgement from one of the authors that "the dairy industry is involved in some part of the study"'.

There are several other papers that purport to show that there is no relationship between dairy and cancer or, worse, that dairy is protective. All the ones that I have read were funded by the dairy lobby. A recent example, funded by the UK dairy industry, a paper by Patricia G. Moorman and Paul D. Terry entitled 'Consumption of Dairy Produce and the Risk of Breast Cancer' has been used to send out the message, through a host of magazines, that dairy is not linked to cancer. Some of the many flaws in the paper are discussed on the website www. cancersupportinternational.com. Unfortunately many epidemiological studies that use metanalysis whereby data from multiple studies are combined and analysed as one data set can be totally confused if biased industry-funded research is included. In my research at Imperial College into environmental pollution from pesticides, for example, I now find it essential first to identify bias and be aware of it before combining datasets. This should be standard practice in all epidemiological studies.

On pages 235–236 I warned about the consequences of the privatisation of science. The *Sunday Times* article I quoted above in relation to the dairy industry makes the same point:[18]

> Of course, commercial science will look to where it's paid. 'CLA research was actually got going by the American meat and dairy industry', says Dr Campbell [Professor T Colin Campbell,], 'and it's very depressing when people start looking into little components of this and that. Let's face it, if dairy products contained all the good things that fruit and vegetables do, we'd be tired of hearing about them by now.'

In the UK, until recently, one of our main cancer-treatment centres defended consuming dairy produce. The leaflet 'After Treatment', produced by the Royal Marsden Hospital and issued to a breast-cancer sufferer in 2002, dismissed dietary therapy and claimed that there was no scientific evidence to support exclusion of dairy products from the diet. Clearly the authors of the leaflet have not read the extensive scientific reviews such as those by Outwater and others[19] and the European Commission[20] or the more recent review by Yu and Rohan[21] or the many, many other scientific references cited in my books.

Many people find it difficult to reconcile the advice given by me and others such as Kradjian with the conflicting advice given by their own doctors, nurses and dieticians. I thought this was mainly just the conservatism of the profession, but according to one source,[22]

> **The dairy industry** has a powerful hold on the nutrition industry in this country [the USA]; it **pays huge numbers of dieticians, doctors, and researchers to push dairy**, spending more than $300 million annually, just at the national level, to retain a market for its products. **The dairy industry has infiltrated schools, bought off sports stars, celebrities, and politicians, pushing all the while an agenda based on profit, rather than public health** [my bold].

My book with Gill Tidey on osteoporosis came under fierce attack in a review published in *Science in Parliament*.[23] Here is an extract from our response[24] which I think sums up the situation.

Our osteoporosis book is based on more than 450 references mainly from peer-reviewed sources and includes seven dietary and eight lifestyle factors so we are always suspicious when someone seizes on the non-dairy message. In the case of the lead reviewer of our book, Susan A. New, her university website indicates that her PhD was funded by a 'nutritional consultative panel UK dairy industry scholarship'.

Our response also notes:

New's consistent track record in raising significant research income. Moreover in 2001 she was awarded the silver medal of the (UK) Nutrition Society, where a senior officer recently confirmed that their funding was from publications, grants and fees for membership – and their membership includes mainly representatives of the food, feed and pharmaceutical industries.

R. M. Kradjian[25] draws attention to the problem of science funded by vested interest. He states,

The issue is clear. Much of our highly varied, desired and profitable food supply has been found to be dangerous. The people who furnish this food and who are enriched by its sale do not want you to know this. They have generously contributed to scientists who have supported and are willing to continue to support their products.

In their response[26] to our criticism of their biased review, New and her co-author stated 'We entirely refute Plant and Tidey's inference that our views have been influenced by any political conflict of interest, which we have always disclosed.' Unfortunately, there was no such disclosure in their review of our book on osteoporosis!

In contrast to the findings of scientists in receipt of funding and honours from the dairy industry, leading non-aligned nutritional scientists generally agree that osteoporosis is linked to high dairy consumption (Chapter Four). To quote John Robbins, author of *Diet for a new America*,[27]

The National Dairy Council has spent tens of millions of dollars to make us think that osteoporosis can be prevented by drinking more milk and eating more dairy products. But the only research that even begins to suggest that the consumption of dairy products might be helpful has been paid for by the National Dairy Council itself.

Let me finish this section with some extracts from reviews of *Your Life in Your Hands* posted on the Amazon.com website. One reviewer, a physician, writes: 'This book is a must read for any breast cancer activist and any health care professional who treats breast cancer in women. It is surprising that the book has not gotten more publicity and attention. I suspect the American dairy industry may have had something to do with that.'

A second writes: 'No wonder the dairy industry hates this book. Others have said this book is as important as Rachel Carson's *Silent Spring*. I agree.'

Cheese is junk food: official

In the UK there are some signs of improvement in the information given to the public, especially from the FSA under its new director Dame Deidre Hutton. New labelling of foods according to the amount of saturated fat, salt and sugar they contain mean that several dairy products will be given a red traffic-light symbol to warn of the high levels of saturated fat they contain. Also, since they are now formally classed as junk food, they will not be allowed to be advertised on television at times when children might be watching. So there have been some successes against the dairy lobby.

The Empire fights back and drops the D word

A recent article noting the growing anti-dairy lobby, especially in the UK, described how the industry intended to fight back with the help of a supermarket chain.[28] Certainly, there seem to be endless dairy advertisements, and cheese and cream are used extensively in TV cooking programmes despite their designation as junk foods. *The Times* recently produced a biased, poorly researched article[29] assuring us that dairy is safe, based on information from the official-sounding British Nutrition Federation. This organisation is, in fact, funded by the Dairy Council, Dairy Crest, Kraft Foods and Nestle UK.[30] Dairy is now sold as functional food, often with no mention that it contains dairy. For example yoghurt has been renamed 'probiotics' and no one mentions milk or dairy in any of the advertisements promoting the stuff. Even *ICON*, the magazine aimed at telling cancer sufferers the latest research findings about cancer, carries advertisements for probiotics without mentioning the D word.[31]

FRUITFUL ORGANIC ARGUMENTS AND THE POISON WITHIN

It is unfortunate that the Food Standards Agency in the past and the Advertising Standards Agency did not pursue the claims of the Dairy Council with the same vigour that they applied against organic food producers.

FALSE CLAIMS[32]

Last year [2001], in an attempt to clamp down on false and misleading claims, the Advertising Standards Authority (ASA) issued guidelines for advertisers on claims about organic food. This was prompted by several complaints received by the ASA about organic claims made by well-known names, including Tesco and the Soil Association. The new guidelines state that:

- Advertisers can't claim that organic food is 'safer' or 'healthier' than conventional food, unless they have convincing evidence that this is the case.
- Organic food can't be described as 'environmentally friendly' or 'sustainable', as all managed food production systems cause some environmental damage.
- Claims that organic food uses no chemicals, pesticides or artificial additives can only be made if this is the case.

Why, for example was the UK Dairy Council allowed to make claims that 'A natural fat [CLAs] found in milk, cheese, yoghurts and butter may soon prove to contain anti-cancer properties', when, as the *Sunday Times* article (*see* p. 346) points out, 'the proportion of CLAs is only 1 in 120 parts of saturated fat; ergo, to come by a significant amount of CLAs, you'd have to eat artery-choking amounts of the fat stuff?'[33]

In Chapter Five I have argued that one of the best ways of limiting the ingestion of toxic man-made substances is by eating organically grown food, ideally produced locally to the standards of the Soil Association.

The following is an edited extract of an article in *Which?* magazine,[34] discussing the advantages of organically produced food:

> One of the most common reasons our shoppers gave for choosing organic food was to avoid pesticides. Organic standards allow the use of some approved pesticides but these are mostly from natural sources. There's little data on pesticide residue levels in organic food, but the government's pesticide residue monitoring programme (see *Which?*, September 2001, p. 24) includes a limited number of organic samples, and residues are rarely found in those tested . . . Processing can significantly reduce the levels of residues. Washing and peeling alone has been shown to reduce levels by 50 to 90 per cent in apples, carrots and potatoes. Cooking and other types of processing involving heat can reduce levels further . . .

Also, by restricting the use of artificial fertilisers and pesticides, organic farmers and agricultural workers reduce the risk of harmful health effects to themselves as well as the risk of environmental damage associated with more intensive pesticide use.

Organic food can contain food additives (E numbers) and processing aids, but the list is more restricted – around 35 additives are approved, compared with hundreds in conventional food. Also they are natural substances such as copper sulphate, which has been around on Earth for millions of years, not man-made molecules invented by man over the last 60 years or so. Artificial sweeteners are also banned in organic food and only natural flavourings and colourings are allowed.

In spite of all the evidence to the contrary, the UK government took action, mainly through the Food Standards Agency, to argue that there are no health benefits to eating organically produced foods. The following is an edited extract from another article in *Which?*[35]

> The health benefits of eating fruit and vegetables are clear. The government wants us to eat at least five portions a day.

To encourage this the Department of Health has introduced the National School Fruit Scheme, with the aim that, by 2004, all schoolchildren aged four to six will be receiving a piece of free fruit daily.

But fruit and vegetables tested still contain pesticide residues. Although most residues fall within legal safety levels, figures show 72 per cent of apples and 81 per cent of pears have residues. And, in December [2001] it was reported that 61 per cent of grapes and 63 per cent of kiwi fruit contained toxic chemicals. Exposure to pesticides may be linked to increasing cancer rates and other health problems – young children, in particular, may be more vulnerable . . .

With these concerns, you'd expect the current and long-standing advice to wash and peel fruit as 'a sensible additional precaution when preparing fruit for small children' to be emphasised or improved. Instead, the FSA wants to ditch the advice because its 'misinterpretation' could imply that 'only organic fruit should be supplied to the National School Fruit Scheme' – according to a leaked memo . . .

Which? thought that the FSA approach wasn't good enough and asked the government to be more transparent about its motives.

According to an article in the *Daily Mail*, John Krebs, the former head of the FSA, was particularly sceptical about the value of organic food, and under his direction the Agency faced claims that it was biased against organic agriculture. Since Dame Deidre Hutton took over, the FSA has funded a lecture by Lord Melchett on behalf of the Soil Association, about the benefits of organic food, introduced a simple but effective traffic-light system to indicate food containing high levels of fat, salt or sugar, and classified cheese and other dairy products such as Greek yoghurt as junk food. The FSA website on organic farming and food now states:

Organic farming is a holistic approach to food production, making use of crop rotation, environmental management and good animal husbandry to control pests and diseases. Processed organic foods use ingredients that are produced organically and organically produced ingredients must make up at least 95 per cent of the food. There are only a limited number of additives used in organic food production. Some key aspects of organic farming are:

1. Restricted use of artificial fertilisers or pesticides.
2. Emphasis on animal welfare, and prevention of ill health, including stocking densities, free range, choice of suitable breeds.
3. Use of conventional veterinary medicines is focused on treating sick animals.
4. Emphasis on soil health and maintaining this through application of manure, compost and crop rotation.

My faith in the FSA has increased greatly since Dame Deidre took over.

But what can possibly be wrong with the organic farming movement? All their stated aims seem to make so much sense. Who could possibly oppose such a movement at a time when there is so much talk of sustainability? Once again one has to look who stands to lose out if we all buy organic. Who has a vested interest in portraying all those of us who back the organic movement as emotional unscientific crackpots? Could it be the pesticide industry – an industry worth millions of dollars a year in the USA alone? Might it be that this industry also tries to subvert the truth and to influence some scientists to act on its behalf?

On 8 December 2006 many scientists were shocked to read an email that claimed that, since the late 1970s, Professor Sir Richard Doll had been in receipt of large sums of money from pesticide manufacturers. The email and the various newspaper articles that appeared at the time included a copy of a letter sent to Sir Richard by George Roush, director of Monsanto's medicine and environmental health department, on 29 April 1986, which read as follows:

Dear Sir Richard
This letter is for the purpose of extending your Consulting Agreement with Monsanto Company dated May 10 1979. The consulting agreement is hereby extended for an additional one-year period beginning June 1 1986 and ending May 31, 1987.

During the one year period of this extension your consulting fee shall be \$1,500 per day. All other terms and conditions of the Consulting Agreement of May 10 1979 shall remain in effect during this extension period.

If the foregoing meets with your understanding and approval please so indicate by executing this letter in duplicate and returning one of the signed duplicates to us.

Yours etc

It has been suggested that Doll donated the money he received to Green College Oxford. Nevertheless, it would have been wise to declare such a serious conflict of interest, especially in the much-quoted paper entitled 'The causes of cancer' published in 1981, only two years after Doll's Monsanto consultancy began. In the paper, pesticides and other chemicals in the environment were said to be responsible for only 1–2 per cent of cancers. Recent re-examination of the Doll and Peto study suggests that it was seriously flawed and that it totally underestimated the numbers of cancers that could be prevented by better regulation of chemicals in the environment. A review of environmental and occupational causes of cancer published in 2005[36] states that 'it is difficult to estimate the impact of Doll and Peto's views especially by those who argue that cleaning up the environment is not going to make much difference to cancer rates.' The review goes on to trace how the Doll and Peto study influenced other scientists, governments and cancer organisations to put relatively little emphasis on pollution – much less than on tobacco smoking and other personal lifestyle choices. This approach, the review suggests, is still hampering the USA from implementing a comprehensive policy on chemicals regulation such as that being introduced in the European Union from 2007, known as REACH.

Of course I would not accuse Sir Richard of dishonesty nor even of bias, but it is worth pondering what would have happened if he had investigated links between pesticides and cancer with the same vigour and intensity that, as a young man, he had brought to bear on investigating the links between lung cancer and cigarette-smoking. It is also worth pondering how many cancers might have been prevented had chemicals been better regulated earlier.

As discussed in Chapters Four and Six, there are increasing numbers of studies that now link cancer to endocrine-disrupting chemicals – which include many pesticide formulations. For more information on links between cancer and harmful substances in the environment you might wish to visit www.cancersupportinternational.com.

TECHNOLOGICAL MEDICINE

A doctor friend of mine describes the UK's National Health Service as the 'National Illness Service'. He is right to do so. In my own subject of environmental chemistry the whole approach would be regarded as an outdated 'end-of-pipe' solution. This approach is now discredited in favour of using a full-life-cycle analysis to avoid problems at all stages, from raw-material extraction, refining and manufacturing to end-of-life disposal of products and beneficial after-use of land.[37] In medicine, such an approach would involve placing far more emphasis on prevention, where prevention means giving people clear, truthful, readily understandable information about healthy diet and lifestyle, and becoming involved in limiting the use of cancer-causing chemicals, especially in food production.

Doctors and nutrition

Many people express concern about how little their doctors know about nutrition. Why do some recommend their patients not to take soya? Do they not know that, in common with other peas and beans, it contains phyto-oestrogens which are protective against breast and ovarian cancer? Why do many doctors fail to advise against consuming dairy, which is packed with dangerous growth factors and animal hormones such as oestrogen up to a thousand times more powerful than phyto-oestrogens? Why do many doctors recommend dairy and calcium supplements, when leading researchers at Harvard showed more than 20 years ago that such concentrated sources of calcium suppress a form of vitamin D that is vital for the immune system to protect against cancer and to protect our bones against osteoporosis? I am afraid that the answer is ignorance of the scientific literature. My son is now a doctor, and so I am aware how full the curriculum is, but far more proper science and far less sociology would be my prescription for producing better informed doctors.

With improved survival rates for cancer, especially breast cancer, and increased interest in the extent to which dietary changes improve outcomes, surprisingly little is known about the effects on cancer survival. Instead of emotional outbursts from some UK doctors against the use of such methods to complement conventional medical treatment of cancer, would it not be better to devise some scientific studies to compare outcomes? Fortunately this has begun for breast cancer, with about six studies being started in the USA.[38]

Doctors and cancer prevention

Unfortunately, in conventional medicine, 'prevention' seems to equate to 'early detection' – a battery of screening tests, a considerable proportion of which involve using ionising radiation or the injection of potentially harmful chemicals.[39]

A report from the Health Development Agency (the NHS body responsible for promoting more healthy lifestyles) entitled *Where's the Research on Preventing and Reducing Ill Health*, states that only 0.4 per cent of studies into such issues as smoking, heart disease and cancer looked at prevention rather than cure.[40] Chaturvedi points out that of those medical students aiming for a lucrative private practice, those opting for studies in prevention are considered academically unsound.[41]

The UK National Cancer Research Institute has produced a detailed breakdown of spending on cancer research. It estimates that more than £250 million from 15 leading charities and government organisations goes towards cancer research in the UK every year,[42] most being spent on the most lethal cancers, including prostate and breast cancer. The study showed that the biggest proportion of spending (41 per cent) goes on basic biological research, followed by research into treatment (22 per cent), while only 16 per cent is spent on researching causes. Research into prevention, care of patients, and survival attracts the least funding. The whole approach merely serves to generate yet more jobs and money in the pharmaceutical, medical-equipment and medical industries that constitute industrial medicine today.

Evidence-based medicine

The industrialisation of medicine increasingly depends on costly drugs and other invasive and often unpleasant treatments, for which 'Evidence-based medicine' is one of the main planks.

Writing in the *BMJ*,[43] Richard Smith discussed evidence-based medicine as a means of answering 'One of medicine's most important – and simplest – questions: "Does a treatment work?"' He continued,

> It has now become almost the only 'gold standard' way of testing different treatments to be sure that you are comparing the same sorts of patients at the same time; that is to 'randomise' the patients to one treatment or another. To exclude 'bias' (which might, for example, lead a doctor to put all the sicker patients into one arm of the trial) neither the doctor nor the patient should know who has got the active treatment, making the trial 'double blind'.
> **Because the benefit from most medical treatments is so small and so hard to detect**, you need very many patients in the trial. Although 'double blind randomised trials' are considered the best way of determining whether a treatment works, **many of them have been poorly conducted and have given misleading results**.[44] [my bold]

The problems of recruitment of appropriate patients to randomised trials have been raised by Corrie, Shaw and Harris.[45] They found that even when a trial was available, eligibility criteria excluded over half of patients. Other serious problems of carrying out meaningful double-blind randomised trials have been described by Wald and Morris.[46] Moreover, results may vary according to the source of funding for the trial (see below). Nevertheless it is data from such trials that often dictate treatment. A review of drug-industry funding for trials of breast-cancer drugs found that 84 per cent of industry-funded studies were positive, compared with 54 per cent of those funded by other sources.[47]

Screening for cancer is extremely lucrative but potentially problematical, often involving ionising radiation or the use of high-powered electromagnetic fields or potentially harmful chemicals.

In an editorial in the *BMJ*,[48] Richard Smith wrote:

> The problems (of scans) lie in medicine's difficulties in defining normality, the devil of 'false positives', and our

limited understanding of the natural history of disease. The commonest way of defining normal is that the measure lies within two standard deviations of the mean. So in a set of measurements from a normal population 5 per cent will be classed as 'abnormal'. The whole body scan will produce hundreds of measurements. So you have almost no chance of emerging as normal . . .

Let us look in more detail at some of the other drivers of end-of-pipe technological medicine.

Doctors and pharmaceutical companies

The real problem of the relationship between doctors and pharmaceutical companies has been summed up by Fuard Lechin as follows:[49]

The practice of Medicine is divided into two camps of doctors engaged in combating disease: scientists and clinicians. The former acquires knowledge about physiology, pathophysiology, pharmacology, neurochemistry, neuroendocrinology, immunology, genetics, biochemistry and many other disciplines. Unfortunately these doctors do not practice medicine.

Conversely many physicians or clinical practitioners possess only superficial knowledge of the above disciplines and so are limited to rudimentary and simplistic diagnostic and therapeutic procedures for suppressing symptoms. They do their best although sadly it is seldom enough.

He concludes that 'while doctors are trained as technicians but not scientists, the pharmaceutical industry but not doctors prescribe treatments to patients.' Also too many doctors are essentially professional human biologists, when we need doctors who understand far more chemistry if they are to work as equals with the pharmaceutical companies rather than simply acting as their agents.

PHARMACEUTICALS – SOME PROBLEMS

The pharmaceutical industry is very profitable (US drug sales grew 12 per cent in 2002, to $220 billion[50]), and hence very powerful. An article entitled 'Drug companies maintain "astounding" profits'[51] states that pharmaceuticals ranked as the most profitable sector in the US annual 'Fortune 500' ranking of America's top industries, released in May 2002. Of course, there is nothing wrong with profitability itself – only with the abuse of the power that profits can bestow.

The *BMJ*, from which I have quoted extensively in this book, now asks all contributors to sign a declaration of conflicts of interests, including funding sources and competing interests. This has allowed the association between such interests and the author's conclusions to be investigated.[52] Financial competing interests are defined as funding by for-profit organisations and other competing interests such as personal, academic or political. The results showed that authors' conclusions were significantly more positive towards the experimental intervention in trials funded by for-profit organisations alone than in trials without competing interests or in trials funded by both profit and non-profit organisations. The association between financial competing interests and authors' conclusions was not explained by the quality of the methods used, the statistical power, the type of experimental intervention, involving pharmaceuticals or non-pharmaceutical approaches or medical speciality. The authors concluded that in cases where financial competing interests had been declared, randomised clinical trials significantly favour experimental interventions. In a poll conducted by the *BMJ* on its website (bmj.com), 96 per cent of the 1479 people who voted would like to see all financial relationships between doctors and drug companies conducted with transparent contracts that are disclosed to patients.[53]

In the US, too, researchers have claimed that most randomised trials of new treatments published in leading medical journals are reported in a potentially misleading way, with statistics designed to make the results more positive than if other statistical tests were used.[54]

The problem seems to have become much worse, at least in the US. Industry supported 62 per cent of biomedical research in the US in 2000, almost double the proportion in 1980; during the same period, government support declined. About a quarter of academic investigators have affiliations to industry that could influence research and publication, according to a review in the *Journal of the American Medical Association*.[55]

Concern about links between the pharmaceutical industry and experts were also raised in a study carried out by researchers in Toronto. They claim that most guidelines on clinical practice are written by experts with undisclosed links to the pharmaceutical industry. In a survey of nearly 200 authors of 44 clinical guidelines, 87 per cent of respondents admitted to financial links with one or more pharmaceutical companies,[56] and one new American company called Time-Concepts LLC is offering doctors $50 (£34) each time they listen to a short sales pitch from a drug company representative.[57]

Another increasing concern is the direct marketing of pharmaceuticals to patients, including via the internet. According to a recent article in the *BMJ*, a fifth of Americans contact their doctor as a result of direct-to-consumer drug advertising.[58]

The drug companies have expressed the wish to 'inform' patients,[59] and the chief executive of the Association of British Pharmaceutical Industries states: 'My feeling, from the pharmaceutical industry, is because we are the providers of medicines that people get from the health service, we should not be excluded [from giving information to patients], provided we do it in an objective way.' He denied suggestions that this might stoke demand for certain drugs.

Fortunately (in my view) moves to allow drug manufacturers to advertise directly to particular groups of patients have been rejected by European Union health ministers.[60] In 2006 the drug company Roche, which produces Herceptin and is the leading maker of anticancer drugs, began funding an organisation called Cancer United. The *BMJ* reported that the involvement of Roche cast a cloud over the launch of the new organisation in Brussels.[61] The organisation is calling for the European Commission to develop a Europe-wide cancer strategy and for all EU governments to implement national plans.

In the UK, the General Medical Council has issued new guidance on the standards expected for research carried out in the National Health Service, universities and the private sector,[62] while the US government[63] has joined the American Medical Association and the drug industry in efforts to control drug-company handouts to the medical profession – but the recommendations are voluntary.

THE CANCER INDUSTRY

A book entitled *Breast cancer: an environmental disease*, published by Unison, Breast Cancer UK and the Women's Environmental Network in 2005 referred to the 'cancer industry'. This was said to be 'a generic term for the ever expanding industry which has grown up around the disease'. The book went on,

It is a vast industry incorporating all services, products, materials and technologies for the orthodox management of the disease.

Given its

- traditional preoccupation with control and management of the disease,
- current preoccupation with new therapies (drug and gene) to meet future demands,
- huge research and financial investment in therapies for a burgeoning future market, and
- awareness that profits for society from primary prevention represent a loss of industry profits,

there would appear to be little hope for the primary prevention of breast cancer becoming a priority for the cancer industry.

Interestingly, the book states that cancer charities work in close association with the cancer industry and that primary prevention is not their aim; and it specifically mentions Breakthrough in this respect. In conclusion, the report states, 'A thriving industry with a guaranteed future, "cancer" is a growth industry in every sense of the word. It would be particularly unlikely that this particular industry would champion a cause that has the potential to undermine its very existence.'

CHARITIES, PATIENT ASSOCIATIONS AND RESEARCH

There is also concern about links between pharmaceutical companies and patient organisations and charities.

Writing in the *BMJ* on the subject of industry funding of patients' support groups, Paola Mosconi wrote that declaration of competing interests is rare in Italian breast-cancer associations. The following is an edited version:[64]

Herxheimer reported and commented on relationships between pharmaceutical companies and consumers' and patients' associations.[65] This is a 'hot' topic: the debate on

transparency of fund raising for voluntary health associations is far from being resolved, and consumers' umbrella
associations have an increasingly important role in discussing health at a European level.

In Italy, at least among the 100 breast-cancer associations
belonging to the Italian forum of Europa Donna, transparency of fund raising is rarely discussed and few data are
available. Using a standardised self-administered questionnaire on the characteristics of breast cancer associations,
information on the sponsorship of 67 of them indicated that
although most of the funds come from individual donations,
one third received funds from pharmaceutical companies.

In the same survey it was found that only five breast-
cancer associations had been open and transparent about
sponsorship by pharmaceutical companies.

These data confirm the concern expressed by Herxheimer
and by Hirst[66] on the independence of consumers' and patients'
associations and support the need for more openness and
transparency about funding from the pharmaceutical industry
and other vested interest groups for organisations participating
in the debate on public health. It should be a requirement that
such conflicts of interest are clearly stated on the home page of
the websites of all charities and patient organisations.

Another article in the *BMJ*[67] tells 'How HRT studies have got
drug firms rallying the troops':

In 2002 the powerful New York based Society for Women's
Health Research, whose 'sole mission is to improve the
health of women through research', held a celebrity gala . . .
entirely underwritten by Wyeth. In a *Washington Monthly*
article entitled 'Hot Flash, Cold Cash', journalist Alicia
Mundy reported that only a few days after the gala the
company donated a quarter of a million dollars to the society.

Several weeks later, in July 2002, [negative findings
about HRT were made public after the huge US Women's
Health Initiative (WHI) study was prematurely halted on
grounds of safety[68]] Wyeth was in a tailspin. They found
support from the society . . . [which, as Mundy observed,]
'seemingly took the side of its donors – and of Wyeth in
particular.' As they fervently downplayed the negative

findings of the WHI study and urged women not to abandon their HRT, the society's staff failed to disclose their substantial links to Wyeth and other drug companies.

It is interesting that a 7 per cent reduction in breast cancer incidence in North America in 2003 has been attributed to reduced use of HRT there.[69]

Another investigation in the USA discovered that three key organisations, the United Seniors Association, the Seniors Coalition, and the 60s Plus Association, have all received substantial contributions in recent years from the drug industry: 'When the pharmaceutical industry speaks these days, many Americans may not be able to recognise its voice. That's because the industry often uses "front groups" that work to advance its agenda under the veil of other interests.'[70]

Let us look at what some charities have said about recent reports linking diet to cancer. In November 2006, scientific researchers in the USA published the results of their findings into the links between red meat and breast cancer, based on studies of the diets of 90,000 women.[71] It was found that women who ate more than one and a half servings of red meat a day had a risk of hormone(oestrogen and progesterone)-receptor-positive cancer almost double that of those who ate three or fewer servings a week. It was suggested that this was caused by hormone residues from growth hormones used on cattle in the US or the presence of heterocyclic amines created during cooking of red meat. In the first (2000) edition of this book I predicted that these would be avoidable risk factors for breast cancer. Dr Cho, in summarising the importance of his teams' findings, stated 'Given that most of the risk factors for breast cancer are not easily modifiable these findings have potential public health implications in preventing breast cancer.' So what did the breast-cancer charities say? Sarah Rawlings of Breakthrough Breast Cancer is quoted as saying 'Very little is known about diet and breast cancer risk because we eat a variety of foods and separating out the effect of an individual food is difficult.' What nonsense! Of course trained scientists such as Dr Cho know how to process and interpret data in relation to confounding factors and as for 'very little is known about diet and cancer' one is tempted to ask if Rawlings reads? Maria Leadbetter of Breast Cancer Care's response was equally helpful and informative! She stated 'The benefits of eating a healthy and varied diet are well established and the biggest risk factors for breast cancer remain gender and age.'

Another report released in January 2007 showed that pre-menopausal women who ate more than 30 g fibre from foods such as wholemeal bread, fruit and vegetables in the diet had a risk of breast cancer half that of women who ate less than 20 g a day. There was again a rather muddled, lukewarm response from Breakthrough Breast Cancer. In contrast, Cancer Research UK was quite positive. They stated, 'It further highlights the importance of eating a healthy diet for reducing the risk of cancer.'

Of course, I am delighted with the results of such studies, confirming as they do all my findings based on analysing the scientific literature and first published in 2000. It is interesting to recall how I was attacked by Breakthrough at the time. Their then chief executive, Delyth Morgan, attacked my findings in interview after interview. I wondered at the time what Breakthrough's agenda was and I still wonder what it is! I have generally found prostate-cancer charities to be rather more enlightened and helpful, and more willing to advise their members on diet and lifestyle. Many now advise against eating dairy.

I have been asked countless times since this book was first published about donations to cancer charities. I recommend that any charitable donations should be given to highly reputable charities. The research charity I would choose is Cancer Research UK, which is headed by a distinguished doctor and, although it errs on the conservative side of issues, can, I think, be trusted. I have started a new charity, Cancer PPrevent, aimed at the primary prevention of cancer by identifying and communicating avoidable risks. The charity is part of Imperial College Trust and is headed by a distinguished cancer biologist, Professor Mustafa Djamgoz, Dr Voulvoulis, who is an expert in endocrine-disrupting substances, and me.

I also commend the charities concerned with caring, such as Macmillan Cancer Relief, Marie Curie Cancer Care, Positive Action Against Cancer and the various hospices. Before giving any donations to cancer charities, do consider what proportion of their funds are devoted to administration, or the acquisition of capital assets such as buildings, the merchandising of consumer goods, and what proportion is actually spent on cancer prevention and/or care. Cancer PPprevent has the best profile in terms of expenditure on administration and buildings relative to money spent on research, but it is still new and poorly funded. Personally I would not give a penny to Breakthrough Breast Cancer.

MEDIA AND ADVERTISING

According to another *BMJ* article, positive reporting bias may occur for several reasons. Beyond the seemingly universal desire to believe in cures, which may underlie some of the bias in such media reports, are corporate interests, the author suggests. Journalists seeking experts for comments often turn to seemingly credible and disinterested groups, such as professional associations, non-profit health groups, and patient organisations. The article goes on to say that many journalists do not realise, or fail to report, that many groups receive substantial funding from vested interests. Hospitals in North America, facing brutal competition, have, the article suggests, started buying contracts with television stations to feature them 'in news reports'. A poll of 300 news directors found that 43 per cent felt that such payments create pressures to exert improper influence. Dr Ivan Oransky, who teaches medical journalism at New York University, believes that the sort of investigative reporting that is standard in political coverage is lacking in medical and science reporting, with too many journalists reporting researchers' assertions uncritically.[72]

A recent development in America is the sponsored news programme, and it may be queried whether these are a new form of paid front for the pharmaceutical industry.[73] What many viewers of these news-magazine-style programmes may not realise is that healthcare companies, including pharmaceutical and biotechnology companies, are paying directly for videos and suggesting the topics to be covered, according to a report in the *New York Times*. That article named a number of senior American broadcasters as having worked for a company funded by pharmaceutical giants to make video material. The celebrity journalists were reportedly paid up to $100,000 for one day's work, broadcast as news on public television stations across the country.

In the UK recently the media have led highly charged emotional campaigns for certain drugs to be made available to sufferers of breast cancer in advance of, or in some cases in spite of, the recommendations of NICE, the National Institute for Health and Clinical Excellence, the body established to provide evidence-based advice to the NHS. In 2005 there was a particularly emotional campaign for breast-cancer sufferers to be prescribed Herceptin (trastuzumab).[74] The drug is a monoclonal antibody that acts on the HER-2 (erbB2) receptor which is over-expressed in about 25 per cent of early-stage breast cancers. Herceptin costs about $70,000 for a full course of treatment and debate has centred on whether the drug should be provided to all patients with early HER-2 cancer or only some, given that about 70 per cent of patients do not respond to treatment and cancer resistance develops rapidly in virtually all patients with little evidence of improved survival. Also the drug is associated with heart problems in up to 7 per cent of patients and this percentage increases when the drug is combined with certain types of chemotherapy.[75] Moreover, as a recent article in the *BMJ* points out, the new guidance from NICE recommending Herceptin in early breast cancer with no additional funding and no suggestions on which other services to cut to fund the drug leaves medical staff to make difficult decisions; the authors of the *BMJ* article describe the situation as 'rationing by media'.[76] I heard none of the complications of using Herceptin, which call for fine clinical judgements, in media reports at the time. They simply gave the impression that by denying patients the drug we were committing them to death. Recent discussions on the BBC suggest that they are more aware of ways in which sufferers can be manipulated now.

That pharmaceutical companies devise clever ways to market their products is hardly surprising, but journalists and others should be more sceptical. They should always ask the key questions, 'Who is funding you or your research?' In an article in the *Guardian* in February 2006 George Monbiot stated that 'academics and the media have failed dismally to ask the crucial question of scientists' claims: Who is paying you.' He cited the example of Professor David Warburton of Reading University working for an organisation called ARISE that described itself as 'a worldwide association of eminent scientists who act as independent consultants', but which obtained more than 90 per cent of its funding from the tobacco industry. He describes how Warburton in an uncontested interview on the Today Programme extolled the calming properties of cigarettes and poured scorn on public health messages, and was unchallenged by any of the UK press except for one article in the *Guardian*.

In general, it has been said, newspapers under-report randomised trials, emphasise bad news from observational studies, and ignore research from developing countries.[77]

WHERE DOES THE FAULT LIE?

Instead of trying to prevent disease (based on good dietary advice), we continue to treat disease with pills and potions, surgery or other expensive invasive methods to suppress symptoms. The communication of problems in our diet and lifestyle that affect our health is typically done poorly – or not at all – and usually without proper, clear advice on how to change our behaviour.

In the first edition of this book I asked why. I raised concerns about wealth creation being more highly regarded than quality of life, and the lack of an adequate knowledge of science in Parliament and the civil service, especially after the privatisation of much science in the late 1970s and 1980s, but I had no idea how serious the problems were. The whole approach to chronic illness avoids antagonising special-interest groups, and it maintains the material wealth of (and jobs in) sectors such as farming, agrochemicals, the food industry, pharmaceutical research and the manufacture of medicines and medical equipment. But would it not be better to communicate facts as they are known, clearly and simply, so that people can make their own choices and prevent disease? Would it not be better to create jobs in sectors working for the well-being of society and the environment, for example, in growing wholesome, nutritious organically produced food, with medical professionals being concerned more with health education, disease prevention and monitoring, as dentists now are, than dishing out pills?

And yet society continues to emphasise the search for cures. The point is well made by a story attributed to Joseph Malins (1895) about a dangerous cliff and the debate whether to erect a fence at the top of the cliff, to prevent people falling off, or keep an ambulance down in the valley:

A collection was made to accumulate aid,
and the dwellers in highway and alley
gave dollars and cents, to provide . . . not a fence,
but an ambulance down in the valley.

'For the cliff is all right if you're careful', they said,
'and if folks ever slip and are dropping,
it isn't the slipping and dropping that hurts,
it's the shock down below when they're stopping.'

So for many a year, as these mishaps occur,
quick forth do the rescuers sally,
to pick up the victims who fall from the cliff
with the ambulance down in the valley.

Then one made a plea: 'It's a marvel to me
that you'd give so much greater attention
to repairing results than to curing the cause;
why, you'd much better aim at prevention.

'For the mischief of course should be stopped at its source.
Come, neighbours and friends, let us rally:
it makes far better sense to rely on a fence
than an ambulance down in the valley.'

'He's wrong in his head', the majority said.
'He would end our entire earnest endeavour.
He's the kind who would shirk this responsible work,
But we will support it for ever.'[78]

OUR LIVES IN OUR HANDS

In the first edition of this book I gave much information to reduce
our individual risk of breast cancer, by changing our Western
lifestyle and showing with our buying power that we don't want
dairy produce, or harmful chemicals in our lives but that we do
want locally grown organically produced food. In the UK, this is
beginning to happen as dairy farms give way to more beneficial
uses of land and the market for organic food keeps on expanding.

TOWARDS A HAPPY ENDING

I am delighted that in the seven years since this book was first
published so many people have told me how helpful they have
found it, and that no credible science has been published to
persuade me to change one word of my advice to breast-cancer
sufferers. Indeed, new research confirms that the dietary and
lifestyle changes first suggested in the book to help prevent and
treat breast cancer are sound. I hope that this new edition will

be used widely to help women to reduce their risk of suffering from breast or ovarian cancer. For those already suffering from these diseases, I hope it will provide help and empowerment to work with your medical professionals to overcome your illness.

ADDITIONS TO MY TEN GOLDEN GUIDELINES

1. Avoid supermarkets whose message is aimed at encouraging us to buy cheap food (I shop for food at Waitrose and Marks and Spencer).

2. Ignore meaningless advice to continue to eat a balanced (Western) diet. As Dr Mary Belshaw MD has pointed out,[79] that was precisely what she was doing when she was diagnosed with breast cancer. Read *The China Study*,[80] *A Diet for a New America*,[81] and *White Lies*,[82] and be even more convinced by the message of this book – and take responsibility and control. You can now buy a video and special glove marketed by Breastsense to help you to examine your breasts more effectively. For every pack sold, the company donates 50p to Cancer PPrevent. Remember that an increasing number of women are surviving breast cancer.

8. Be especially sceptical about pills and potions, including vitamins and mineral supplements, especially if there are no clinical trials, and about the use of treatments such as photodynamic therapy in private clinics. Ask for data on outcomes and check with your GP. If the clinic cannot provide you with such data think very carefully before proceeding.

9. Try to find counselling. The charity, Positive Action against Cancer, provides a free service.

10. Visit the website, www.cancersupportinternational.com, and consider joining. It contains no-nonsense information about cancer to help you take control, instead of anodyne establishment statements typical of many other websites. It also has an excellent discussion forum where members can share their experiences and knowledge, and also offer support and encouragement to each other.

Let us all try to spread the word. 'Public opinion when it is truly aroused, can be unstoppable.' John Humphrys, *The Great Food Gamble*, Hodder and Stoughton, 2001.

In the first edition of the book (*see* p. 244) I advised, 'Keep reminding yourself that it is possible to overcome even advanced cancer. I know because I did it.' I should now add *and I now know many others who have done the same.*

Case Studies of People on the Plant Programme

Since I wrote the original edition of Your Life in Your Hands *in 2000 I have continued my research into cancer, including the link with nutrition – especially dairy foods – which has also led me to write several other books. More recently I left the British Geological Survey to concentrate on my work on the environment, nutrition and human health as a professor at Imperial College, London. I also work at the Cancer Support Clinic in London and helped launch a website www.cancersupportinternational.com to raise awareness of the link between diet and other avoidable risk factors and cancer, as well as diseases such as heart disease and osteoporosis.*

When I was diagnosed with cancer, and throughout my illness, it was very important to me to hear how other people had coped successfully with their cancer. This new edition therefore includes several case studies written by my friends and patients describing their experiences with the Plant Programme and how it affected their diagnosis, treatment, recovery and their lifestyle. Each story is told in the individual's own words and from their own unique perspectives and I hope they help you by providing support through your own experiences or those of your friends and relatives.

DR MARY BELSHAW

In July 2004, I found a lump on the outer edge of my right breast whilst in bed. I had felt pre-menstrual tenderness for several months and had experienced a tendency to lumpiness in the outer edges of both breasts for many years. The latter I self-diagnosed as fibroadenosis of the breasts. Suddenly, instead of the diffuse lumpiness, I felt a distinct firm and irregular lump about 2cm in diameter, and on exploring further I found a firm small gland in the right axilla.

My mind immediately went into overdrive and I feared the worst. I cried when I imagined my worst fears which were breast cancer with widespread metastasis and an inevitable premature death. Harry would be left without a mother and my husband Chris would be bereft.

I am a GP and my son was just 6 years old. I lost my own father when I was only 12, and an elderly aunt had died in her

70s of breast cancer within 3 weeks of the diagnosis. I had also seen young patients die of the condition in the course of my work.

I saw my GP two days later and had an ultrasound scan, mammogram and biopsy of the lump shortly afterwards. Five days later whilst on holiday the surgeon rang and told me in a very matter-of-fact way that I had breast cancer. (As though I had been prepared and was expecting this news.) I was not prepared! I went into shock and had great difficulty in coping. I was 45 years old, felt in perfect health, and had just been told I had breast cancer!

Whilst on holiday I told my six-year-old son about the cancer and was able to clear up his misunderstanding that this meant I was 'very, very ill'. Harry had also observed a significant change in our behaviour with too much hugging and kissing! I was very relieved when he coped very well with the news and we had in parts a normal holiday.

A few days later I began to feel 'very, very ill' due to pelvic and abdominal pains, loss of appetite and nausea. I was convinced again that I had widespread metastasis and that I would be admitted to heaven speedily via palliative care before even getting home. It later transpired that these symptoms were due to irritable bowel syndrome and stress. Medical knowledge has disadvantages as well as advantages, as I've learnt during the course of my illness!

I decided to accept all conventional treatment offered to me for the sake of my family and especially Harry. I was lucky enough to need only a simple lumpectomy and also had all the glands removed from the right axilla. My surgeon offered a mastectomy but I was aware that this would not improve my prognosis and I strongly didn't want disfiguring surgery if it could be avoided. I then had six months of intensive chemotherapy (as part of the Tango trial which included a Taxane), three weeks of radiotherapy and twelve months of treatment with Herceptin. Herceptin was given intravenously every three weeks and was funded privately because the NHS wasn't funding Herceptin at the time. I experienced no significant side effects with the Herceptin treatment.

Like Jane, I had a rollercoaster ride. During the course of my treatment I experienced two very sad, stressful close bereavements. This and the intensive nature of the chemotherapy treatment made the first twelve months of my treatment a very stressful period. I needed a great deal of psychological support to cope with the diagnosis, the harrowing way in which I received my results and prognosis, and also the side effects of the chemotherapy.

I decided to explore all adjuvant complementary therapies that I felt would help reduce the risk of recurrence. In addition to adopting the Jane Plant programme I also started to take various herbs and good quality vitamins, and have regular reiki treatment and homoeopathy, which I believe helps support my immune system. I have also taken up yoga and used a relaxation tape to help me cope with stress. A very positive attitude, ignoring the scary statistics, and support from positive women in support groups also helped me a great deal. In short, I moved within three months from a position of fear and pessimism to feeling in control, hopeful and positive about the future.

My tumour was a stage 2, Grade 3, 2 cm sized oestrogen and progesterone negative and Herceptin positive adenocarcinoma, which had spread to 4 out of 13 lymph glands. The tumour had not spread beyond the local lymph glands.

My first question after being given the diagnosis was what could I do to help myself, and in particular whether a change in my diet might help reduce my risk of a recurrence. I wasn't surprised when I was told there was no evidence that it would help and the breast care nurses recommended I continue with a 'healthy balanced diet'. However, this made no sense at all to me as I had developed my cancer whilst eating a so called 'healthy balanced diet'.

For many years I had eaten what was generally considered to be a healthy diet, with more than five portions of fruit or vegetables a day, low-fat dairy products and a typical Western mix of fresh and convenience pre-prepared foods. I felt in good health and did regular exercise in the form of walking, swimming and gardening.

Around 10 days after my surgery I had a Eureka moment when by chance I found Jane Plant's book in a local bookshop. I had been sent lots of information from the breast care nurses about breast cancer and had also read medical textbooks on the subject. I found most of this information made very depressing reading. I decided to browse for some books written for lay people and hoped to find practical and uplifting accounts of coping with breast cancer. Jane Plant's book 'Your Life in Your Hands' stood out. It is both inspiring and impressively well researched and well referenced.

I read it quickly and was gripped by her story. I strongly related to her account of the emotional highs and lows of the illness. But above all I felt exhilarated about the fact that I could do something myself to make a difference to the outcome of my illness.

Reading Jane's book and adopting her programme turned things around for me psychologically very quickly. I felt in control and physically I gained energy, lost around a stone in weight (dropping from a size 14 to a size 12 dress size in around 6 weeks) and felt great. My breasts also lost the lumpiness present since my early 20s and felt soft and were no longer tender. All my previous chronic minor problems have also cleared up, including mild asthma, eczema and a tendency to frequent colds. My cholesterol is very good at 3.5 and despite having an abrupt and premature menopause I experienced no menopausal symptoms, except for a brief period during chemo-therapy. I also found I tolerated the chemotherapy fairly well and was able to take my son to school and do exercise.

Over the course of the next eighteen months I read lots of well-researched books on cancer and diet/lifestyle. All the books I have read give similar advice about lifestyle changes and especially diet being important to help recover from and prevent a recurrence of breast cancer.

My reading caused me to radically reassess my views about cancer. I now believe that breast and other cancers are caused by a sick metabolism due to the modern Western diet. The treatment, therefore, requires a change in the diet for a cure. I am convinced that adjuvant diet and life style changes will radically reduce the risk of both new cancers and of breast cancer recurrence. The dietary changes need to be for life because breast cancer can recur at any time, even 20 or more years after the initial disease. Being dairy-free is important because the hormones in milk are very powerful even when present in only very small amounts. My experience in patient support groups supports the view that women who adopt the Jane Plant programme do better than those who make no changes in their diet. Sadly, taking only your doctor's advice and doing nothing else is not the best course of action. I know from my own training that doctors' knowledge about nutrition is extremely limited and little advanced from GCSE biology level. As a GP I now recommend this diet to all my patients with breast or prostate cancer.

I have more faith in my diet and holistic approach than the conventional treatments, though the latter are essential to remove the bulk of the tumour. It's now 2½ years since my diagnosis and I feel very well. I am confident about the future and do not live in fear of a recurrence.

My oncologist looks more cheerful each time I see him too. I've taken my life in my own hands and prefer the way it is now. I owe a great deal of thanks to Jane Plant for having the courage to write up her experience and researching the evidence for the link with diet and breast cancer. I wholeheartedly recommend Jane Plant's diet which is very safe, and has proven benefits for the prevention of heart and bone disease and is beneficial for general health and wellbeing. You have nothing to lose by adopting it and – like me, Jane, and many hundreds of women – what you gain could be your life.

© Dr Mary Belshaw, 2007

MARCIA'S STORY

Looking back, I was a text book case – breast cancer waiting to happen. A thirty-something woman, running two businesses, a home and family, too busy making money to worry about the proper nourishment of my body . . .

I lived on low-fat cottage cheese, yoghurts, milky drinks and takeaway sandwiches filled with glop! I'd get home at night and throw a cheesy minced-beef diet meal into the microwave and console myself with the fact that I took multi-vitamins and supplements.

Then my world came crashing down. In August 2005, I went to my GP with what looked like eczema in my left nipple. I was referred to a wonderful lady consultant breast surgeon. I asked for her specifically because I own ladies' clothes shops and I see so much of the results of breast cancer in the fitting rooms. The local support group was our pet charity, we raised thousands for them and I'd seen this woman's work. But I had never heard of the link between breast cancer and dairy.

My mammogram was clear! The ultra-sound was clear too, and I skipped out of the hospital. Only the core biopsy results to come in five days' time, and surely they would be fine.

But they weren't.

I had a grade two, ER positive, Her-2 positive tumour behind my left nipple. So much for mammograms!

My consultant suggested breast-conserving oncoplasty (a slight breast reduction incorporating the removal of the cancer). It meant operating on the healthy breast too, but she would give me a full breast lift at the same time. I awoke from my surgery relieved and pleased with the results.

Nine days later my world crashed again: five out of the nine lymph nodes removed were infected with the cancer. I would have to undergo six strong chemotherapy sessions before my planned twenty radiotherapy sessions.

I lay in my bed imagining looking like someone from a concentration camp. I stroked my elbow-length hair in despair and cried at shampoo ads on the TV. My fancy clothes, jewellery and sports car meant nothing to me now. The world I used to live in seemed a long way away.

I asked my mother to call my second cousin (who'd been diagnosed with breast cancer the previous year) to see if she had any advice for me. She came (God bless her) the next day with Jane's new book, given to her by her oncologist at the Royal Marsden in London.

The book changed everything! It gave me hope that I could overcome this awful disease and, moreover, it gave me some control in treating it.

My oncologist, however, was very dubious. He told me that I needed dairy food to maintain strong bones and I would suffer without it. I told him, 'Hippopotamuses and elephants didn't eat dairy foods and they had better bones than I'd ever have!'

He told me categorically that I would lose my hair. I said that my diet suggested that I may be able to keep it if I drank fresh juices that were high in folic acid. He smiled wryly and told me that I would definitely lose my hair.

I burned the midnight oil reading the book. I was in a sort of breast cancer bubble, isolated from my regular life. This new life involved bone scans, liver scans and MRI scans with weeks of waiting, worrying and pondering on life and death in between.

Having studied science to a respectable level in school, I assessed the evidence and decided to go with the book. Each day I drank carrot juice, apple and fennel juice and melon juice – ½ pint each mixing them with other fresh fruit and vegetables. I threw out all dairy produce and processed food and replaced it with (much tastier) organic fruit and veg, wholesome cereals, seeds, dried fruits, olive oil, herbs and eastern spices. I made delicious soups, salads, spag bols and chillis (made from TVP). I took kelp tablets, brewer's yeast, selenium ACE and omega 3 and 6 oils every day.

I sat through chemo with a lady who'd been on a non-dairy diet and had been scared by the recent soya/phyto-oestrogen controversy. She went back to milk and her cancer re-occurred, hence she was sat with me having her second cycle of chemo. I gave her Jane's book, and she was overwhelmed that no one had informed her properly about this.

I hung on to Jane's book for dear life (literally!). As the weeks passed and the chemo sessions came and went, the doctors and nurses started to take more notice of the mad woman with the melon juice – my eyes sparkled, my hair grew thicker and my skin looked ten years younger (in spite of the chemo).

Apart from a little sickness on the day I had it, my list of side effects was nil. Don't get me wrong, I knew it was in me, but I kept to the plan, and the plan stayed true to me.

It's still early days for me. I only finished my treatment a few months ago, but I will say this – breast cancer has changed me and my family. It devastates so many lives. My husband, parents, brother and sister have all suffered too because of it.

I am dedicated to making sure that all people facing this have access to the information that I had. I now supply the hospital with Jane's book to give out to new patients. They gladly do it because they can't believe how well I came through my treatment. Indeed, I heard two weeks ago that a lady with advanced breast cancer who was given a few months to live had started the diet and has now been told that her tumours are shrinking. How wonderful! It is so vital to pass this information on. I cannot rest in my bed knowing that every day new families are facing a devastating future because of this disease and our lack of information on it.

I was lucky my cousin had access to it and gave it to me, and I will make it my mission to pass it on to a thousand more!

Thank you dear Jane for making this precious information available to us.

THE STORY OF DEBBIE HORSFIELD

In June 2005 I booked myself a general health MOT. I was pronounced fit, healthy and in great shape. A week later I was called back for a 'routine' repeat mammogram. There had been no lump, but something tiny had shown up on the first mammogram which they wanted to check out. The second mammogram was inconclusive so I had ultrasound and then a biopsy 'just to be on the safe side'. The medical staff were calm and reassured me that it was 'probably nothing'. I also convinced myself that it would be a false alarm. A week later I was told that it was cancer.

My initial response was shock and dread. I have four children aged twelve, fourteen, sixteen and eighteen and all I could think of was whether I would live to see them grow up. My mum had died of breast cancer at the age of 59 and I just kept thinking 'ten years, just give me ten years'.

From the moment of diagnosis everything seemed to happen very quickly. I saw a consultant and was booked for surgery within eight days.

The operation was apparently straightforward and the prognosis was excellent. It was during the days after I came out of hospital that I had the space to start to think about what had happened and how to respond to it. I don't believe in things being random. It was clear that despite my generally healthy lifestyle, something had caused the cancer – and although it had turned out to be grade one, Stage 1 and 'indolent' (i.e. small, slow-growing and hadn't spread), I knew that it hadn't got there by accident.

At my first check-up after surgery I asked the consultant whether we are any nearer to knowing what causes cancer. He talked of 'environmental factors' – anything from chemicals in the environment to pesticides on food. I asked more questions – he said he could tell that I was pretty well-informed about health, exercise and nutrition and that I favoured a proactive approach to my own well-being. He mentioned – almost casually – a book that he said I might be interested in. It was a title which had already been recommended to me by two other people – *Your Life In Your Hands*.

I bought it immediately and read it cover-to-cover, almost at a single sitting. At first I read in disbelief (I remember exclaiming 'Oh my God, this is unbelievable!' then later, 'Wow, this makes total sense'). By the end I was hopping mad! Why did we not know this stuff already? Why hadn't we been told?

Suddenly it all seemed so obvious. Why, for example, were we drinking the milk of another species? Of course cow's milk is designed to grow baby cows, not to feed fully-grown humans! But I'd always loved my cappuccinos, and I'd totally bought into the myth that natural yoghurt is good for you.

I put down the book and I adopted the Plant Programme immediately. It made total sense to me, and a lot of it (bar cutting out dairy) I was already doing. I didn't even find it hard. I think the shock of having cancer gave me a mental clarity I hadn't possessed before.

People often say 'Isn't it awful to think that you can never have milk or cream or butter ever again?' but, for me, it's a no-brainer. If you believe, as I do, in the validity of Jane's claims, there's no contest. Safeguard your health or eat a cheese sandwich? Where's the dilemma?

For me one of the key – but unexpected – results of reading Jane's book was coming to a better understanding of the effects of stress. Despite having a pretty demanding job and a very full home life with my husband and four children, I'd never thought of my life as particularly stressful. I soon realized that stress can come in many forms – mental, physical, emotional, nutritional and environmental. I set about informing myself more fully of its effects, and began to reduce (drastically) my exposure to it.

For instance, when I discovered how much oestrogen there is in normal tap water, I had a reverse-osmosis water filter fitted. When I counted up how little time off I'd taken in the previous five years, I took six months off and completely reassessed my priorities. I made a list of things I love doing: spending time with my children, fell-walking with my husband, family holidays in the sun, family holidays in the snow, watching Manchester United, singing loudly, learning a new skill (currently snowboarding!). And I started doing them. Frequently.

I'm aware that I'm very lucky – my cancer wasn't aggressive, it was tiny and I didn't need chemotherapy. But it was a wake-up call, and I'm eternally grateful for what I've learned – and continue to learn daily – from the process.

THE STORY OF HARRY CASTLE

I was chief executive of a worldwide mining consultancy, non-executive chairman and deputy chairman of two large public sector bodies and a member of the local University Council. I am now retired from my former consulting engineering role.

In 1995 I received an honorary doctorate at one of our newer universities and in 1999 received the CBE for my contribution to science and business. At that time I and my wife Joan were very happy and (slightly) proud of our children and grandchildren and our 46 years together. We were fit and well and had regular health checks which showed no signs of impending problems.

In March 2000 there was a dramatic and rather disturbing change. I had been chatting with friends at the golf club about health and the usual tests. One of my friends said he had tests on blood pressure, cholesterol, diabetes etc. and PSA (which indicates the health of the prostate). I'd never heard of this but asked my GP to include this in my next blood tests. The GP did so reluctantly, as I'd not indicated problems with any of my natural urinary functions. On the 20 February 2000 the results were returned to the GP with a PSA reading in the mid-20s, which is high. The GP recommended further tests and consultations with the local consultant urologist. These confirmed that I had prostate cancer, which was, as he described it 'a little over the average in malignant intensity'.

This was quite a considerable shock. I'd always considered myself healthy and began to ask what are, perhaps, all the usual questions: What are the chances of cure? How far has the cancer gone? What are the next steps for me? How long will I live?

There followed a period of intense anxiety. I was uncertain about the further test programme, worried by delays in getting the final diagnosis and an acceptable treatment regime, apprehensive about the success or otherwise of the recommended treatment and concerned about both the immediate and long-term side effects of the treatment.

The further tests, mainly scans, ultrasound, biopsies and blood analysis indicated that the cancer had not spread significantly but surgery was unlikely to be successful. As the alternative, a programme of hormone treatment and radiotherapy was indicated.

During this period I mentioned my problem to Professor Jane Plant with whom I had a professional relationship at the British Geological Survey. Jane explained about her research work into breast cancer, her personal experiences and the relationship between diet and the control of the spread of the illness. She said that a book of her findings would be published shortly but, in the meantime, I should stop eating all dairy products, beef, old meats and red wine. As substitutes she recommended the following: vegetables and fruits, particularly those coloured red, orange and yellow; young meats in small quantities, for example chicken, turkey, veal, lamb, rabbit etc.; soya products such as soya milk and tofu; fish and organic eggs. I could also have beer and the occasional whisky.

She emphasised that food supplements were probably necessary if I were to stick strictly to the diet; she mentioned kelp, brewers yeast and selenium.

I was convinced by the scientific merits of Jane's research and have continued to follow these recommendations, supplemented by those in the book, *The Plant Programme*, written by her and Gill Tidey. I've discussed these with my consultant oncologist, who is convinced of the diet's powers of prevention, but has not yet been persuaded of the role which diet can play in cancer treatment. He recognises, however, the very satisfactory progress which I've made in keeping the cancer under control for the last seven years.

The treatment which I undertake is now restricted to three monthly Zoladex injections. I have few, if any, side effects and my PSA value is 0.03 which is healthy. The oncologist's nine-monthly physical examination now indicates 'there is no sign of the prostate cancer'.

I am satisfied that following Jane Plant's dietary regime has helped significantly in the cancer treatment. I am fully fit, playing golf (almost) as well as ever, with a handicap of fourteen, not bad for someone over 75. Joan and I are happy again and look on the experience of dealing with cancer in a very positive light. My recommendation to all fellow cancer patients is to keep a sense of humour and be cheerful and positive. I recall, during one of my radiotherapy sessions, one of the supervisory staff saying 'What's all this fun and enjoyment about? Don't you know this is the National Health Service?'

THE STORY OF FELICITY HELLIER

'It's not your lucky day, you've got cancer.'

'Thanks for that – and you're certainly not blessed with a bedside manner,' I thought as I was told my diagnosis, but fortunately our paths did not cross again. It was not a complete blow in the solar plexus, as I knew the year before that I had early signs of tumour activity. This had been picked up in a specific blood test following a mammogram which had been said to give the 'all clear' after I had found a pea-sized lump in my left armpit. Although my surgery had been informed of this, they felt confident in the mammogram result. My breast tissue was still dense, which can mean that tests are not as accurate as they are after the menopause, when one becomes less of a Pamela Anderson.

It was at this time I saw Professor Plant's book. The story was inspiring and her argument extremely compelling. My diet was completely overhauled, no dairy – I have been known to eat a complete Brie cheese – no animal fats, no simple sugars. I followed this and six months on, another blood test and my tests were virtually back to normal. Great.

Sadly, as I have always had a great passion for the sins of life, I started back on dairy and sugars with a vengeance. Another six months later I found a ripple in my left breast, and that was it. I was back on a roller coaster of mammograms and biopsies, which left me looking as if I had been in the ring with Mike Tyson. The result was two ductal carcinomas. Although they were small, action had to be taken.

The National Health Service was very good. I was so lucky to have a world-renowned surgeon who specialised in breast cancer and reconstruction. He was a compassionate and dedicated man. After the surgery, which consisted of a mastectomy on my left breast and reconstruction using my back muscle, as well as having six lymph glands removed, I can honestly say I had no pain, no complications and the staff at the hospital were fantastic. One day I was even given hummus on pitta bread – who says the National Health doesn't listen? I came out full of admiration for what they do with their limited resources; even though I passionately believe that the key word is 'prevention' as Jane Plant so clearly tells us.

I decided to take the National Health Gift Pack as I called it: surgery, chemotherapy and radiotherapy. This was a difficult decision as I'm not and never have been conventional, but I took it for the sake of my family. I have three young children, Florence, Hamish and Robert, the youngest only nearly five at the time, and a very dear husband, Paul, plus an elderly mother. I did not want anyone to say 'If you had only'.

I sailed through the chemotherapy without nausea or tiredness thanks to Jane's diet minimising the side effects. My hair became thin, so a friend and I had a jolly day choosing a National Health wig at a very helpful salon, then she shaved my head – very cathartic. As I am quite dark, I decided to make it more fun and go mousy-blonde. The effect, I felt, was a cross between Dick Emery and a transvestite, but everyone else loved it and a lot of people who did not know the history thought it was my hair. It is so amazing the way the National Health Service provided all this.

Finally, I had my ovaries zapped with Zoladex and a new nipple reconstructed with skin from my side. I tried some aromatase inhibitors to reduce oestrogen levels but stopped them as the side effects of joint inflammation were not good. Fortunately, I have a very committed and compassionate oncologist who understands my aversion to carrying on this treatment and now I do not take any orthodox medication.

During this period I followed, and I continue religiously to follow, Jane's programme. It is easy to use, comprehensive, and the recipes cater for a huge range of tastes: simple, classical, Far Eastern, plus experimental. My eyes have been reopened to some completely new foodstuffs which I would never have thought of trying before. The whole house is continually being bombarded with wonderful aromas and friends are regularly asking for the recipes. The joy of it is the simplicity, once you have the theory you can adapt other old favourite recipes and, when going out, it is simple to work around other menus.

Apart from ensuring you stay on the planet a lot longer, with Jane's Plant Programme you look and feel so good. Another interesting factor is that my asthma, which has plagued me since my late teens, has virtually disappeared. Jane's diet has cleared all the congestion out and I am very blessed to have found two brilliant yoga teachers, Deborah and Steve, who have helped me to breathe correctly and strengthen my system.

On Jane Plant's guidance I monitor my pH levels. Cancer thrives on sugars, fats and salt. Keeping one's system more alkaline than acid is vitally important. Jane also advised me to use natural progesterone to help keep my hormones balanced.

I would like to express a huge debt of gratitude to Jane Plant – who I see several times a year and who continues to plot my course of good health, plus is always there to answer my questions. I am blessed to have this special friendship. Jane is a courageous person to have found another route away from the pressures of the pharmaceutical industries – globally the third richest and the most protected – and the guarded bastions and practices of orthodox medical practice.

I would like to thank some unique and special people for their loving support and friendship. Jo Bartlett, Natalie Digweed, David Dunnett, Sonia Gubb, Sarah Hinmann and Helen Tanner.

This quotation from Parthasarathi Rajagopalachari epitomises my cancer:

> we, in our folly, in our fear of death, fail to understand that which represents a new journey, a new page on which to write, and thus to believe in a new beginning for ourselves . . .'

© Felicity Hellier, 2006

THE STORY OF GEORGE HARDY

At the age of 53 I appeared to be in very good health, despite the fact that all my life I had detested fruit and veg and loved Chinese takeaways and Indian curries, which I always ate with chips.

However, a few days before my 54th birthday, towards the end of March 2005, I decided to see my doctor because I was tired of being tired. I had been getting up three or four times every night to pass water. My initial thoughts were that this was caused by too many cups of tea before bedtime, but even cutting down made no difference. My GP sent me for a blood test, the result of which was to change my life forever.

The doctor's receptionist rang me a few days later to say that the doctor wanted to see me urgently. At my appointment, he sat me down and showed me the blood test results, with the PSA level (the number of Prostate Specific Antigens in my blood) boldly circled. At this point I had no idea what on earth PSA was. When he explained that my level of 182 was sky high and I was to be referred immediately to a urologist, something clicked into place and I asked him outright if it was prostate cancer. He refused to speculate.

Within days I was with the urologist, who, after examining me, pronounced that he was 99.9 per cent certain that I really did have what I had feared. He booked me in for a cystoscopy on 14 April. The biopsy showed cancerous cells that had spread to tissues next to the prostate. I was in trouble.

At this point, I have to mention that the urologist was very pessimistic and when I asked him my survival chances, he reckoned I had two or three, maybe even five years to live. That day I decided to learn all I could about prostate cancer and fight like I'd never fought before.

As soon as I got home I sat at the computer and began searching every website concerned with prostate cancer. It didn't take me very long to find references to the work of Professor Jane Plant. The more I read, the more it seemed to make such good sense. I can honestly say, the whole non-dairy theory shone out like a beacon.

I was very, very interested. In a short time I'd become familiar with such things as isoflavones, lignans, genistein, daidzein etc. In short, through following up my research after Jane had aroused my interest, I knew an awful lot about phytoestrogens and what a tremendous ally they would be in my battle.

Without any hesitation I ordered three of Jane's books: *Your Life In Your Hands*, *The Plant Programme* and *Prostate Cancer: Understand, Prevent and Overcome*. They became my constant companions. I now had an arsenal to fight with.

Within four weeks of diagnosis I started the diet she recommends for those with active cancer. I actually found the diet very easy to live with, although at first my wife and I had no idea what half of the ingredients even looked like! Eventually it became routine. I have stuck rigidly to all Jane's recommendations, even never using Cellophane wrapping and totally avoiding all processed foods. I go as far as to wash my hair with baby shampoo and bathe using only Simple Soap.

I must admit that I've added a few supplements too, although most of them I'd come across for the first time in her books – things such as red clover blossoms, saw palmetto and soya isoflavones. I also have at least 30mg of golden linseed daily.

Two weeks after my cystoscopy I started hormone therapy (Zoladex), and have been told I must stay on this for a full three years. In September 2005 I started radiotherapy and have completed 37 treatments. I am absolutely certain that because of my diet I have avoided many side effects of both treatments. The hormone therapy has caused no hot flushes, no weight gain and no enlarged or tender breasts.

During the radiotherapy I suffered no bowel problems whatsoever, I lost not a single hair, and I had no irritation at all in any place the beam was aimed. The only discomfort was an increased frequency of urination for a time, and quite a few tired days. Because I frequent internet forums for prostate cancer sufferers from around the world, I know for a fact that, comparably, I've had a much easier time than most during my treatments.

My latest PSA level was 0.2 on 5 January 2006. It was also pointed out to me that my blood was healthier than it had been in many years.

To conclude, the diet has certainly improved my quality of life and I'm sure my chances of survival too. In fact, my oncologist has told me that if he were in the same position as me, he would follow exactly the same path I have taken.

© George Hardy, 2006

THE STORY OF GWEN SUNDERLAND

Professor Jane Plant's book *Your Life in Your Hands* meant exactly that to me at a time when I was devastated, confused and more importantly facing my mortality. That is the impact that the diagnosis of cancer has on you.

Prior to my diagnosis I had been visiting my GP quite frequently with very bad leg cramps, weight gain which I had never experienced before and a problem with my smear tests due to extreme dryness. Everyone, including myself, put it down to the menopause, I was that age.

I was diagnosed with ovarian cancer with metastases (Stage 3) in September 2002. In February 2004 I was informed that, if I did not continue with the regime of chemotherapy, I had only months to live. I made the decision that, however long I had left, I would preserve my quality of life. Most members of my family had died with one sort of cancer or another (including ovarian) and now it was my turn to face this disease, and I was determined (after the initial shock) to fight it. The diagnosis is a big wake-up call to change your life and lifestyle. It is important that you reclaim power and take some control over your own life.

The most difficult part of having ovarian cancer was that I could find very little encouraging and helpful information on the subject. Most of it was about statistics which I found very negative. Ovarian cancer is called the 'silent one' due to the fact that there are few symptoms until the disease has progressed too far.

I was introduced to Professor Jane Plant's book through my homeopath who had another client who had been impressed by the diet in her fight against breast cancer. I started the diet immediately and was impressed not only by the research that Professor Plant had done but with her journey with breast cancer. I decided that, though ovarian cancer is not the same, it's caused by a similar gene to breast and prostate cancer and if it worked for her then why not me? I had nothing to lose and everything to gain.

The diet is easy to adapt to after you get over cutting out a lot of your favourite foods. I now look at cheese and think it looks like a lump of fat and it smells awful to me. I loved fruit so the juicing was not a problem. The biggest problem is getting all the food down you in a day, and you have to be prepared to give enough time each day to prepare fresh food. It soon becomes a way of life, however.

We are very lucky in the area where I live; we have an organic shop and also a café with organic produce. Following the diet was, therefore, made easier and as a treat I could go out to eat knowing that my diet was adhered to.

Part of my journey was the shock at having to wait six weeks for my operation after the diagnosis. I opted to go private even though the cost would put a lot of strain on us financially. The bonus of going private was that the chef at the BUPA Hospital supported my diet, even using organic ingredients. I was in for six days, and this helped me maintain my positive attitude.

Professor Plant's book is not only about the diet but also about the toxicity of our lifestyle today and she explains the reasons why you need to address them all, including oestrogen in plastic, resins in tooth fillings, hair colourings, and monitoring your pH levels.

The most important thing to me about Professor Jane Plant is that she is 'walking the talk' and that is good enough for me.

I feel she had to have this cancer in order to analyse the diet and toxins and help others in a similar situation. She is genuinely coming from the heart and from her personal experience to help people. This diet is a way of life for me now and will be for however long I am here. I pass on my knowledge to other cancer patients whenever I am asked; indeed my story has encouraged people who have not been diagnosed with this disease to look at their diet and lifestyle.

I follow a strict regime of other alternative therapies to support the diet. I did briefly make the diet more restrictive under another doctor's instructions but I later went back on Professor Plant's diet. I am writing my own story to encourage people that there is another way, that is how strongly I feel about my alternative regime.

People are always amazed when they see me, how well I look and also how much energy I have. Many people are amazed that I have an illness and are shocked when I tell them about my diagnosis. But more importantly I feel well and look forward to every day and make plans for my future, something I did not think I had.

© Gwen Sunderland, 2006

THE STORY OF JANET LINES

My breast cancer first came to light in September 2001 when I discovered a lump in my armpit while taking a bath. I was due to see my doctor on another matter, so mentioned this to him at the time and he gave me a thorough examination. He found a lump at the bottom of my right breast. A letter was immediately sent off to the Nottingham City Hospital and I was called to the clinic for examination and to have biopsies taken. The results showed that I had a large tumour.

In October I was given a mastectomy and several lymph nodes were taken out. I was in hospital for a few days and then sent home to recuperate for about six weeks before further treatment began. The only problem I had during this time was the build-up of fluid around the operation site, which had to be drained off every three to four days. This was fairly usual, but very uncomfortable. I had to visit the hospital on about eight occasions for the drainage to be carried out.

In December I started my chemotherapy sessions. My treatment was supposed to be once every three weeks, but this rarely happened as my blood count was usually too low and I had to wait another week each time to be well enough to take the drugs. I eventually finished the sessions towards the end of April. I didn't find it as gruelling as I thought it might be and never had any of the sickness or mouth ulcers that I had been warned might happen. I always felt tired in between the sessions, but that was expected. One of the worst things was losing my hair, which happened in between the first and second courses and, although I knew it would happen, I felt quite devastated. However, once most of it had gone, I got my daughter to cut off all the remaining 'tufty' bits and then got used to wearing my wig, which I must admit was very good and very difficult to tell from the real thing. One of the real horrors was seeing myself in the mirror first thing in the morning with no hair, very little in the way of eyebrows, and looking extremely pale – much like an alien!

Though my chemotherapy had dragged out, my consultant was keen to start the radiotherapy course and I was given 25 sessions over May and June, which involved going in every day apart from weekends and the days when the equipment was serviced. I felt that the hospital had become my second home. The one good thing was that very soon after the chemotherapy had finished my hair started to grow back, slowly at first, and after a few months became quite thick again and is now back to normal.

It was good to finally finish the treatment, although I must admit I had the feeling that I was now on my own. After a few months I returned to work, although I reduced my hours, and at last I felt I was getting back to normal. I use my spare time in a more leisurely way now and try not to get stressed.

I knew Jane Plant through working at the same organisation and was aware of her personal battle against breast cancer and her research into alternative measures to beat the disease. Her findings showed real evidence of a much lower incidence of breast cancer in countries that consumed much less dairy produce. After my diagnosis I decided that I would try to help myself as much as possible by eating healthily and also following the dairy-free diet. I felt that you sometimes have to take your life into your own hands and try to do as much as possible to help yourself. By avoiding processed foods and dairy products and only using fresh ingredients, I thought I would give my body a much better chance of recovering and I have felt much healthier. I didn't find it particularly difficult to change my eating habits and adapt my cooking and it has now become a way of life. The main thing is that I actually feel that I am taking the responsibility for my own well being. I believe it gives me a very positive outlook to hope that I can change things for the better and I would certainly recommend this approach to others.

© Janet Lines, 2006

THE STORY OF JILL MILLER

Breast cancer is possibly one of the biggest fears women face, the statistics are extremely high and although there are measured improvements to mortality over the last decade, many women will die from what is considered to be a 'rich Western disease'. One in nine women will receive a breast cancer diagnosis and as a consequence will be terrified of the future and the outcome.

I was diagnosed with breast cancer in 1993 and subsequently had a mastectomy. I was stunned when the consultant told me I had cancer. I automatically equated the dreaded word with death. The fear came over me in waves, at the most unexpected moments, and began to take over my days and nights. I sought counselling to help me come to terms with the changes in my body as well as my life.

I have led a very active life since then, coping with the intermittent fear and anxiety about the return of the cancer, and juggling work and play. Since 1994, I have founded a charity, Positive Action on Cancer, which is a free professional counselling service for people affected by a cancer diagnosis; and co-founded a theatre company, Little Gift Theatre Company, whose play *Time Bomb*, about the realities of living with breast cancer, performs to health professionals throughout the UK.

I always considered myself to be a healthy eater, but I started to reassess my diet when one of my daughters introduced me to the concept of a non-dairy diet, advocated by Jane Plant in her book *Your Life in Your Hands*. I bought Jane's book and read it avidly. It made so much sense. It was heartening to read Jane's personal account of her journey with cancer. Her theory that the dairy-free diet of certain cultures leads to a lower incidence of breast cancer, makes so much sense. All of this information is backed up by sound scientific knowledge and a determination to provide people with this pioneering information.

It is enlightening to learn that there are so many great sources of calcium we can incorporate into our diets, dairy is not the only source. Taking dairy from my diet has made a great difference to my health and that of my husband. After a kidney stone and several urine infections, my husband's PSA was revealed, by chance, to be very high. His GP at the time was surprised to find that it was drastically reduced after only three months of cutting dairy out of his diet.

I am pleased that Jane continues to put her neck on the line and encourage people to be mindful of what they put into their bodies.

© Jill Miller, 2006

THE STORY OF JULIA THOMAS

I was 43 when I discovered I had breast cancer in 2003. At the time I was the CEO of a children's charity based in Bristol. I had just started IVF treatment for the first time and I was thrilled to find I was pregnant and I was feeling well and excited.

I was between nine and ten weeks into the pregnancy when I found the lump. It was in my right breast and about the size and hardness of a pea. I went to my GP. I wasn't particularly concerned at the time; I thought it was something to do with the pregnancy. The GP thought it wasn't serious but to be on the safe side she referred me to the specialist Breast Cancer Unit at Hereford County Hospital. I was lucky to get an appointment within the week. I went along with my husband, expecting to be told there was no problem, but I saw a surgeon who took a needle biopsy. I was given a local anaesthetic so it didn't hurt and I was told the results would be available in two days. But then I asked the surgeon what she thought it was and she said she was 90 per cent sure it was breast cancer – she was quite blunt as surgeons often are. My husband and I were introduced to a Breast Care Nurse but we did not take much in at the time – we were both too shocked.

We went back two days later, when the surgeon confirmed it was breast cancer. We agreed dates for an operation, it had to be at least twelve weeks into my pregnancy. We asked the breast cancer nurse if there was anything I could do in the meantime to help myself. She said no and not to pay any attention to special diets. I felt this was a very negative response, not what I wanted to hear. I decided I didn't want to see her again.

I decided to use my private insurance cover, and was referred to another surgeon. He confirmed that I would have a lumpectomy rather than mastectomy. At that point I heard through my sister-in-law, Catherine, who worked at Imperial College about her colleague there – Professor Jane Plant and her books *Your Life in Your Hands* and *The Plant Programme* about breast cancer. Catherine sent us a copy of each book, which I read and decided to follow. I found them interesting but initially a bit complicated – especially the scientific background – but John, my husband, read them and was very enthusiastic. This gave him a way of helping me and being actively involved in my care.

When I was at twelve weeks of my pregnancy, I had the lumpectomy and my lymph nodes were removed. My surgeon felt, I think, that I should not proceed with the pregnancy. I did not want to terminate the pregnancy but John wanted to do the best for me. Ten days after the surgery I returned to see the surgeon for the results. Again this surgeon, though nice, was blunt and said I had six lymph nodes out of thirteen affected. He also said there was only a 20 per cent chance of me being alive in 10 years, he felt I should terminate the pregnancy as I had to start my chemotherapy treatment immediately.

I was devastated, I wanted my baby so much. We saw the oncologist the same day and he spent an hour with us. He agreed to research the best combination of chemo treatments hopefully to protect the baby. I saw a doctor specialising in foetal medicine who scanned the baby and confirmed all was well at this point. One week later my oncologist had decided on the best course of treatment in view of my cancer and my pregnancy. I started the treatments during the sixteenth week of my pregnancy. I reacted badly, initially, to the anti-sickness drug and I also picked up an infection because of my low white cell count, but I bounced back quickly. I had four chemo treatments, then I had Charlie at thirty-four weeks; six weeks premature by Caesarean section. I then had two weeks off and began my other four chemo treatments. It was at this point I found out I had HER-2 positive cancer. My oncologist said this was not particularly good.

I felt very down, but Catherine arranged for me to have lunch with Jane. The whole experience of being in London, especially seeing Jane in person helped enormously. The fact Jane seemed so well was encouraging. Jane said, 'Oh, yes, HER-2 positive that's fine. It's just a different growth factor to the normal IGF-1', and she knew of other women with this type of cancer doing well on her regime. Apart from being extremely tired because of the chemo, pregnancy and subsequent birth of Charlie, I felt really well.

I had fifteen radiotherapy sessions after the chemo but I found these worse than chemo, maybe because I was very tired. I therefore introduced a little organic meat into my diet although no dairy – indeed I will never eat it again. I used to drink cups of milky tea endlessly, a lot of cheese on toast and at least one yoghurt a day. I don't miss any of it. Towards the end of my treatments I heard about a new drug called Herceptin and was delighted to find my insurer was happy to cover one year's treatment.

I have just had my latest six-monthly check up and everything seems fine at the moment. Indeed my oncologist encouraged me to tell my story. At this point I told him I had been on Jane's diet and would be contributing my story to her new book, and he thought it was 'brilliant'.

I certainly think that Jane's diet helped me with both my chemo and pregnancy and is helping to keep me healthy. I intend to keep it up for the rest of my life and that is no hardship. The food is delicious and we enjoy cooking and eating it. Charlie is now six months old. He is the apple of his mother, father and Auntie Catherine's eye. He was born with all his hair and is a normal, healthy and wonderful little boy.

I don't consider that I have ever been ill. Certainly I never felt ill. Looking back it all seems frightening but really just something I could well have done without.

Jane's diet can't possibly do you any harm so I think people have everything to gain by going on it.

© Julia Thomas, 2006

THE STORY OF LIANE BALDOCK (CONTINUED)

Since I wrote my story in Jane's first book, I can really only say that six years later (and now nine years since my diagnosis with breast cancer) I am still here, and have recently been 'discharged' from the breast cancer clinic. I no longer need to go for annual check-ups, just once every two years for a mammogram.

I still keep off dairy products as much as possible, but am not as rigid about this when away from home as I was initially. I never managed to follow the rest of Jane's diet of nuts, seeds, pulses, tofu etc. as I had always hated nuts and seeds and found tofu quite disgusting! After a lot of trial and error I discovered one brand of soya milk which was quite palatable (So Good low fat) and still use that, but do sometimes now eat yoghurt and cheese. Since moving from Leicester to Devon I now eat far more fish (probably three or four times a week) as there is such a wide variety of fresh fish down here that I had never even heard of before. I also eat a lot of locally produced organic fruit juices particularly those produced by Heron Valley, and vegetables, plus occasionally some ready-cooked meals made by Red Earth Kitchen which are made locally and using local produce without any artificial preservatives and just frozen in order to preserve them.

I continue to take coenzyme Q10, but have reduced the amount from the 400mg/day I took while undergoing treatment and for the first five years afterwards, to around 120mg/day, partly because it is so expensive! I also continue to take a calcium supplement to replace what I no longer get from milk, cream, butter, etc.

From my own experience I can only say that I was badly let down by my GP in Leicester and the private health sector where I first sought help, because nine years ago the long wait for an initial NHS referral to a breast consultant was unacceptable. My advice nowadays would be to insist on an early referral (within fourteen days) or, if going privately, to make absolutely certain that the consultant you go to also works in an NHS dedicated breast care clinic. This was my biggest mistake – the surgeon I consulted privately was a general surgeon and was not attached to the local NHS breast care unit (although I knew he had done breast cancer surgery). Once onto the NHS 'system' I had the very best of treatment in the minimum of time – possibly because by then the NHS had recognised the blunders made by my GP and the general surgeon and were doing whatever possible to minimise the effects and avoid being sued (which I was advised to do, but did not).

Since moving down to Devon the team at Derriford Hospital, who took over my annual check-ups, have given me every care. This did mean removal of a suspect lymph node which turned out thankfully to be benign, which caused me a lot of anguish and trauma at the time – but better safe than sorry. When I found two small lumps in my other breast two years ago, I was seen within 48 hours and monitored regularly with ultrasound scans as they diminished in size, until they had totally disappeared of their own accord.

The only other advice I would give is to try always to have something in the future to focus on achieving and to look forward to, be it a concert or outing with friends or a weekend break. Initially it should be something only a few weeks ahead, but then as time goes on and you are getting better, make it further ahead. I was determined to see the total eclipse of the sun in 2001 from the Zambesi Valley and for two years this was my big focus, so when I finally climbed on the plane at Heathrow the sense of achievement was tremendous and for the first time I began to believe that I was actually going to live.

© Liane Baldock, 2006

THE STORY OF MARGARET SHEPHERD

In February 2000 I spent many happy hours gardening, but, after digging, I kept feeling very uncomfortable. In March I had a scare with my right breast when it started bleeding from the nipple. I had minor surgery to remove a blocked milk duct. At this time I turned 57. Six weeks later I was still feeling unwell, but put it down to the anaesthetic. Then, in June, my husband and I went out to celebrate our 35th wedding anniversary. I hardly ate a thing as I was feeling so bloated and that night my husband suggested I see a doctor – I looked pregnant.

I saw the Doctor the next day. He examined me and was concerned so sent me for a scan, which I had the next day. I had to have a full bladder for the scan, which I found agonising. As a result of the scan I was told I had a growth the size of a grapefruit on my ovary. I saw the specialist a week later and was told it was ovarian cancer, and that it had probably spread to my bowel. I was devastated – my whole world had collapsed. Fortunately I had taken with me a friend who was staying with us on holiday from Australia. Up to this stage, I hadn't told my husband it might be 'nasty' so as not to worry him. My friend and the Gynaecological Nurse Specialist were wonderful.

I had a full hysterectomy less than a month after I first went to the doctor. The first thing I remember when I came round from the anaesthetic was my husband standing there with a broad smile on his face and saying 'It's alright, it hasn't gone to your bowel.' I was so relieved and felt I could cope with everything else.

My husband and I had been invited to a wedding in New Zealand in February 2001, so, while recuperating, I rang our friends to explain why we might not be able to attend. My friend immediately told me to buy Professor Jane Plant's book *Your Life in Your Hands* (it was popular in New Zealand) and to go dairy-free.

On reading Professor Plant's story I was full of admiration for her determination to beat breast cancer. The Plant Programme gave me something to focus on throughout the chemotherapy as I not only went dairy-free, but went vegan the day I started chemotherapy. Although I hadn't eaten red meat for about twenty years, I still found it daunting going dairy-free and having to read every single label and to find alternatives, but I was fortunate that I had done a vegan cookery course many years previously, which was so helpful.

Perhaps the very fact that I had eaten so much dairy food over the previous twenty years – I had eaten yoghurt and cottage cheese with few exceptions daily – was part of the reason why I got ovarian cancer . . . It was probably also reading a chapter written by Dr Daniel Cramer in the *Lancet* about ovarian cancer that convinced me that Professor Jane Plant had truly identified something very important and relevant to cancer growth.* From then on I was determined to stay dairy-free. I also went to a nutritionist to check I wouldn't be deficient in anything and she recommended I take supplements of vitamin B6, folic acid, selenium and vitamin E (all vegan), linseed and lecithin. My blood levels were fine for each session of chemotherapy, and to this day I still take the supplements.

* See Dr Daniel Cramer 1989, *Lancet* 2, 66–71.

I am convinced the diet helped me through chemotherapy. I had six sessions of chemotherapy at three-weekly intervals and on the whole felt fit and well and had lots of energy. That was with the exception of feeling sick, once suffering aching joints, and itching all over for a couple of days after the first chemo session. I always made a point of taking it easy for a couple of days after each session, and was then back to normal.

When I went to see my oncologist for a check up on completion of my chemotherapy course he told me that my Ca125 cancer count had halved after the first chemo session, which was a good sign. I am convinced not only that the chemo killed the cancer cells but that the diet starved them, so the cells were attacked on two fronts. After my chemo finished I gradually introduced poultry and fish into my diet but, to this day, five and a half years later, I am still dairy-free.

We made it to New Zealand for the wedding which was just the most incredible tonic of all. On seeing my oncologist for my five-year check-up, he discharged me. How we celebrated!

I'd like to say thank you not only to my husband, friends and oncologist, who were all so supportive, but a very special thank you to Professor Jane Plant and The Plant Programme which I believe greatly contributed to my recovery.

© Margaret Shepherd, 2006

THE STORY OF MARY RAMBAUT

I am a 56-year-old woman whose family has a history of breast cancer. My mother was diagnosed with the disease and underwent a mastectomy in the 1950s; she was aged 53 at the time. She survived without reccurrence of the disease and died of a stroke at 85. My eldest sister was diagnosed with the disease approximately ten years ago, had a lumpectomy and, because of a small quantity of suspicious cells found in the lump, she underwent radiotherapy, and has been fine since. She was not treated with chemotherapy nor was she given Tamoxifen. I suspect my mother and my eldest sister had the same type of tumour.

My second eldest sister was diagnosed four years ago in April 2002 with ductile infiltrating carcinoma Type 4, Stage 1 with no hormone receptors. She had a double mastectomy and unfortunately a pulmonary embolism post-operatively. The disease rapidly spread to her spine six months later. She was started on chemotherapy and radiotherapy and she died eighteen months later. I went to South Africa to see her after my own treatment was completed and nursed her till she passed away. This was an extremely daunting and stressful time for me as I kept thinking: How long before I land up like this?

I was diagnosed in March 2002 with ductile infiltrating carcinoma Type 4 Stage 2, only months before my sister. This was a delayed diagnosis as the mammogram I had in February had been negative.

I underwent a right mastectomy in April 2002, followed by chemotherapy for three months then radiotherapy to the chest wall for a period, followed by six months of further chemotherapy. I recovered well and thought this was behind me for a while. Eighteen months later, in December 2004 I started having lower back pain and a scan showed a lytic lesion on my lumbar 3 vertebra. I underwent radiotherapy on areas of the spine. In March 2005 my blood results were fine so I decided to go to Perth for radiowave treatment. I underwent the treatment and returned to Sydney. It was of no use as my blood markers went up after my return and in July I was diagnosed with further bone metastases and liver tumours. I underwent radiotherapy to the spine and then commenced chemotherapy for six months.

It was the month before I started treatment that I read on the Internet about Dr Jane Plant's book. I was looking at food connections and cancer – I had already adopted eating organically and had reduced the animal fats in my diet and was juicing vegetables and eating a healthy diet. I was looking healthy and working full time. I thought when I read about Jane that I should look into it, so bought the book and omitted the dairy completely.

The Plant Programme is relatively easy to follow especially if you take the view that dairy is poison. I had started following the idea of only eating fish a couple of times a week. I ate no red meat, except for the occasional small amount of young lamb and no chicken at all as they are all female and have hormones naturally occurring in them which I don't want to put in my body. This is the same with beef as the butcher cannot tell you whether it is male or female. Not a single milk product of any kind has passed my lips in the past eight months. If you buy prepared foods, which I don't, you have to read the label carefully as often dairy has been added to them in some form or other.

Since I started the diet my blood results and scans have been excellent. I have just completed eight rounds of chemotherapy over the past six months and the final results will be known in two weeks' time. I was given only a 30 per cent chance of the chemotherapy treatment working but I was close to remission at the last blood test.

I do believe that what Dr Plant has written in her book makes perfect sense and is not just some crackpot idea. I have been a teacher of nursing for too long to get involved in some wacky ideas of treatment. The diet is so good and I have lost some excess weight that I couldn't shift, as I always ate cheese, yoghurt and ice cream and drank plenty of skimmed milk.

Most of us that want to live gave the cigarettes away a long, long time ago. You can only live, laugh and have fun and do what you can to keep healthy and alive and if dairy is out you can discover plenty of alternatives.

© Mary Rambaut, 2006

THE STORY OF ROGER BACON

My journey with prostate cancer started when I went to see my GP about a totally unrelated problem that required a blood test. As I was approaching fifty, my GP thought it might be a good opportunity to include a PSA test (to test the number of Prostate Specific Antigens in my blood), and about a week later I got a phone call from the surgery asking me to make an appointment. The result had shown my PSA was 19.6 (the normal reading should be around 3). My doctor said this was high and he was going to refer me to a consultant. I had no idea at the time what a PSA test was, what it stood for, what the prostate's function was and how all this was going to change my life.

That was eight years ago and since then I've learned a lot about the prostate and all the problems it causes men. The PSA test does not prove you have cancer, a high reading merely indicates there may be something wrong with the prostate. The consultant urologist I was referred to examined me and said he could not make a diagnosis without a biopsy being done, as this can usually determine if there is a prostate problem. I really hadn't taken in at that time the full seriousness of the situation and when I returned to see him a week or so after having the biopsy tests, I fully expected him to say there wasn't a problem, and to apologise for putting me through all the inconvenience.

The biopsy results showed that four out of six samples taken were cancerous, so it was fairly advanced and, as prostate cancer is slow growing, I probably unknowingly had cancer when I was 45 or even younger. I was shocked. My consultant suggested there and then that I choose one of three treatments: I could either watch and wait, have hormone therapy or have surgery. Knowing very little about anything to do with the prostate, still in a state of shock from hearing the word cancer and with no support group to turn to, I went with his recommendation of surgery (radical prostatectomy) as my best hope of survival. I had private medical insurance and following an MRI scan and bone X-rays that proved clear, I had open surgery to remove the prostate.

My surgery went well and recovery was quick, at the time I was a physically fit 49 year old. I was in hospital less than a week and returned home with a catheter. When this was removed I was fortunate that I was able to control my bladder within about five days and after a few months I returned to work.

I had been given some information about the prostate, but wanted to know more, particularly about the cause, ongoing prevention and, for my son's sake, hereditary factors. I soon learned that diet can play a major role in preventing cancer, and upped my intake of vegetables and fruit. I stopped eating chicken, which was the only meat I did eat and increased my intake of fish, seeds and nuts for omega 3 and 6 oils.

Then, about two years after my operation, my wife read an article in the *Daily Mail*, about a woman who had had advanced breast cancer and had beaten it by following a non-dairy diet. The article was written by Professor Jane Plant and she had published a book called *Your Life in Your Hands* which described how she eventually managed to overcome her cancer through diet change.

We managed to obtain a copy of the book and read the diet programme with interest along with her references to prostate cancer. I was already eating a lot of the foods, but to cut out *all* dairy was something else! I had a sweet tooth and loved my cream cakes and the thought of giving up cheese, which was part of my everyday diet, horrified me.

However, on reading Professor Plant's story in great detail, it convinced me that I should try and follow her programme. I started by reducing my dairy intake and finding alternatives that I found acceptable; milk was easy to lose, along with yoghurts and ice cream, all replaced with soya alternatives. Cheese was more difficult and I compromised by reducing my intake. I had to be careful with my diet as I had suffered acute pancreatitis, following which I had my gall bladder removed, so spicy hot foods were definitely off the menu.

My consultant said that following the operation I needed to stay clear of cancer for five years before I could say I had beaten it. My PSA readings were monitored every six months. After about the third of these readings they slowly started to rise – 0.2, 0.3, 0.5, then 0.7. A re-growth of the cancer had occurred. My consultant was reluctant to wait any longer, and, as the last reading jumped 40 per cent in six months, he recommended a course of radiotherapy treatment in the summer of 2001. I was targeted with radiation beams every day for four weeks, in the hope of destroying the cancer cells. The treatment is totally painless and just involves lying perfectly still while the machine circulates around you delivering the amount of radiation prescribed. There can be side effects, but all I felt was tiredness by the fourth week and an upset stomach.

This re-growth made me more determined that I should fight this disease and give up the last remaining dairy-based food products that I was eating, in order to maximise my chances of staying cancer-free, as my treatment options were diminishing fast. Should the cancer return after this second form of treatment, I could only have hormone therapy, which is used to contain rather than cure.

I have followed a dairy-free diet based closely on Professor Plant's since 2001 and find the programme and recipes very adaptable and easy to follow. I take selenium ACE, which is recommended in her books and my PSA readings have been monitored every six months and remain as low as they can be (0.01). I have remained in good health since adopting Professor Plant's diet and feel fitter, with more energy.

I am a founder member of a prostate cancer support group, which I helped set up in Somerset, information about the group

and prostate problems can be found on www.somersetpros-
tatecancer.org.uk, and Professor Plant's books are available in
the group's library. Hardly a meeting goes by without a
discussion on diet and I always recommend the advantage of
following The Plant Programme to other members of the group.

© Roger Bacon, 2006

THE STORY OF SHEILA SALMON

I was diagnosed with lobular breast cancer late in the year 2000.
I was told that it had been found in most of the lymph nodes
under my arm and was showing signs of spreading. It was a
shocking and depressing start to Christmas. I was told that I
must have had it for several years even though I was not
overweight, had breast-fed three children, did not smoke, drank
in moderation and ate an apparently healthy diet.

A friend who had been through a similar experience got in
touch and suggested that I read Jane's book as it had been a
great help to her. I am extremely grateful. Once I had started I
found it very hard to put down and vividly remember reading
it until the early hours of the morning. I found her ideas and
approach inspirational and it gave me the focus that I desperately needed; it also motivated me to do as much as I could to
help myself while being treated by the medical profession. I
underwent a radical mastectomy due to the nature and extent
of the cancer, followed by chemotherapy and radiotherapy.
Following Jane's advice I changed to a vegan diet and remained
vegan for a year after the diagnosis. I juiced endlessly and still
do, although I have to admit that I am not as consistent and
diligent as I used to be.

My oncologist, who knew of this book, treated my approach
with considerable scepticism but I was not to be swayed. As my
cancer was oestrogen positive he strongly recommended that I
take Tamoxifen, which I did with reluctance. Happily I have
had no side effects at all. At the start I made the error of not
looking at the ingredients, which contained lactose, but a
supportive pharmacist has since ensured that I have a lactose-
free brand.

A non-dairy diet has been easy to follow and, when eating
out, I have found pubs and restaurants extremely helpful and
accommodating. Friends have likewise been very supportive. I

feel healthy, have plenty of energy and in addition to remaining free of cancer so far, I no longer have unpleasant sinus problems which used to trouble me.

My diet remains largely vegan, although I also enjoy fish, occasional organic chicken and locally sourced lamb. I now prefer soya to cows' milk, eat plenty of tofu as long as it is marinated or flavoured, and consume far more fruit and vegetables than I did before my diagnosis.

I owe a huge debt to Jane for helping me to get through the past few years. Not eating dairy is a small price to pay for a healthy life which I feared would be taken away from me.

Notes

PREFACE TO FOURTH EDITION

1. Plant, Jane and Tidey, Gill, 2002. *The Plant Programme*. Paperback edition. Virgin Books; Plant, Jane and Tidey, Gill, 2005. *Eating for Better Health*. Virgin Books.
2. Kradjian, Robert D., 1994. *Save Yourself from Breast Cancer*. Berkley Publishing.
3. Plant, Jane and Tidey, Gill, 2003. *Understanding, Preventing and Overcoming Osteoporosis*. Virgin Books.

WELCOME

1. Selected causes of death: by gender and age. Office for National Statistics; General Register Office for Scotland; Northern Ireland Statistics and Research Agency. 1997.
2. Deaths: selected causes (International Classification) and sex, 1971 onwards (England and Wales): *Health Statistics Quarterly*, 04. 1998
3. http://who-pcc.iarc.fr/
4. Trichopoulos, Dimitrios, Li, Frederick, P., and Hunter, David J, 1996. What Causes Cancer? *Scientific American*, Special Issue, What you need to know about Cancer, September, 275, 3, 80–85.

CHAPTER ONE

1. Plant, Jane A. and Moore, P.J., 1979. Geochemical mapping and interpretation in Britain. *Phil. Trans. Roy. Soc.*, London, B288, pp. 95–112.
2. Plant, Jane A., Smith, D., Smith, B. and Williams, L., 2000. Environmental Geochemistry at the Global Scale. Geological Society Special Issue.
3. Dewey, John F., 1999. *Geoscientist* 9, 6 June, Society Awards, pp. 2–4.
4. Blair's war on cancer is a sham, say top doctors. *Independent On Sunday*. 14 November 1999.
5. Rennie, J. and Rusting, R., 1996. Making Headway Against Cancer. *Scientific American*, Special Issue, What you need to know about Cancer, September, 275, 3, 56–9.
6. Peto, R. and others, 2000. Smoking, Smoking Cessation and Lung Cancer in the UK since 1950. *British Medical Journal*, 321, 323–9.
7. Raleigh, V.S., 1999. World Population and Health in Transition. *British Medical Journal*, 319, 981–4.

8. Packham, D.E., 1999. Impacts of Commercialisation and Privatisation on Capabilities for Scientific Advice, Oracles or Scapegoats? IPMS Conference notes, October.

See also: Packham, David and Tasker, Mary, 1997. Industry and the academy – a Faustian contract. *Industry and Higher Education*, April, 85–90.

9. See the World Health Organisation's International Agency for Research on Cancer website: http://who-pcc.iarc.fr/

10. Physicians Committee for Responsible Medicine: PCRM Update of Winter 1991.

11. Cancer Research Campaign Factsheet 6.2, 1996.

12. Depression is very common – over two million people a year report symptoms. If you are a sufferer, first try to identify if it is caused by real problems. If it is, get practical help in sorting them out – the Citizen's Advice Bureau is an excellent source of free advice on financial and legal problems and Samaritans or friends can often help you to address emotionally based problems and help you to work towards methods of coping. MIND, the mental health charity also offers good advice. In one of its recent booklets (MIND 1999. Depression – don't let it get you down. MIND and Pharmacy Healthcare; Mind Information, 15–19 Broadway, London E15 4BQ; Pharmacy Healthcare scheme, 1 Lambeth High Street, London SE1 7JN) about depression, it states that 'pills are for symptoms, talking is for problems'. You should also ensure you eat a good, nutritious diet, the brain needs proper nutrition, and avoid exposure to artificial pesticides especially organophosphates (*see* Chapter 6) and excessive alcohol consumption. If you do have serious depression however, it is important to seek medical help. Although modern anti-depressants have side effects in some patients, it is better to take them than suffer from serious depressive illness.

13. *The Times*, 7 February 1998.

14. Cox, Peter and Brusseau, Peggy, 1992. *Superliving A Beginner's Guide to Medspeak*, Vermillion.

15. Boots the Chemist, 1998. *Breast Awareness – an essential guide*. Be enlightened, not frightened. Published in association with the charity Breast Cancer Care.

16. *Sunday Correspondent*, 26 November 1989.

17. Alternative Therapy, British Medical Association, 1986.

18. *New Scientist* 'article' 27 August 1987.

19. Vickers, A. and Zollman, C., 1999. ABC of complementary medicine: Acupuncture. *British Medical Journal*, 9 October, 973–976.

20. Gerson, M., 1958. *A Cancer Therapy: Results of Fifty Cases*, Gerson Institute, California.

Forbes, Alec, 1984. *The Bristol Diet*, Century.

21. Greenwald, P., 1996. Chemoprevention of Cancer. *Scientific Amercan*, Special issue: What you need to know about Cancer, vol. 275, 3, pp. 96–100 and see also the World Health Organisation's International Agency for

Research on Cancer website: http://who-pcc.iarc.fr/ and see also the British National Formulary, 1998.

22. See, for example, section on cytotoxic (cell poisoning) drugs in the British National Formulary, 1998.

CHAPTER TWO

1. Weinberg, Robert A., 1996. How Cancer Arises. *Scientific American*, Special Issue, What you need to know about Cancer, September, 275, 3, 62–70.

2. Pollack, M.N. and others, 1998. IGF-1 Risk Factor for Prostate Cancer. *Science*, 279, 563–566.
   Pollack, M.N., Huynh, H.T., and Lefebvre, S.P., 1992. Tamoxifen reduces serum insulin-like growth factor 1 (IGF-1). *Br Cancer Res Treat*, 22, 91–100.
   Pollack, M.N., Polychronakos, C., Yousefi, S., and Richard, M., 1988. Characterisation of insulin-like growth factor-1 (IGF-1) receptors of human breast cancer cells. *Biochem Biophy Res Commun*, 154, 1, 326–331.

3. Oliff, Allen, Gibbs, Jackson, B. and McCormick, Frank, 1996. New Molecular Targets for Cancer Therapy. *Scientific American*, Special Issue, What you need to know about Cancer, September, 275, 3, 144–149.

4. Weinberg, Robert A., 1996. How Cancer Arises. *Scientific American*, Special Issue, What you need to know about Cancer, September, 275, 3, 62–70.

5. Jain, R.K., 1994. Barriers to Drug Delivery in Solid Tumours. *Scientific American*, July, 271(1), pp. 58–65.

CHAPTER THREE

1. Trichopoulos, Dimitrios, Li, Frederick, P. and Hunter, David J., 1996. What Causes Cancer? *Scientific American*, Special Issue, What you need to know about Cancer. September, 275, 3, 80–85.

2. Boots the Chemist, 1998. *Breast Awareness – an essential guide*, Be enlightened, not frightened. Published in association with the charity Breast Cancer Care.

3. Trichopoulos, Dimitrios, Li, Frederick, P. and Hunter, David J., 1996. What Causes Cancer? *Scientific American*, Special Issue, What you need to know about Cancer. September, 275, 3, 80–85.

4. Holland, J.C., 1996. Cancer's Psychological Challenges. *Scientific American*, Special Issue, What you need to know about Cancer, September, 275, 3, 158–161.

5. http://www.who.int/nut/malnutrition_worldwide.htm

6. *Cancer Incidence in Five Continents*, 1997. Vol. V11, published by the IARC (International Agency for Research on Cancer).

7. *Cancer Incidence in Five Continents*, 1997. Vol. V11, published by the IARC (International Agency for Research on Cancer).

8. Kliewer, E.V. and Smith, K.R., 1995. Breast cancer mortality among immigrants in Australia and Canada. *Journal of Natl Cancer Institute*, 87, 15, 1154–1161. See also Cancer Research Campaign, 1996, Factsheet 6.2, Breast Cancer – UK.

9. Campbell, T.C. and Junshi, C., 1994. Diet and chronic degenerative disease perspectives from China. *Am. J Clin. Nutr*, 59, Suppl., 11,535–11,615.

10. Rohan, T.E., McMichael, A.J. and Bagbursi, P.A., 1988. A population-based case control study of diet and breast cancer in Australia. *Am. J. Epidemio*, 128, 478–489; Howe, G.R., Hirobata, T., Hislap, T.G. and others., 1990. Dietary factors and risk of breast cancer, combined analysis of 12 case-control studies. *J. Natl Cancer Inst.*, 8, 561–569; Willet, Walter C. and others, 1987. Dietary fat and the risk of breast cancer. *N. Engl J. Med.*, 316, 22–28; Jones, D.Y., Schatzkin, A., Green, S.B. and others., 1987. Dietary fat and breast cancer in the National Health and Nutrition Examination Survey epidemiological follow-up study. *J Natl. Cancer Inst.*, 79, 465–471.

11. Trichopoulos, Dimitrios, Li, Frederick, P. and Hunter, David J., 1996. What Causes Cancer? *Scientific American*, Special Issue, What you need to know about Cancer, September, 275, 3, 80–85.

12. Cramer, D.W. and others, 1989. Galactose consumption and metabolism in relation to the risk of ovarian cancer. *Lancet*, 2, 66–71.

13. Stocks, P., 1970. Breast cancer anomalies. *British Journal of Cancer*, 24, 633–643.

14. Maruchi, N. and others, 1977. Relation of food consumption to cancer mortality in Japan, with special reference to international figures. Gann, 1977; 68, 1–13.

CHAPTER FOUR

1. Cox, Peter and Brusseau, Peggy, 1995. *LifePoints For Kids*. Bloomsbury.

2. Statistical Abstracts of the US, 1994 edition.

3. Willett, W.C. and others, 1996. Strategies for Minimizing Cancer Risk. *Scientific American*, Special Issue, What you need to know about Cancer, 275:3, pp. 88–95.

4. Akre, James, ed., 1989. *Infant feeding: the physiological basis*. WHO Bulletin, OMS Supplement, Vol. 67, and Lawrence, Ruth A., 1994. *Breastfeeding: A guide for the medical profession*. Fourth Edition, Mossby, USA.

5. Lawrence, Ruth A., 1994. *Breastfeeding: A guide for the medical profession*. Fourth Edition, Mossby, USA.

6. Lawrence, Ruth A., 1994. *Breastfeeding: A guide for the medical profession*. Fourth Edition, Mossby, USA.

7. Akre, James, Ed., 1989. *Infant feeding: the physiological basis*. WHO Bulletin, OMS Supplement, Vol. 67; and Lawrence, Ruth A., 1994. *Breastfeeding: A guide for the medical profession*. Fourth Edition, Mossby, USA.

8. Akre, James, Ed., 1989. *Infant feeding: the physiological basis*. WHO Bulletin, OMS Supplement, Vol. 67, and Lawrence, Ruth A., 1994. *Breastfeeding: A guide for the medical profession*. Fourth Edition, Mossby, USA.

9. Akre, James Ed., 1989. *Infant feeding: the physiological basis*. WHO Bulletin, OMS Supplement, Vol. 67, and Lawrence, Ruth A., 1994. Breastfeeding: A guide for the medical profession. Fourth Edition, Mossby, USA.

10. American Academy of Pediatrics Committee on Nutrition (1992). The use of whole cows' milk in infancy. *Pediatrics*, 89, 1105–1109.

11. Anyon, C.P. and Clarkson, K.G., 1971. A cause of iron-deficiency anaemia in infants. *N.Z. Med. J.*, 74, 24–25.

12. Clyne, P.S. and Kulczycki, A. 1991. Human breast milk contains bovine IgG. Relationship to infant colic? *Pediatrics*, 87(4), 439–444.
    Wilson, J.F., Lahey, M.E. and Heiner, D.C., 1974. Studies on iron metabolism. V. Further observations on cow's milk-induced gastrointestinal bleeding in infants with iron-deficiency anaemia. *J. Pediatr*, 84, 335–344.

13. Pugh, R.H., 1981. Allergy to Cows' Milk Protein. *Health Visitor*, Vol. 54, 231–233.

14. Scott, F.W., 1990. Cow milk and insulin-dependent diabetes mellitus: is there a relationship? *Am J Clin Nutr*, 51, 489–491.

15. Bahna, S.L., 1987. Milk allergy in infancy. *Ann Allergy*, 59, 131.

16. Dunea, G., 1982. Beyond the Etheric. *Br. Med. J.*, 285, 428–429.

17. Kretchmer, N., 1981. The Significance of lactose intolerance. In: Paige, D.M. and Bayless, T.M., Eds., *Lactose Digestion: Clinical and nutritional implications*, Johns Hopkins University Press.

18. Chiodini, R.J. and Hermon-Taylor, J., 1993. The thermal resistance of Mycobacterium paratuberculosis in raw milk under conditions simulating pasteurisation. *J. Vet. Diagn. Invest.*, 5, 629–631 and Grant, I.R., Ball, H.J., and Rowe, M.T., 1996. Inactivation of Mycobacterium paratuberculosis in cows' milk at pasteurisation temperatures. *Appl. and Env. Microbiology*, 62, 631–636.

19. The Institute of Food Science & Technology Position Statement, 1998. *Food Science & Technology Today*, 12 (4), 223–228, September. http://www.ifst.org/hottop23.html

20. *Financial Times* for the weekend 20–21 November 1999.

21. The Institute of Food Science & Technology Position Statement http://www.ifst.org/hottop2.html. Hard copies available from IFST, 5 Cambridge Court, 210 Shepherds Bush Road, London, W6 7NJ.

22. EU Directive 70/524 February 1999.

23. US FDA websites: http://vm.cfsan.fda.gov/~ear/m190-11.html; http://vm.cfsan.fda.gov/~ear/

24. Ingersoll, Bruce, 1990. Technology and Health: FDA Detects Drugs in Milk but Fails to Confirm Results. *Wall Street Journal*, 6 February pB6; Ingersoll, Bruce, 1990. Politics and Policy: GAO Says FDA Can't Substantiate Claims About Milk. *Wall Street Journal*, 21 November pA16; and Ingersoll, Bruce, 1990. Technology & Health: FDA Plans a Nationwide Test of Milk for Antibiotics, Other Drug Residues. *Wall Street Journal*, 28 December p10.

25. European Commission, Scientific Committee on Veterinary Measures relating to Public Health, 1999. *Report on Public Health Aspects of the Use of Bovine Somatotropin*, 15–16 March.

26. Outwater, J.L. and others, 1997. Dairy Products and Breast Cancer: the IGF-1, estrogen and bGH hypothesis, *Medical Hypotheses*, 48, 453–461.

27. The *Guardian*, 13 July 1999.

28. McCusker, R.H., 1998. Controlling insulin-like growth factor activity and the modulation of insulin-like growth factor binding protein and receptor binding. *J. Dairy Sci.*, 81, 1790–1800.

29. The Institute of Food Science & Technology Position Statement http://www.easynet.co.uk/ifst/hottop8a.htm

30. Eppard, P.J. and others, 1985. Effect of dose of bovine growth hormone on milk consumption: alpha-lactalbumin, fatty acids and mineral elements. *J. Dairy Science* Vol. 68(11), pp. 3047–3054. See also Cohick, W.S. and others, 1992. Regulation of insulin-like growth factor-binding proteins in serum and lymph of lactating cows by somatotropin. *Endocrinology*, 130(3), pp. 1508–1514.

31. Mepham, T.B. and others, 1994. Safety of Milk from Cows Treated with Bovine Somatotropin. *Lancet*, 334, November 19, 1445–1446 and Mepham, T.B. and Schonfield, P.N., 1995. *Health Aspects of BST Milk*, prepared for the International Dairy Federation Nutrition Week conference in Paris, France, June 1995.

32. Simpson and others, http://www.nal.usda.gov/ttic/tektran/glimpse/data/000007/75/0000077539.html

33. Miller, M.A., Hildebrand, J.R., White, T.C., Hammond, B.G., Madson, K.S., and Collier, R.J., 1989. Determination of insulin-like growth factor-1 (IGF-1) concentrations in raw pasteurised and heat treated milk. *Journal of Dairy Science*, 72, Supplement 1, 186–187.

34. Hankinson, Susan E. and others, 1998. Circulating concentrations of insulin-like growth factor-1 and risk of breast cancer. *Lancet* 351, 9113, 9 May, 1393–1396.

35. Chan and others, 1998. Plasma IGF-1 and Prostate Cancer Risk: A Prospective Study. *Science*, 279, January.

36. Pollack, M.N., Huynh, H.T. and Lefebvre, S.P., 1992. Tamoxifen reduces serum insulin-like growth factor 1 (IGF-1). *Br Cancer Res Treat*, 22, 91–100.

37. Pollack, M.N. and others, 1998. IGF-1 Risk Factor for Prostate Cancer. *Science*, 279, 563–566.

38. Chan and others, 1998. Plasma IGF-1 and Prostate Cancer Risk: A Prospective Study. *Science*, 279, January.

39. Holly, Jeff, 1998. Insulin-like growth factor-1 and new opportunities for cancer prevention. *Lancet*, 351, 9113, 9 May, 1373–1375.

40. Epstein, Samuel S., 1996. Unlabelled Milk from Cows Treated with Biosynthetic Growth Hormones: A Case of Regulatory Abdication. *International Journal of Health Services*, 26, 1, 173–185.

41. Outwater, J.L., Nicholson A. and Barnard N., 1997. Dairy products and breast cancer: the IGF-1, estrogen, and bGH hypothesis. *Medical Hypotheses* 48, 453–461.

42. Leonard, Rodney E., 1995. Codex at the Crossroads: Conflict on Trade Health. *Nutrition Week*, Vol. 25, No 26, 14 July, pp. 4–5. *Nutrition Week* is

published by the Community Nutrition Institute, 910 17th Street, N.W., Suite 413, Washington DC 20006.

43. The European Commission. Health and Consumer Protection. Scientific Committee on Veterinary Measures relating to Public Health – Outcome of discussions. http://europa.eu.int/comm/dg24/health/sc/scv/out19_en.html

44. D'Ercole, J.A., Underwood, L.E. and Van Wyk, J.J., 1977. Serum Somatomedin-C in hypopituaritism and in other disorders of growth. *J. Pediatr*, 90, 3, 375–381. See also Cullen, K.J. and others, 1990. Insulin-like growth factor receptor expression and function in human breast cancer. *Cancer Research*, vol. 50, pp. 48–53.

45. De Leon, D.D., Wilson, D.M., Powers, M. and Rosenfeld, R.G., 1992. Effects of insulin-like growth factors (IGFs) and IGF receptor antibodies on the proliferation of human breast cancer cells. *Growth Factors*, 6, 327–336.

46. Peyrat, J.P., Bonneterre, J. and Hecquet, B. and others, 1993. Plasma insulin-like growth factor 1 (IGF-1) concentrations in human breast cancer. *Eur J Cancer*, 29A, 4, 492–497.

47. Peyrat, J.P., Bonneterre, J. and Hecquet, B. and others, 1993. Plasma insulin-like growth factor 1 (IGF-1) concentrations in human breast cancer. *Eur J Cancer*, 29A, 4, 492–497.

48. Musgrove, E.A. and Sutherland, R.I., 1993. Acute effects of growth factors on T471 breast cancer cell cycle progression. *Eur J Cancer*, 29A, 16, 2273–2279.

49. Heldrin, C.N. and Westermark, B., 1984. Growth factors: mechanism of action and relation to oncogenes. *Cell*, 37:9, 20.

50. Macaulay, V.M., 1992. Insulin-like growth factors and cancer. *Br J Cancer*, 65, 311–320.

51. Underwood, L.E., D'Ercole, J.A. and Van Wyk, J.J., 1980. Somatomedin-C and the assessment of growth. *Ped Clin N Amer*, 27, 4, 771–782, and Perdue, J.F., 1984. Chemistry, structure and function of insulin-like growth factors and their receptors: a review. *Can J Biochem Cell Bio.*, 62, 1237–1245.

52. Outwater, J.L., Nicholson, A. and Barnard, N., 1997. Dairy products and breast cancer; the IGF-1 estrogen, and bGH hypothesis. *Medical Hypotheses*, 48, 453–461.

53. The European Commission. Health and Consumer Protection. Scientific Committee on Veterinary Measures relating to Public Health – Outcome of discussions. http://europa.eu.int/comm/dg24/health/sc/scv/out19_en.html

54. Council on Scientific Affairs, American Medical Association, Biotechnology and the American Agricultural Industry, 1991. *Journal of the American Medical Association* (JAMA), 265, 11, 20 March, p. 1433.

55. Mepham, T.B. and Schonfield, P.N., 1995. Health Aspects of BST Milk, prepared for the International Dairy Federation Nutrition Week conference in Paris, France, June 1995.

56. Challacombe, D.N. and Wheeler, E.E., 1994. Safety of milk from cows treated with bovine somatotropin. *Lancet*, 344, 17 September, p. 815.

57. Sell, C., Rubin, R. and Baserga, R., 1995. Insulin-like growth factor I (IGF-I) and the IGF-I receptor prevent etoposide-induced apoptosis. *Cancer Research*, Jan 15, 55(2), 303–306.

58. Burton, Jeanne L. and others, 1994. A review of bovine growth hormone. *Canadian Journal of Animal Science*, 74, 167–201.

59. Xian, C., 1995. Degradation of IGF-1 in the Adult Rat Gastrointestinal Tract is limited by a Specific Antiserum of the Dietary Protein Casein. *Journal of Endocrinology*, 146, 2, 1 August, p. 215, and Thornburg, W. and others, 1984. Gastrointestinal absorption of epidermal growth factor in suckling rats. *American Journal of Physiology*, 246, G80–G85.

60. Outwater, J.L., Nicholson, A. and Barnard, N., 1997. Dairy products and breast cancer; the IGF-1 estrogen, and bGH hypothesis. *Medical Hypotheses*, 48, 453–461.

61. Haraguchi, S., Good, R.A., Engelman, R.W. and Day, N.K., 1992. Human prolactin regulates transfected MMTV LTR-directed gene expression in a human breast-carcinoma cell line through synergistic interaction with steroid hormones. *Int J Cancer*, 52, 923–33.

62. Clevenger, C.V., Chang, W.P., Ngo, W., Pasha, T.L., Montone, K.T. and Tomaszewski, J.E., 1995. Expression of prolactin and prolactin receptor in human breast carcinoma. Evidence for an autocrine/paracrine loop. *Am J Pathol*, 146, 695–705.

63. Vonderhaar B.K., 1989. Estrogens are not required for prolactin induced growth of MCF-7 human breast cancer cells. *Cancer Lett*, 47, 105–110.

64. http://www.shef.ac.uk/uni/academic/a-c/csi/1997/pir2.html

65. Lochnan, H.A. and others, 1995. Functional activity of the human prolactin receptor and its ligands. *Mol. Cell. Endocrinol*, 114, 91–99.

66. http://mammary.nih.gov/reviews/tumorigenesis/Vonderhaar001/slides/introduction.html

67. Struman, I., Bentzien, F., Lee, H., Mainfroid, V., D'Angelo, G., Goffin, V., Weiner, R.I. and Martial, J.A., 1999. Opposing actions of intact and N-terminal fragments of the human prolactin/growth hormone family members on angiogenesis: an efficient mechanism for the regulation of angiogenesis. *Proc. Natl Acad Sci USA*, 96, 1246–1251.

68. http://www.eurekalert.org/releases/upmc-bcc061699.html

69. Lawrence R., 1994 *Breastfeeding – A Guide to the Medical Profession*, Fourth edition, Mossby, USA.

70. e.g. http://www.inter-medico.com/prolactn.html

71. Lawrence, R., 1994. Breastfeeding: A Guide for the Medical Profession. Fourth edition, Mossby, USA.

72. Poggi, S.H., Skinner, H. Catherine W. and others, 1998. Using scanning electron microscopy to study mineral deposits in breast tissues. *American Mineralogist*, 83, 1122–1126.

73. Lee, J.R., 1996. *Natural Progesterone*. John Carpenter Publishing, Oxfordshire, 113pp.

74. Wolford, S.T. and Argoudelis, C.J., 1979. Measurement of Estrogens in Cow's Milk, Human Milk and Dairy Products. *J. Dairy Sci.*, 62(9), 1458–63.

75. Outwater, J.L., Nicholson, A. and Barnard, N., 1997. Dairy products and breast cancer; the IGF-1 estrogen, and bGH hypothesis. *Medical Hypotheses*, 48, 453–461.

76. The European Commission. Health and Consumer Protection. Scientific Committee on Veterinary Measures relating to Public Health – Outcome of discussions. 1999. Report on Public Health Aspects of the Use of Bovine Somatotropin. http://europa.eu.int/comm/dg24/health/sc/scv/out19_en.html

77. Allen, N.E., and others, 2000. Hormones and Diet: Low Insulin-like Growth Factor-1 but Normal Bioavailable Androgens in Vegan Men. *Brit. J. Canc.*, 83 (1), 95–97.

78. Chan, J.C., and others, 1998. Plasma IGF-1 and Prostate Cancer Risk: A Prospective Study. *Science* 279, January.

79. Kradjian, R.D., 1994. *Save Yourself from Breast Cancer*, Berkley Books, New York.

CHAPTER FIVE

1. Wright, K., 1996. A plea for prevention. *Scientific American*, September. (Inset p99 in article by Greenwald 1996, see below ref. 20).

2. Collaborative Group on Hormonal Factors in Breast Cancer, 1996. *Lancet*, 347, 1713–1727.

3. http://www.who.int/nut/malnutrition_worldwide.html

4. *The Times*, 2 November 1999.

5. Riggs, B.L., Wahner, H.W., Melton, L.J. 3rd, Richelson, L.S., Judd, H.L. and O'Fallon, W.M., 1987. Dietary calcium intake and rates of bone loss in women. *J Clin Invest*, Oct, 80, 4, pp. 979–982.

6. Hegsted, D.M., 1986. Calcium and Osteoporosis. *J Nutr*, 116, 2316–2319.

7. Kim, J.B., 1990. Fractured truths. *Bestways* v18, n2, p26(7).

8. Kim, J.B., 1990. Fractured truths. *Bestways* v18, n2, p26(7).

9. http://www.who.int/nut/malnutrition_worldwide.html

10. Dietary Reference Values for Food Energy and Nutrients for the United Kingdom. Department of Health, 1991.

11. Dietary Reference Values for Food Energy and Nutrients for the United Kingdom. Department of Health, 1991. Page 139 table 22.2.

12. Havala, S. and Dwyer, J., 1988. Position of the American Dietetic Association: Vegetarian Diets – technical support paper. *J Am Diet Assoc*, 88:3 352–355.

13. Barnard, N., 1993. *Food for life*, Harmony Books.

14. 'Research Advances in Osteoporosis', 1990. Conference by the National Osteoporosis Foundation, the National Institutes of Health, and the Ameri-

can Society of Bone and Mineral Research, Arlington, Virginia, USA February.

15. Heaney, R.P. and Weaver, C.M., 1990. Calcium absorbability from kale. *Am J Clin Nutr*, 51, 656–657.

16. Breslau, N.A., Brinkley, L., Hill, K.D. and Pak, C.Y., 1988. Relationship of animal protein-rich diet to kidney stone formation and calcium metabolism. *J Clin Endocrinol Metab*, Jan, 66, 1, pp. 140–146.

17. Heaney, R.P. and Recker, R.R., 1982. Effects of nitrogen, phosphorus, and caffeine on calcium balance in women. *J Lab Clin Med*, Jan, 99, 1, pp. 46–55.

18. Pritchard, K.I. and others, 1996. Increased thromboembolic complications with concurrent tamoxifen and chemotherapy in a randomized trial of adjuvant therapy for women with breast cancer. *Journal of Clinical Oncology*, vol. 14 (10), 2731–2738.

19. Gooderham, M.J., Adlercreutz, H., Sirpa, T.O., Wahala, K. and Holub, B.J., 1996. A Soy Protein Isolate Rich in Genistein and Daidzein and its Effects on Plasma Isoflavone Concentrations, Platelet Aggegation, Blood Lipids and Fatty Acid Composition of Plasma Phospholipid in Normal Men. *J. Nutr.*, 126, 2000–2006.

20. Greenwald, Peter, 1996. Chemoprevention of Cancer. *Scientific American*, Special Issue, What you need to know about Cancer, September, 275, 3, 96–99.

21. Kurzer, M.S. and Xu, X., 1999. Dietary Phytoestrogens. *Annual Reviews of Nutrition*, Vol. 17, pp. 353–381.

22. Shurtleff, William and Aoyagi, Akiko, 1975. *The Book of Tofu*. Autumn Press Inc.

23. Kurzer, M.S. and Xu, X., 1999, Dietary Phytoestrogens. *Annual Reviews of Nutrition* Vol. 17, pp. 353–381.

24. UK Ministry of Agriculture, Fisheries and Food advice as reported in the *Sunday Times*, 1999.

25. Willet, W.C., 1994. Micronutrients and cancer risk. *Am J Clin Nutr*, 59, (suppl), 1162S–5S. See also: Willett, Walter C., Colditz, Graham A. and Mueller, Nancy A., 1996. Strategies for Minimising Cancer Risk. *Scientific American*, Special Issue, What you need to know about Cancer, September, 275, 3, 88–95.

26. Greenwald, Peter, 1996. Chemoprevention of Cancer. *Scientific American*, Special Issue, What you need to know about Cancer, September, 275, 3, 96–99.

27. Levy, J., Bosin, E., Feldman, B., Giat, Y., Miinster, Danilenko, M. and Sharoni, Y., 1995. Lycopene is more potent inhibitor of human cancer cell proliferation than either A-carotene or B-carotene. *Nutr. Cancer*, 24, 257–266.

28. Nagasawa, H., Mitamura, T., Sakamoto, S. and Yamamoto, K., 1995. Effects of lycopene on spontaneous mammary tumour development in SHN virgin mice. *Anticancer Res*, 15, 1173–1178.

29. Willett, Walter C., Colditz, Graham A. and Mueller, Nancy A., 1996. Strategies for Minimising Cancer Risk. *Scientific American*, Special Issue, What you need to know about Cancer, September, 275, 3, 88–95.

30. Ortega, R.M. and others, 1996. Functional and Psychic Deterioration in Elderly People may be aggravated by folate deficiency. *J. Nutr.*, 126, 1992–1999.

31. Phipps, W.R., Martini, M.C., Lampe, J.W., Slavin, J.L. and Kurzer, M.S., 1993. Effect of flax seed ingestion on the menstrual cycle. *J Clin Endocrinol Metab.*, 77, 5, November, 1215–1219.

32. www.flax.com.fda

33. Greenwald, Peter, 1996. Chemoprevention of Cancer. *Scientific American*, Special Issue, What you need to know about Cancer, September, 275, 3, 96–99.

34. Coghlan, Andy, 1999. Crunch Time for Cancer. *New Scientist*, 13 November, 264, 2212.

35. Pinto, J.T., Qiao, C.H., Xing, J., Rivlin, R.S., Protomastro, M.L., Weissler, M.L. and Heston, W.D.W., 1999. Effects of garlic thioallylic derivatives on growth, glutathione concentration, and polyamine formation of human prostate carcinoma cells in culture. *Am. J. Clin. Nutr.* See also: Li, G., Qiao, C.H., Lin, R.I., Pinto,J., Osborne, M.P. and Tiwari, R.K., 1995. Antiproliferative effects of garlic constituents in cultured human breast cancer cells. *Oncology Rpts.*, 2, 787–791.

36. http://www.3mistral.co.uk/garlic/cancer.htm   see   also: http://www.mskcc.org/rande/pharmacology/189.html

37. Greenwald, Peter, 1996. Chemoprevention of Cancer. *Scientific American*, Special Issue, What you need to know about Cancer, September, 275, 3, 96–99.

38. Doll, R. and Peto, R., 1981. *The causes of cancer: quantitative estimates of avoidable risks of cancer in the United States today*. New York: Oxford University Press.

39. Lang, T. and Clutterbuck, C., 1991. *P is for Pesticides*, Ebury Press, Random Century Group, 256p.

40. McMichael, A.J., 1993. *Planetary Overload – Global Environmental Change and the Health of the Species*. Cambridge University Press.

41. Lang, T. and Clutterbuck, C., 1991. *P is for Pesticides*, Ebury Press, Random Century Group, 256p.

42. http://www.radian.com/standards and http://ro-systemsnet/atrazine.html

43. Stevens and others, 1994. http://www-oem.ucdavis.edu~beaumont/Agrichem/herbicides/triazine/triazine.html see also: Stevens, J.T. and Sumner, D.D., 1991. Herbicides, in *Handbook of Pesticide Toxicology, Vol. 3. Classes of Pesticides*, Toronto: Academic Press Inc, 1317–1408. See also *Environmental Endocrine Disrupters: A handbook of property data*, 1999.

44. http://who-pcc.iarc.fr/

45. Hambridge, K. M., Casey, C. E. and Krebs, N. F., 1986. Zinc, In: *Trace Elements in Human and Animal Nutrition*, Fifth Edition, Mertz, W., Ed. Academic Press, Inc, London.

46. McCusker, R.H., 1998. Controlling Insulin-Like Growth Factor Activity and the Modulation of Insulin-Like Growth Factor Binding Protein and Receptor Binding. *J Dairy Sci*, 81, 1790–1800.

47. Simpson and others. Effect of exogenous estradiol on plasma concentrations of somatotropin, insulin-like growth factor 1, insulin-like growth factor-binding protein activity, and metabolites in ovariectomised Angus and Brahman cows. http://www.nal.usda.gov/ttic/tektran/glimpse/data/000007/75/0000077539.html

48. The *Globe and Mail* 31 July 1999.

49. Hendler, S.S., 1990. *The Doctors' Vitamin and Mineral Encyclopaedia*, Simon and Schuster, New York.

50. Hetzel, B.S. and Maberly, G.F., 1986. Iodine, In: *Trace Elements in Human and Animal Nutrition*, Fifth Edition, Mertz, W., Ed. Academic Press, Inc, London.

51. Eskin, B.A., Shuman, R., Krouse, T., Merion, J.A., 1976. Rat mammary gland atypia produced by iodine blockade with perchlorate. *Cancer Res*, 35(9), 2332–2339. See also Eskin, B.A., 1978. In: *Inorganic and Nutritional Aspects of Cancer*. Schrauzer, G.N., ed., 293–304, Plenum Press, New York. This reference is quoted in Crouse, Robert G., Pories, Walter J., Bray, John T. and Mauger, Richard L., 1983. Geochemistry and Man: Health and Disease 1. Essential Elements. In: *Applied Environmental Geochemistry*. Thornton, I., Ed. London, Academic Press, 267–308.

52. Johnson, C., 1999, Environmental controls in iodine deficiency disorders (IDD), *Earthworks*, 9 November, p. 3, British Geological Survey.

53. Simopoulos, A.P., 1991. Omega-3 fatty acids in health and disease and in growth and development. *Am J Clin Nutr.*, 54, 438–463.

54. Simopoulos, A.P., 1991. Omega-3 fatty acids in health and disease and in growth and development. *Am J Clin Nutr.*, 54, 438–463. See also Fernandes, G. and Venkatraman, J.T., 1993. Role of omega-3 fatty acids in health and disease. *Nutr. Res.*, 13, S19–S45.

55. Reported in the London *Evening Standard*, 17 March 1989. See also Willet, W. C., 1994. Micronutrients and cancer risk. *Am J Clin Nutr*, 59, (suppl), 1162S–1165S.

56. Hunter, David J. and Willett, Walter C., 1993. Diet and Body Build: Diet, Body Size and Breast Cancer, *Epidemiologic Reviews*, 15, 1, 110–132.

57. Ingram, A.J. and others, 1995. Effects of a Flaxseed and Flax Oil Diet in a Rat – 5/6 Renal Ablation Model. *American Journal of Kidney Disease*, February 25, 2, 320–329.

58. Obermeyer, W.R., Musser, S.M., Betz, J.M., Casey, R.E., Pohland, A.E. and Page, S.W., 1995. Chemical studies of phytoestrogens and related compounds in dietary supplements – flax and chaparral. *Proceedings of the Society for Experimental Biology and Medicine*. See also Obermeyer, W.R., Warner, C.,

Casey, R.E. and Musser, S., 1993. Flaxseed lignans isolation metabolism and biological effects. *Fed Am Soc Exp Biol, J.*, A863.

59. Dupont, J., White, P.J., Johnston, K.M. and others, 1989. Food safety and health effects of canola oil. *J Am Coll Nutr., 8*, 360–375.

60. Kohlmeier, L. and others, 1997. Adipose tissue trans fatty acids and breast cancer in the European Community Multicenter Study on Antioxidants, Myocardial Infarction, and Breast Cancer, *Cancer Epidemiol. Biomarkers prev.*, 6, 9, 705–710.

61. Koletzko, B., 1992. Trans fatty acids may impair biosynthesis of long-chain polyunsaturates and growth in man. *Acta Paediatr.*, 81, 302–306.

62. Trichopoulos, Dimitrios, Li, Frederick, P. and Hunter, David J, 1996. What Causes Cancer? *Scientific American*, Special Issue, What you need to know about Cancer, September, 275, 3, 80–85.

63. Forbes, Alec, 1984. *The Bristol Diet*, Century.

64. Ingram, A.J., Parbtani, A., Clark, W.F, Spanner, E., Huff, M.W., Philbrick, D.J. and Holub, B.J., 1995. Effects of flaxseed and flax oil diets in a rat-5/6 renal ablation model. *Am J Kidney Dis.*, February, 25, 2, 320–329.

65. Lee, S. and others, 1999. Monitoring of Drinking Water in terms of Natural Organic Matter and Disinfection By-products. Proc 2nd Intern. Symp. On Advanced Env. Monitoring, Kwangju, Korea.

66. Herrick, D., 1996. Cryptosporidium and Giardia: Should you be concerned? *Water Well Journal*, 50, 4, 49, 44–46.

67. Jankun, Jerzy, Selman, Steven H., Swiercz, Rafal and Skrzypczak-Jankun, Ewa, 1997. Why drinking green tea could prevent cancer. *Nature*, 387, 15 June, p. 561 see also: Greenwald, Peter, 1996. Chemoprevention of Cancer. *Scientific American*, Special Issue, What you need to know about Cancer, September, 275, 3, 96–99.

68. Jankun, Jerzy, Selman, Steven H., Swiercz, Rafal and Skrzypczak-Jankun, Ewa, 1997. Why drinking green tea could prevent cancer. *Nature*, 387, 15 June, p. 561.

69. Campion, K., 1986. *Vegetarian Encyclopaedia*, Century Hutchinson Ltd, London.

70. Jankun, Jerzy, Selman, Steven H., Swiercz, Rafal and Skrzypczak-Jankun, Ewa, 1997. Why drinking green tea could prevent cancer. *Nature*, 387, 15 June, p. 561.

71. http://research.kib.ki.se/e-uven/public/51419.html

72. Lockwood, K., Moesgaard, S., Hanioka, T. and Folkers, K., 1994. Apparent partial remision of breast cancer in 'high risk' patients supplemented with nutritiional antioxidants, essential fatty acids and coenzyme Q_{10}. *Mol aspects Med*, 15, Suppls, 231–240.

Lockwood, K., Moesgaard, S. and Folkers, K., 1994. Partial and complete regression of breast cancer in patients in relation to dosage of coenzyme Q_{10}. *Biochemical and Biophysical Research Communications*, 199, 3, March 30, 1504–1508.

Lockwood, K., Moesgaard, S., Yamamoto, T. and Folkers, K., 1995. Progress on therapy of breast cancer with vitamin Q_{10} and the regression of metastases. *Biochemical and Biophysical Research Communications*, 212, 1, 172–177.

CHAPTER SIX

1. Gerhard Schrauzer, Ph.D., of the University of California cited in *Better Nutrition*, Nov, 1989, v51, no. 11, p. 14(2).

2. *Redbook*, April, 1989, v172, n6, p. 96(5).

3. Spallholz, J.E., Stewart, J.R., 1989. Advances in the role of minerals in immunobiology. Center for Food and Nutrition, Texas Tech University, Lubbock 79409. *Biol Trace Elem Res Mar*, 19 (3) pp. 129–151.

4. *Archives of Environmental Health*, September/October 1976.

5. Knekt, Paul, and others, 1988. Selenium Deficiency and Increased Risk of Lung Cancer. Abstract of paper read at the Fourth International Symposium on Selenium in Biology and Medicine, Tubingen, West Germany, July.

6. Reinhold, U., and others, 1988. Selenium Deficiency and Lethal Skin cancer. Abstract of paper read at the Fourth International Symposium on Selenium in Biology and Medicine, Tubingen, West Germany, July.

7. Lockwood, K., Moesgaard, S., Hanioka, T. and Folkers, K., 1994. Apparent partial remission of breast cancer in 'high risk' patients supplemented with nutritional antioxidants, essential fatty acids and coenzyme Q_{10}. *Mol Aspects Med*, 15, Suppls, 231–40. See also: Lockwood, K., Moesgaard, S. and Folkers, K., 1994. Partial and complete regression of breast cancer in patients in relation to dosage of coenzyme Q_{10}. *Biochemical and Biophysical Research Communications*, 199, 3, 30 March, 1504–1508. See also: Lockwood, K., Moesgaard, S., Yamamoto, T. and Folkers, K., 1995. Progress on therapy of breast cancer with vitamin Q_{10} and the regression of metastases. *Biochemical and Biophysical Research Communications*, 212, 1, 172–177.

8. Monographs on the Evaluation of the Carcinogenic Risk of Chemicals to Man, 1982. Geneva: World Health Organization, International Agency for Research on Cancer, 1972–present. (Multivolume work). V29 p. 282.
See also Osihi, Shinshi, 1990. Effects of phthalic acid esters on testicular mitochondrial functions in the rat. *Archives of Toxicology*, March, V64 n2 p. 143(5).

9. Holland, J C., 1996. Cancer's Psychological Challenges. *Scientific American*, Special Issue, What you need to know about Cancer, September, 275, 3, 158–161.

10. Heason, P., *Deep Relaxation* available from 37 Tollerton Lane, Tollerton, Nottingham.

11. Based on Holland, J C., 1996. Cancer's Psychological Challenges. *Scientific American*, Special Issue, What you need to know about Cancer, September, 275, 3, 158–161.

12. Trichopoulos, Dimitrios, Li, Frederick, P. and Hunter, David J., 1996. What Causes Cancer? *Scientific American*, Special Issue, What you need to know about Cancer, September, 275, 3, 80–85.

13. Levy, Len, 1998, Biomed II: Exposure to low-level benzene, p. 76. In: *Institute for Environment and Health*, Annual Report, 100pp.

14. Pearson, J.K., 2000. *The Air Quality Challenge*, American Society of Automotive Engineers and HMSO.

15. North Atlantic Treaty Organisation, 1988. International Toxicity Equivalency Factor (I-TEF) method of risk assessment for complex mixtures of dioxins and related compounds. Pilot study on international information exchange on dioxins and related compounds. CCMS Report Number 176, Environmental Protection Agency, Washington DC, USA.
    Department of Health, 1995. Statement by the Committee on Toxicity of Chemicals in Food, Consumer Products and the Environment on the US EPA draft health assessment document for 2,3,7,8-tetrachlorodibenzo-*p*-dioxin (TCDD) and related compounds. Dept of Health, London.

16. EPA Dioxin Reassessment Summary, 1994 4/94 – Vol. 1, CERI/ORD Publication Centre, USEPA.

17. MAFF, 1997. Dioxins and PCBs in retail cows' milk in England. *Food Surveillance* No. 136, December, Ministry of Agriculture, Fisheries and Food, London.

18. Tanabe, S., 1988. PCB Problems in the Future: Foresight from Current Knowledge. *Environmental Pollution*, 50, 5–28.

19. Department of the Environment, 1989. Dioxins in the Environment. *Pollution Paper*, No. 27, HMSO, London.

20. MAFF, 1997. Dioxins and Polychlorinated Biphenyls in Fish Oil Dietary Supplements and Licensed Medicines. *Food Surveillance Information Sheet*, No 106, Ministry of Agriculture, Fisheries and Food, London.

21. MAFF, 1996. Dioxins in Human Milk. *Food Surveillance Information Sheet*, No 88, Ministry of Agriculture, Fisheries and Food, London.

22. MAFF, 1996. Polychlorinated Biphenyls in Food – UK Dietary Intakes. *Food Surveillance Information Sheet*, No 89, Ministry of Agriculture, Fisheries and Food, London.

23. *Environmental Endocrine Disruptors: A Handbook of Property Data*, John Wiley and Sons.

24. Shin, K.J. and others, 1999. Development of a bioassay system for identification of Endocrine Disrupters. Proc 2nd Intern. Symp. On Advanced Env. Monitoring, Kwangju, Korea.

25. Soto, A.M. and others, 1992. An in culture bioassay to assess the estrogenicity of xenobiotics. In: *Chemically-induced alterations in sexual and functional development. The wildlife/human connection*. Vol. 21, Colborn T.C. Clement ed., Princeton Scientific Publishing, 295–309. See also: Soto, A.M. and others, 1995. The E-SCREEN assay as a tool to identify estrogens: An update

on estrogenic environmental pollutants. In: *Estrogens in the Environment, Environmental Health Perspectives*, 113–122.

26. Davis, Devra Lee, Axelrod, Deborah, Osborne, Michael P. and Telang, Nitin T., 1997. Environmental influences on Breast Cancer Risk, World Resources Institute, Washington, DC, USA, *Science and Medicine*, May/June.

27. Colborn, T., Dumanoski, D. and Myers, J.P., 1996. *Our Stolen Futures*, Dutton, Penguin Books, USA.

28. Dyson, T., 1999. Prospects for feeding the world. *British Medical Journal*, 319, 988–991.

29. Reuters, 8 October 1998.

30. McMurry, Laura M., Oethinger, Margaret, Levy, Stuart B., 1998. Triclosan targets lipid synthesis. *Nature*, 394, 6693, 531–532.

31. Trichopoulos, Dimitrios, Li, Frederick, P. and Hunter, David J, 1996. What Causes Cancer? *Scientific American*, Special Issue, What you need to know about Cancer, September, 275, 3, 80–85.

CHAPTER SEVEN

1. Campbell, T.C. and Junshi, C., 1994. Diet and chronic degenerative disease perspectives from China. *Am. J Clin. Nutr*, 59, Suppl., 11,535–11,615.

2. Packham, D.E., 1999. Impacts of Commercialisation and Privatisation on Capabilities for Scientific Advice, Oracles or Scapegoats? IPMS Conference notes, October.

3. Packham, D.E., 1999. Impacts of Commercialisation and Privatisation on Capabilities for Scientific Advice, Oracles or Scapegoats? IPMS Conference notes, October.

4. Association of University Teachers. *Efficiency Gains or Quality Losses?* 1996 (Based on DfEE and Welsh Office figures).

5. Bok, D., 1990. In: *Universities and the Future of America*, Duke University Press, Durham NC.

6. Glantz, S.A., 1996. *Times Higher Education Supplement*, 6 September, p. 15. and Glantz, S.A., Slade, J., Bero, L.A., Hanauer, P. and Barnes, D.E., 1996. *The Cigarette Papers*, University of California Press.

7. Packham, D.E., 1999. Impacts of Commercialisation and Privatisation on Capabilities for Scientific Advice, Oracles or Scapegoats? IPMS Conference notes, October. See also: Packham, David and Tasker, Mary, 1997. Industry and the academy – a Faustian contract. *Industry and Higher Education*, April, 85–90.

8. Packham, D.E., 1999. Impacts of Commercialisation and Privatisation on Capabilities for Scientific Advice, Oracles or Scapegoats? IPMS Conference notes, October. See also: Packham, David and Tasker, Mary, 1997. Industry and the academy – a Faustian contract. *Industry and Higher Education*, April, 85–90.

9. Jasanoff, S., 1997. Civilization and madness: the great BSE scare of 1996. *Public Understand. Sci.*, 6, 221–232.

10. McMichael, A.J. and Powles, J.W., 1999. Human numbers, environment, sustainability and health. *British Medical Journal*, 319, 9 October, 977–80.

UPDATE TO CHAPTER ONE

1. www.nlm.nih.gov/medlineplus/ency/article/002919.htm
2. McKenna, Claire, 2002. UK has highest reduction in deaths from lung and breast cancer. *BMJ*, 325, 63.
3. Irwig, Les, 2006. Evaluating new screening tests for breast cancer. *BMJ*, 332, 678–679.
4. Anon, 2006. Screening for breast cancer. *BMJ*, 332, 499–500.
5. e.g. www.nlm.nih.gov/medlineplus/ency/article/002919.htm
6. e.g. Baum, M., 2000. Survival and reduction in mortality from breast cancer – Impact of mammographic screening is not clear (Letter). *BMJ*, 321, 1470.
7. Spurgeon, David, 2002. Annual mammography in women in their 40s does not cut death rate. *BMJ*, 325, 563.
8. Spurgeon, David, 2002. Annual mammography in women in their 40s does not cut death rate. *BMJ*, 325, 563.
9. Josefson, Deborah, 2002. Breast self-examination does not improve cancer survival. *BMJ*, 325, 793.
10. Zackrisson S. and others, 2006. Rate of over-diagnosis of breast cancer 15 years after end of Malmo mammographic screening trial; follow up study. *BMJ*, 332, 689–692.
11. Anon, 2006. Screening for breast cancer. *BMJ*, 332, 499–500.
12. Symonds, R. Paul, 2002. Cancer biology may be more important than diagnostic delay. *BMJ*, 325, 774.
13. Spurgeon, David, 2002. Annual mammography in women in their 40s does not cut death rate. *BMJ*, 325, 563.
14. www.cancerscreening.nhs.uk/breastscreen
15. White, Caroline, 2002. 'Unacceptable' errors found in breast screening process. *BMJ*, 324, 933.
16. UK National Radiological Protection Board. www.nrpb.org/radiation_topics/risks/exposure.htm
17. Irwig, Les, 2006. Evaluating new screening tests for breast cancer. *BMJ*, 332, 678–679.
18. www.well-connected.com/rreports/doc06full.html
19. www.well-connected.com/rreports/doc06full.html
20. Keyomarsi, K., Tucker, S.L., Buchholz, T.A., Callister, M., Ding, Y., Hortobagyi, G.N., Bedrosian, I., Knickerbocker, C., Toyofuku, W., Lowe, M., Herliczek, T.W., and Bacus, S.S., 2002. Cyclin E and Survival in Patients with Breast Cancer. *N Engl J Med*, 347, 1566–1575.
21. Yancik, R. and Ries, L.A., 1994. Cancer in older persons. Magnitude of the problem – how do we apply what we know? *Cancer*, 74 (7 Suppl), 1995–2003.
22. Silliman, R.A. and Baeke, P., 1998. Breast cancer in the older woman. In: Balducci, L., Ersher, W.B. and Lyman, G.H., *Comprehensive geriatric oncology*. Amsterdam: Harwood.

23. Welch, H.G., Albertson, P.C., Nease, R.F., Bubolz, T.A. and Wasson, J.H., 1996. Estimating treatment benefits for the elderly: the effect of competing risks. *Ann Intern Med*, 124, 577–584.

24. Holmes, F.F., 1994. Clinical course of cancer in the elderly. *Cancer Control*, 1, 108–114.

25. Nixon, A.J., Neuberg, D., Hayes, D.F., Gelman, R., Connolly, J.L., Schnitt, S. and others, 1994. Relationship of patient age to pathological features of the tumor and prognosis for patients with stage I or II breast cancer. *J Clin Oncol*, 12, 888–894.

26. Balducci, Lodovico and Phillips, D. Melissa. 1998. Breast cancer in older women. *American Family Physician*, October 1, 1998. www.aafp.org/afp/981001ap/balducci.html

27. www.well-connected.com/rreports/doc06full.html

28. Medical Report: Prostate Cancer. *ICON*, 2002, 1 (5), 8–10.

29. Waxman, Jonathan, 2001. *The Prostate Cancer Book*. London: Vermillion.

30. http://www.nccn.org/patient_gls/_english/_prostate/

31. http://www.nccn.org/patient_gls/_english/_prostate/

32. Hart, D. and Wall, 2004. UK population dose from medical examinations. *European Journal of Radiology*, 50 (3), 285–291; Brenner, D.I. and others, 2001. CT scanning of children has been calculated to increase their lifetime risk of cancer. *American Journal of Roentology*, 176, 289–296.

33. http://www.nccn.org/patient_gls/_english/_prostate/

34. http://www.cancer.org

35. Spurgeon, David, 2003. Advanced scanning techniques help doctors stage prostate cancer. *BMJ*, 326, 1418.

36. *New England Journal of Medicine*, 2003, 348, 2491–2499.

37. http://www.nccn.org/patient_gls/_english/_prostate/

38. Fisher, B. and others, 2002. Twenty year follow-up of a randomised trial comparing total mastectomy, lumpectomy and lumpectomy plus irradiation for the treatment of invasive breast cancer. *New England Journal of Medicine*, 347 (16), 1233–1241.

39. Fisher, B., Bryant, J., Dignam, J.J., Wickerham, D.L., Mamounas, E.P., Fisher, E.R., Margolese, R.G., Nesbitt, L., Paik, S., Pisansky, T.M., Wolmark, N., 2002. Tamoxifen, radiation therapy, or both for prevention of ipsilateral breast tumor recurrence after lumpectomy in women with invasive breast cancers of one centimeter or less. *J Clin Oncol*, 20 (20), 4141–4149; www.ncbi.nlm.nih.gov:80

40. Fisher, B., Anderson, S., Bryant, J., Margolese, R.G., Deutsch, M., Fisher, E.R., Jeong, J.H. and Wolmark, N., 2002. Twenty-year follow-up of a randomised trial comparing total mastectomy, lumpectomy, and lumpectomy plus irradiation for the treatment of invasive breast cancer. *N Engl J Med*, 347 (16), 1233–1241; www.ncbi.nlm.nih.gov:80

41. Gottlieb, Scott. Lumpectomy is as effective as mastectomy for breast cancer. *BMJ*, 325, 921.

42. www.nlm.nih.gov/medlineplus/ency/article/002919.htm

43. www.nlm.nih.gov/medlineplus/ency/article/002919.htm

44. www.cancer.org/docroot/cri/content/cri_2_6x_breast_reconstruction_afte
    r_mastectomy_5.asp

45. Bartelinkh and others, 2001. Recurrence rates after treatment of breast
    cancer with standard radiotherapy with or without additional radiation. *New
    England j med*, 345 (19), 1378–1387.

46. http://cis.nci.nih.gov/fact/7_16.htm

47. Morrow, Monica and Gradishar, William, 2002. Recent Development: Breast
    Cancer. *BMJ*, 324, 410–414.

48. Coombes, R.C. and others, 2006. American Society of Clinical Oncology,
    Annual Meeting, Atlanta Georgia, June 2006.

49. Gralow, Julie R., 2002. Bisphosphonates as adjuvant treatment for breast
    cancer. *BMJ*, 325, 1051–1052.

50. www.gene.com/gene/products/information/oncology/herceptin;
    www.herceptin.com/herceptin/physician/pi.htm

51. www.herceptin.com/herceptin/physician/pi.htm

52. Anon, 2006. Patient is to appeal High Court ruling on breast cancer drug.
    BMJ, 332–443.

53. Barrett, A. and others, 2006. How much will herceptin really cost? *BMJ*, 333,
    1118–1120.

54. *Daily Mail*, Monday, 9 October, 2006.

55. www.ahrq.gov/news/press/pr2002/brchempr.htm

56. http://cis.nci.nih.gov/fact/7_16.htm

57. Gottlieb, Scott, 2002. Tamoxifen may increase risk of uterine sarcoma. *BMJ*,
    325, 7.

58. http://cis.nci.nih.gov/fact/7_16.htm

59. Mayor, Susan, 2002. Anastrozole shows promise for early breast cancer.
    BMJ, 324, 1539

60. www.gene.com/gene/products/information/oncology/herceptin;
    www.herceptin.com/herceptin/physician/pi.htm

61. http://cis.nci.nih.gov/fact/7_45.htm

62. www.ahrq.gov/news/press/pr2002/brchempr.htm

63. *New Scientist*, 20 January, 2007.

64. Editorial, *New Scientist*, 31 March, 2007.

65. Josefson, Deborah, 2002. Doctors warned to be wary of new drugs. *BMJ*,
    324, , 1113.

66. Garattini, Silvio and Bertele, Vittorio, 2002. Efficacy, safety, and cost of new
    anticancer drugs. *BMJ*, 325, 269–271.

67. www.cancer.gov/

68. Modified after: Chemotherapy and You: A Guide to Self-Help During Cancer
    Treatment. Information about what to expect during chemotherapy and
    what patients can do to take care of themselves during and after treatment.
    NIH Publication #99-1136; www.cancer.gov/cancerinfo/chemotherapy-and-
    you (There are, however, other recommendations in this booklet with
    which I do not agree.)

69. Smith, I. and Chue, S., 2006. Medical treatment of early breast cancer. *BMJ*,
    332, 162–181.

70. Allison, R. and others, 2006. *Photodiagnosis and photodynamic therapy*, 3, 139–146.

71. Fritsch, C. and Ruzika, T., 2003. Fluorescence diagnosis and photodynamic therapy of skin diseases atlas and handbook. Vien: Springer-Verlag.

72. Coulter, Angela, 2003. Killing the goose that laid the golden egg. *BMJ*, 326, 1280.

73. Coulter, Angela, 2003. Killing the goose that laid the golden egg. *BMJ*, 326, 1280.

74. Ernst, E., 2003. Herbal medicines put into context. *BMJ*, 327, 881–882.

75. Waxman, Jonathan, 2001. *The Prostate Cancer Book*. London: Vermillion.

76. Dyer, Owen, 2003. Aspirin could be used to prevent cancer. *BMJ*, 326, 565.

77. Flower, Rod, 2003. What are all the things that aspirin does? *BMJ*, 327, 572–573.

78. UK limits use of aspirin by under 16s. *BMJ*, 2002, 324, 1294.

79. Astralagus. *ICON*, 2002, 1 (3), 23.

80. Bartram, T., 1998. *Bartram's encyclopedia of herbal medicine*. Robinson publishing.

81. Campbell, T.C. and Campbell, T.M., 2006. *The China Study*. Benbella Books.

82. Greenwald, Peter. 2002. Cancer chemoprevention. *BMJ*, 324, 714–718.

UPDATE TO CHAPTER TWO

1. Clarke, M.F. and Becker, M.W., 2006. Stem cells: the real culprits in cancer? *Scientific American*, July 2006, 53–59.

2. Study reveals how growth factors affect human stem cells. www.hhmi.org/news/melton.html

3. Murray, R.K., Granner, D.K., Mayes, P.A. and Rodwell, V.W., 1990. *Harper's Biochemistry*. Appleton and Lange Norwalk, CT, p. 653.

4. Woolf, Neville, 1998. *Pathology, Basic and Systemic*. W.B. Saunders Publishing Co., Chapter 28, p. 274, Figure 28.

5. www.intouchlive.com/cancergenetics/onco.htm

6. Ludwig, T., Fisher, P., Ganesan, S. and Efstratiadis, 2001. Tumorigenesis in mice carrying a truncating BRCA1 mutation. *Genes and Development*, Vol. 15 (10), 1188–1193.

7. Xu, X., Wagner, K.U., Larson, D., Weaver, Z., Li, C., Ried, T., Hennighausen, L., Wynshaw-Boris, A. and Deng, C.X. 1999., Conditional mutation of BRCA1 in mammary epithelial cells results in blunted ductal morphogenesis and tumour formation. *Nature Genetics*, Vol. 22 (1), 37–43.

8. Paull, T.T, Cortez, D., Bowers, B., Elledge, S.J. and Gellert, M., 2001. Direct DNA binding by BRCA1. *Proceedings of the National Academy of Sciences of the USA*, Vol. 98 (11), 6086–6091.

9. Jensen, R.A., Thompson, M.E., Jetton, T.L., Szabo, CI., van der Meer, R., Helou, B., Tronick, S., King, M-C., Page, D.L. and Holt, J.T., 1996. BRCA1 is secreted and exhibits properties of a granin. *Nature Genetics*, 12, 303–308; www.mc.vanderbilt.edu/cancer/research/roster/jensen.html

10. Struewing, J.P., Abeliovich, D., Peretz, T., Avishai, N., Kaback, M.M., Collins, F.S. and Brody, L.C., 1995. The carrier frequency of the BRCA1 185delag mutation is approximately 1 percent in Ashkenazi-Jewish individuals. *Nature Genetics*, 11, 198–200; http://rex.nci.nih.gov/massmedia/backgrounders/ashkenazi.html

11. Roa, B.B., Boyd, A.A., Volcik, K. and Richards, C.S., 1996. Ashkenazi Jewish population frequencies for common mutations in BRCA1 and BRCA2. *Nature Genetics*, 14, 185–187; Oddoux, C., Struewing, J.P., Clayton, C.M., Neuhausen, S., Vrody, L.C., Kaback, M., Haas, B., Norton, L., Borgen, P., Jhanwar, S., Golgar, D., Ostrer, H. and Offit, K., 1996. The carrier frequency of the BRCA2 6174delT mutation among Ashkenazi Jewish individuals is approximately 1%. *Nature Genetics*, 14, 188–190; http://rex.nci.nih.gov/massmedia/backgrounders/ashkenazi.html

12. www.mercola.com/2002/apr/27/sv40.htm

13. Hursting, S.D., Slaga, T.J., Fischer, S.M., DiGiovanni, J. and Phtang, J.M., 1999. Mechanism-based cancer prevention approaches: targets, examples, and the use of transgenic mice. *Journal of the National Cancer Institute*, 35, 2031–2038.

14. Cheeseman, K.H. and Slater, T.F., 1993. *Free Radicals in Medicine*. Churchill Livingston.

15. Cheeseman, K.H. and Slater, T.F., 1993. *Free Radicals in Medicine*. Churchill Livingston.

16. Stewart, H.J., 1989. Clinical experience in the use of antioestrogen tamoxifen in the treatment of breast cancer. *Proceedings of the Royal Society of Edinburgh*, 95B, 231–237.

17. Miller, W.R., 1997. Aromatase inhibitors and breast cancer. *Cancer Treatment Reviews*, 23, 113–131.

18. Dao, T.L., Sinha, D.K., Nemato, T. and Patel, J., 1982. Effects of estrogens and progesterone on cellular replication of human breast tumours. *Cancer Research*, 42, 359–362.

19. Conte, P.F., Fraschini, G. and Dewinko, B., 1985. Estrogen induced expansion of the growth fraction in receptor negative human breast cancer. *Journal of Steroid Biochemistry*, 23, 1169–1172.

20. Miller, W.R. and Langdon, S.P., 1997. Hormonal, growth factor and cytokine control of breast cancer. In: *Biology of Female Cancers*, pp. 43–60. Langdon, S.P., Miller, W.R. and Berchuck, A. (editors). New York: CRC Press.

21. Miller, W.R., 1991. Oestrogens and breast cancer: biological considerations. *British Medical Bulletin*, 47, 470–483.

22. Yu, H. and Rohan, T., 2002. Role of the insulin-like growth factor family in cancer development and progression. *J Natl Cancer Inst*, 92, 1472–1489.

23. Rose, Steven, with Mileusnic, Radmila, 1999. *The Chemistry of Life*. Fourth (revised) edition. Penguin Books.

24. Voet, Donald and Voet, Judith, 1995. *Biochemistry*. Second edition. John Wiley & Sons, Inc.

25. Jiang, Wen G., Matsumoto, Kunio and Nakamura, Toshikazu (editors), 2001. *Growth Factors and their Receptors in Cancer Metastasis*. Dordrecht: Kluwer Academic Publishers.

26. Yu, H. and Rohan, T., 2002. Role of the insulin-like growth factor family in cancer development and progression. *J Natl Cancer Inst*, 92, 1472–1489.

27. Yu, H. and Rohan, T., 2002. Role of the insulin-like growth factor family in cancer development and progression. *J Natl Cancer Inst*, 92, 1472–1489.

28. E.g. www.ucop.edu/srphome/bcrp/progressreport/abstracts/innov/3CB-0186.html

29. Yu, H. and Rohan, T., 2002. Role of the insulin-like growth factor family in cancer development and progression. *J Natl Cancer Inst*, 92, 1472–1489.

30. www.preventcancer.com/pdf/InsulinGrowth266.html

UPDATE TO CHAPTER THREE

1. www.dep.iarc.fr/globocan/database.pdf

2. WHO International Agency for Research on Cancer (IARC), IARC Cancer Epidemiology Database. GLOBOCAN 2000. Cancer incidence, mortality and prevalence worldwide. Ferlay, J., Bray, F., Piesci, P. and Parkin, D.M. (editors). www.dep.iarc.fr/globocan/database.pdf

3. American Cancer Society. Modelled data: cancer facts and figures, 2006.

4. www.cancerresearchuk.org

5. www.cancerresearchuk.org

6. www.cancerresearchuk.org

7. Pike M.C., Kolonel, L.N., Henderson, B.E., Wilkens, L.R., Hankin J.H., Feigelson, H.S., Wan, P.C., Stram, D.O. and Nomura, A.M., 2002. Breast cancer in a multiethnic cohort in Hawaii and Los Angeles: risk factor-adjusted incidence in Japanese equals and in Hawaiians exceeds that in whites. *Cancer Epidemiol Biomarkers Prev*, 11 (9), 795–800.

8. www.hawaii.edu/crch/ProfileKolonel.htm

9. www.yoursurgery.com/ProcedureDetails.cfm?BR=3&Proc=36

10. American Cancer Society. Modelled data: cancer facts and figures, 2006.

11. Worldwide Cancer Mortality Statistics, ASR(w) for Annual Mortality per 100,000 by sex and age group. http://www.depd.iarc.fr/who/menu.htm

12. Yancik, R. and Ries, L.A., 1994. Cancer in older persons. Magnitude of the problem – how do we apply what we know? *Cancer*, 74 (7 Suppl), 1995–2003.

13. Silliman, R.A. and Baeke, P., 1998. Breast cancer in the older woman. In: Balducci, L., Ersher, W.B. and Lyman, G.H. *Comprehensive geriatric oncology*. Amsterdam: Harwood.

14. Welch, H.G., Albertson, P.C., Nease, R.F., Bubolz, T.A. and Wasson, J.H., 1996. Estimating treatment benefits for the elderly: the effect of competing risks. *Ann Intern Med*, 124, 577–584.

15. Campbell, T. Colin, Campbell, Thomas M. II, Robbins, John and Lyman Howard, 2006. *The China Study: The Most Comprehensive Study of Nutrition Ever Conducted and the Startling Implications for Diet, Weight Loss and Long-term Health.* Benbella Books.

16. Dobson, R., 2006. Breast cancer incidence rises in contaminated areas 10 years after explosion at Chernobyl reactor. *BMJ*, 332, 567.

17. Jakes, R.W. and others, 2002. Mammographic parenchymal patterns and self-reported soy intake in Singapore Chinese women. *Cancer Epidemiological Biomarkers Prev*, 11, 608–613.

18. www.cancer.org;   www.cancer.org/docroot/CRI/content/CRI_2_4_2X_ What_are_the_risk_factor s_for_breast_cancer_5.asp

19. Dobson, R., 2006. Diethylstilbestrol increase risk of breast cancer death. *BMJ*, 333, 64.

20. www.cancer.org/docroot/CRI/content/CRI_2_4_2X_What_are_the_risk_ factor s_for_male_breast_cancer_28.asp

21. www.dep.iarc.fr/globocan/database.pdf

22. WHO International Agency for Research on Cancer (IARC), IARC Cancer Epidemiology Database. GLOBOCAN 2000. Cancer incidence, mortality and prevalence worldwide. Ferlay, J., Bray, F., Piesci, P. and Parkin, D.M. (editors). www.dep.iarc.fr/globocan/database.pdf

23. Campbell, T.C. and Junshi, C., 1994. Diet and chronic degenerative disease perspectives from China. *American Journal of Clinical Nutrition*, 59, Suppl., 11,535–11,615.

24. Jakes, Rupert W., Duffy, Stephen W., Ng, Fook-Cheong, Gao, Fei, Ng, Eng-Hen, Seow, Adeline, Lee, Hin-Peng and Yu, Mimi C., 2002. Mammographic Parenchymal Patterns and Self-reported Soy Intake in Singapore Chinese Women. *Cancer Epidemiology Biomarkers & Prevention*, 11, 608–613.

25. Statistical Abstracts of the US, 1994 edition.

26. T. Colin Campbell, quoted in www.milksucks.com/osteo.html; Robbins, John, 1987. *A Diet for a New America*. Stillpoint Publishing; McDougall, John, 2000. *The McDougall Program for Women*; Plant, Jane and Tidey, Gill, 2003. *Understanding, Preventing and Overcoming Osteoporosis*. Virgin Books.

27. IARC Cancer Epidemiology Database. GLOBOCAN 2000, Cancer incidence, mortality and prevalence worldwide. Ferlay, J., Bray, F., Piesci, P. and Parkin, D.M. (editors). www.dep.iarc.fr/globocan/database.pdf.

28. Frassetto, L.A., Todd, K.M., Morris, R.C., Jr and Sebastian, A., 2000. Worldwide incidence of hip fracture in elderly women: relation to consumption of animal and vegetable foods. *Journal of Gerontology: Medical Sciences*, 55A, 10, M585–M592.

UPDATE TO CHAPTER FOUR

1. Jakes, Rupert W., Duffy, Stephen W., Ng, Fook-Cheong, Gao, Fei, Ng, Eng-Hen, Seow, Adeline, Lee, Hin-Peng and Yu, Mimi C., 2002. Mammographic Parenchymal Patterns and Self-reported Soy Intake in Singapore Chinese Women. *Cancer Epidemiology Biomarkers & Prevention*, 11, 608–613.

2. Pringle, H., 1998. Neolithic agriculture: reading the signs of ancient animal domestication. *Science*. 282, 1448.

3. Thomas M and others, 2007. *Proc Nat Acad Sci*.

4. Latham, M.C., 1997. Human nutrition in the developing world, Rome, 1997. FAO Food and Nutrition Series No 29, Cornell University, Ithaca, NY.

5. Butler, J., 2006. *White lies*. Vegetarian and Vegan Foundation.

6. AbuGhazaleh, A.A. and others, 2004. CLA increases in milk when cows fed fish meal and extruded soybeans for an extended period of time. *Journal of Dairy Science*, 87 (6), 1758–1766.

7. Petit, H.V., 2002. Digestion, milk production, milk composition, and blood composition of dairy cows fed whole flax seed. *Journal of Dairy Science*, 85 (6), 1482–1490.

8. Wahle, K.W. and others, 2004. CLAs: are they beneficial or detrimental to health? *Progress in Lipid Research*, 43 (6), 553–587.

9. Willett, W.C. and Stampfer, M.J., 2007. Rebuilding the food pyramid. *Scientific American*, Special edition on diet and health, February 2007, 12–21.

10. The Royal Society, 2000. Endocrine-disrupting chemicals. *Document* 06/00. The Royal Society.

11. Butler, J., 2006. *White lies*. Vegetarian and Vegan Foundation.

12. Qin, L.Q. and others, 2004. Estrogen: one of the risk factors in milk for prostate cancer. *Medical Hypotheses*, 62 (1), 133–142.

13. Hartman, S. and others, 1998. Natural occurrence of steroid hormones in food. *Food Chemistry*, 62, 7–20.

14. Butler, J., 2006. *White lies*. Vegetarian and Vegan Foundation.

15. Ganmaa, D. and Sato, A., 2005. Possible role of female sex hormones in milk from pregnant cows in the development of breast, ovarian and corpus uteri cancers. *Medical Hypotheses*, 65 (6), 1028–1037.

16. DEFRA, 2005. *Agriculture in the UK, 2004*. Norwich, UK: HMSO.

17. Campbell, T.C. and Junshi, C., 1994. Diet and chronic degenerative disease perspectives from China. *Am J Clin Nutr*, 59, Suppl., 11,535–11,615.

18. Charatan, Fred, 2003. Book Review: Fat Land: How Americans Became the Fattest People in the World, by Greg Critser. *BMJ*, 326, 229.

19. Charatan, Fred, 2003. Book Review: Fat Land: How Americans Became the Fattest People in the World, by Greg Critser. *BMJ*, 326, 229.

20. Charatan, Fred, 2003. Book Review: Fat Land: How Americans Became the Fattest People in the World, by Greg Critser. *BMJ*, 326, 229.

21. Grosvenor, C.E. and others, 1992. Hormones and growth factors in milk. *Endocrine Reviews*, 14 (6), 710–728.

22. http://www.dhn.csiro.au/crctissue.html

23. http://www.13.waisays.com/cancer2.htm

24. le Huerou-Luron, I. and others, 1998. Source of dietary protein influences kinetics of plasma gut regulatory peptide concentration to feeding in preruminant calves. *Comparative Biochemistry and Physiology: A – Molecular and Integrative Physiology*, 119 (3), 817–824.

25. Koldovski, O. and others, 1995. Milk-borne hormones: possible tools of communication between mother and suckling. *Physiological Research*, 1995, 44 (6), 349–351; Koldovsky, O. and others, 1994. Hormonally active peptides in human milk. *Acta Paediatrica* Suppl., 402, 89–93; Lehy, T. and others, 1990. Promoting effect of bombesin on the cell proliferation in the rat endocrine pancreas during the early post natal period. *Regulatory Peptides*, 27 (1), 87–96; Pollack, P.F., 1989. Effects of enterally- and parenterally-administrated bombesin on intestinal luminal tryptic activity and protein in the suckling rat. *Experienta*, 45 (4), 385–388; Lazarus, L.H. and others, 1986. An immunoreactive peptide in milk contains bombesin-like bioactivity. *Experienta*, 42 (7), 822–823; Jahnke, G.D. and others, 1984. A bombesin immunoreactive peptide in milk. *Proc Natl Acad Sci USA.*, 81 (2), 578–582.

26. Berseth, C.I. and others, 1990. Postpartum changes in pattern of gastrointestinal regulatory peptides in human milk. *Am J Clin Nutr*, 51 (6), 985–990.

27. Burns, D.M. and others, 1999. Breast cancer cell-associated endopeptidase EC24.11 modulates proliferative response to bombesin. *British Journal of Cancer*, 79 (2), 214–220; Bold, R.J. and others, 1998. Bombesin stimulates in vitro growth of human breast cancer independent of estrogen receptor status. *Anticancer Research*, 18 (16A), 4051–4056; Miyazaki, M. and others,

1998. Inhibition of growth of MDA-MB-231 human breast cancer xenografts in nude mice by bombesin/gastrin-releasing peptide (GRP) antagonists RC-3940-II and RC-3095. *European Journal of Cancer*, 34 (5), 710–717; Nelson, J. and others, 1991. Bombesin stimulates proliferation of human breast cancer cells in culture. *Br. J. Cancer*, 63 (6), 933–936; Giacchetti, S. and others, 1990. Characterization, in some human breast cancer cell lines, of gastrin-releasing peptide-like receptors which are absent in normal breast epithelial cells. *Int J Cancer*, 46 (2), 293–298; Weber, C.J. and others, 1989. Gastrin-releasing peptide, calcitonin gene-related peptide, and calcitonin-like immuno-reactivity in human breast cyst fluid and gastrin-releasing peptide-like immunoreactivity in human breast carcinoma cell lines. *Surgery*, (6), 1134–1139 (disc.1139–1140).

28. Markwalder, R. and others, 1999. Gastrin-releasing peptide receptors in the human prostate: relation to neoplastic transformation. *Cancer Research*, 59 (5), 1152–1159; Festuccia, C. and others, 1998. In vitro regulation of pericellular proteolysis in prostatic tumor cells treated with bombesin. *Int. J. Cancer*, 75 (3), 418–431; Krongrad, A. and others, 1997. Endopeptidase 24.11 activity in the human prostate cancer cell lines LNCaP and PPC-1. Urological Research, 25 (2), 113–116; Jungwirth, A. and others, 1997. LHRH antagonist Cetrolix (SB-75) and bombesin-antagonist RC-3940-II inhibit the growth of androgen-independent PC-3 prostate cancer in nude mice. *Prostate*, 32 (3), 164–172; Larran, J. and others, 1996. In vitro characterization of bombesin and calcitonin on the proliferation of PC3, DK145 and LNCaP cancer prostatic cell lines. International Journal of Developmental Biology, 1996 (Suppl. 1), 275S–276S; Aprickian, A.G. and others, 1996. Bombesin specifically induces intracellular calcium mobilization via gastrin-releasing peptide receptors in human prostatic cancer cells. *Journal of Molecular Endocrinology*, 16 (3), 297–306; Bologna, M. and others, 1989. Bombesin stimulates growth of human prostatic cancer cells in vitro. *Cancer*, 63 (9), 1714–1720; Wasilenko, W.J. and others, 1996. Effects of the calcium influx inhibitor carboxyamido-triazole on the proliferation and invasiveness of human prostate tumor cell lines. *Int J Cancer*, 68 (2), 259–264.

29. Takeyama, M. and others, 1989. Enzyme immunoassay of gastrin-releasing peptide (GRP)-like immunoreactivity in milk. *Int J Pept Protein Res*, 34 (1), 70–74.

30. Ducroc, R. and others, 1995. Immunoreactive substance P and calcitonin-gene-related peptide (CGRP) in rat milk and in human milk and infant formula's. *Am J Clin Nutr*, 62 (3), 554–558.

31. Lembeck, F. and others, 1979. Substance P as neurogenic mediator of antidromic vasodilation and neurogenic plasma extravasation. *Arch Pharmacol*, 310 (2), 175–183.

32. Khare, V.K. and others, 1998. The neuropeptide/mast cell secretagogue substance P is expressed in cutaneous melanocyticlesions. *Journal of Cutaneous Pathology*, 25 (1), 2–10.

33. Ducroc, R. and others, 1995. Immunoreactive substance P and calcitonin-gene-related peptide (CGRP) in rat milk and in human milk and infant formula's. *Am J Clin Nutr*, 62 (3), 554–558.

34. Faulkner, A., 1998. Insulin-like growth factor 1 concentrations in milk and plasma after growth hormone treatment. *Biochemical Society Transactions*, 26 (4), 386; Silanikove, N. and others, 1998. Metabolic and productive response of dairy cows to increased ion supplementation at early lactation in warm weather. *Journal of Dairy Research*, 65 (4), 529–543; Ginjala, V. and others, 1998. Determination of transforming growth factor-beta 1 (TGF-beta 1) and insulin-like growth factor-1 (IGF-1) in bovine colostreum samples. *Journal of Immunoassay*, 19 (2–3), 195–207; Schober, D.A. and others, 1990. Perinatal expression of type 1 IGF receptors in porcine small intestine. *Endocrinology*, 126 (2), 1125–1132.

35. Rao, R.K. and others, 1998. Luminal stability of insulin-like growth factor-1 and -2 in developing rat gastrointestinal tract. *Journal of Pediatric Gastroenterology and Nutrition*, 26 (2), 179–185.

36. Parisot, J.P. and others, 1999. Altered expression of the insulin-like growth factor-1 receptor in a tamoxifen-resistant human breast cancer cell line. *Br J Cancer*, 79 (5–6), 693–700; Sciacca, L. and others, 1999. Insulin receptor activation by insulin-like growth factor-2 in breast cancers: evidence for a new autocrine/paracrine mechanism. *Oncogene*, 18 (15), 2471–2479; Grothey, A. and others, 1999. The role of insuline-like growth factor and its receptor in cell growth transformation, apoptosis, and chemoresistance in solid tumors. *Journal of Cancer Research and Clinical Oncology*, 125 (3–4), 166–173; Perks, C.M. and others, 1999. Activation of integrin and ceramide signalling pathways can inhibit the mitogenic effect of insulin-like growth factor-1 (IGF-1) in human breast cancer cell lines. *Br J Cancer*, 79 (5–6), 701–706; de Cupis, A. and others, 1998. Responsiveness to hormone, growth factor and drug treatment of a human breast cancer cell line: comparison between early and late cultures. *In Vitro Cellular and Developmental Biology – Animal*, 34 (10), 836–843; Kobari, M. and others, 1998. The inhibitory effect of an epidermal growth factor receptor specific tyrokinase inhibitor on pancreatic cancer cell lines was more potent than inhibitory antibodies against the receptors for EGF and IGF-1. *International Journal of Pancreatology*, 24 (2), 85–95; Gooch, J.L. and others, 1998. Interleukin 4 inhibits growth and induces apoptosis in human breast cancer cells. *Cancer Res*, 58 (18), 4199–4205; Choki, I. and others, 1998. Osteoblast-derived growth factors enhance adriamycin-cytostasis of MCF-7 human breast cancer cells. *Anticancer Res*, 18 (16A), 4213–4224; Jackson, J.G. and others, 1998. Insulin receptor substrate-1 is the predominant signalling molecule activated by insulin-like growth factor-1, insulin, and interleukin-4 in estrogen receptor-positive human breast cancer cells. *Journal of Biological Chemistry*, 273 (16), 9994–10003; Westley, B.R. and others, 1998. Interactions between the oestrogen and IGF signalling pathways in the control of breast epithelial cell proliferation. *Biochemical Society Symposium*, 63, 35–44; Surmacz, E. and others, 1995. Overexpression of insulin receptor substrate 1 (IRS-1) in the human breast cancer cell line MCF-7 induces loss of estrogen requirements for growth and transformation. *Clinical Cancer Research*, 1 (11), 1429–1436.

37. Untergasser, G. and others, 1999. Proliferative disorders of the aging human prostate: involvement of protein hormones and their receptors.

Experimental Gerontology, 34 (2), 275–287; Xu, Z.D., 1999. Hammerhead ribozyme-mediated cleavage of the human insulin-like growth factor-2 ribonucleic acid in vitro and in prostate cancer cells. *Endocrinology*, 140 (5), 2134–2144; Marelli, M.M. and others, 1999. Luteinizing hormone-releasing hormone agonists interfere with the antagonic activity of the insulin-like growth factor system in androgen-dependent prostate cancer cells. *Endocrinology*, 140 (1), 329–334; Lamharzi, N. and others, 1998. Growth hormone-releasing hormone antagonist MZ-5-156 inhibits growth of DY-145 human androgen-independent prostate carcinoma in nude mice and suppresses the levels and mRNA expression of insulin-like growth factor-2 in tumors. *Proc Natl Acad Sci USA*, 95 (15), 8864–8868; Wang, Y.Z. and others, 1998. Sex hormone-induced prostatic carcinogenesis in the noble rat: the role of insulin-like growth factor-1 (IGF-1) and vascular endothelial growth factor (VEGF) in the developement of cancer. *Prostate*, 35 (3), 165–177.

38. He, Y., 1999. Comment on the Association between Insulin-Like Growth Factor-I (IGF-I) and Bone Mineral Density: Further Evidence Linking IGF-I to Breast Cancer Risk. *Journal of Cellular Endocrinology and Metabolism*, 84, 1760.

39. Perks, C. M. and Holly, J.M.P., 2000. Insulin-Like Growth Factor Binding Proteins (IGFBPs) in Breast Cancer. *Journal of Mammary Gland Biology and Neoplasia*, 5, 75–84.

40. Murphy, M.S. and others, 1998. Growth factors and the gastrointestinal tract. *Nutrition*, 14 (10), 771–774; Buts, J.P., 1998. Bioactive factors in milk. (in French.) *Archives de Pediatrie*, 5 (3), 298–306.

41. Shen, W.H. and others, 1998. Stability and distribution of orally administered epidermal growth factor in neonatal pigs. *Life Sciences*, 63 (10), 809–820; Rao, R.K. and others, 1998. Bovine milk inhibits proteolytic degradation of epidermal growth factor in human gastric and duodenal lumen. *Peptides*, 19 (3), 495–504; McCuskey, R.S. and others, 1997. Effect of milk-borne epidermal growth factor on the hepatic microcirculation and Kupfer cell function in suckling rats. *Biology of the Neonate*, 7 (3), 202–206; Oguchi, S. and others, 1997. Growth factors in breast milk and their effect on gastrointestinal developement. *Chang Hua Min Kuo Hsiao Erh Ko I Hsuek Tsa Chih*, 38 (5), 332–337.

42. Salomon, D.S. and others, 1999. Cripto: a novel epidermal growth factor (EGF)-related peptide in mammary gland developement and neoplasia. *Bioessays*, 21 (1), 61–70; Chou, Y.C. and others, 1999. Induction of mammary carcinomas by N-methyl-N-nitrosurea in ovariectomized rats treated with epidermal growth factor. *Carcinogenesis*, 20 (4), 677–684; Kurtz, A. and others, 1998. Local control of mammary gland differentation: mammary-derived growth inhibitor and pleiotrophin. *Biochemical Society Symposium*, 63, 51–69; Taylor, M.R. and others, 1997. Lactadherin (formerly BA46); a membrane-associated gycoprotein expressed in human milk and breast carcinomas, promotes Arg-Gly-Asp (RGD)-dependent cell adhesion. *DNA and Cell Biology*, 16 (7), 861–869.

43. Zhau, H.J. and others, 1996. Androgen-depressed phenotype in human prostate cancer. *Proc. Natl. Acad. Sci. U.S.A.*, 93 (26), 15152–15157.

44. Thornburg, W. and others, 1984. Gastrointestinal absorption of epidermal growth factor in suckling rats. *American Journal of Physiology*, 246, G80–G85.

45. www.prostatepointers.org/cmyers/pf0696.html

46. Gaull, G.E. and others, 1985. Significance of growth modulators in human milk. *Pediatrics*, 75 (2), 142–145.

47. Delgrange, E. and others, 1997. Sex related differences in the growth of prolactinomas : a clinical and proliferation marker study. *Journal of Clinical Endocrinology and Metabolism*, 82 (7), 2102–2107.

48. Vonderhaar, B.K., 1998, Prolactin: The forgotten hormone of human breast cancer. *Pharmacology and Therapeutics*, 79 (2), 169–178; Das, R. and others, 1996. Involvement of SHC, GRB2, SOS and RAS in prolactin signal transduction in mammary epithelial cells. *Oncogene*, 13 (6), 1139–1145; Mershon, J. and others, 1995. Prolactin is a local growth factor in rat mammary tumors. *Endocrinology*, 136 (8), 3619–3623; Ginsberg, E. and others, 1995. Prolactin secretion by human breast cancer cells. *Cancer Res*, 55 (12), 2591–2595; Fuh, G. and others, 1995. Prolactin receptor antagonists that inhibit the growth of breast cancer cell lines. *J Biol Chem*, 270 (22), 13133–13137.

49. Leav, I. and others, 1999. Prolactin receptor expression in the developing human prostate and in hyperplastic, dysplastic, and neoplastic lesions. *American Journal of Pathology*, 154 (3), 863–870; Horti, J. and others, 1998. A phase 2 study of bromocriptine in patients with androgen-independent prostate cancer. *Oncology Reports*, 5 (4), 893–896; Franklin, R.B. and others, 1997. Prolactin regulation of mitochondrial aspartate aminotransferase and proteinkinase C *Molecular and Cellular Endocrinology*, 127 (1), 19–25; Janssen, T. and others, 1996. In vitro characterization of prolactin-induced effects on proliferation in the neoplastic LNCaP, DU145, and PC3 models of the human prostate. *Cancer*, 77 (1), 144–149; Janssen, T. and others, 1995. Organ culture of human tissue as study model of hormonal and pharmalogical regulation of benign prostatic hyperplasia and of prostatic cancer. (frans) *Acta Urol Belg*, 63 (1), 7–14; Oliver, R.T. and others, 1995. New directions with hormone therapy in prostate cancer: possible benefit from blocking prolactin and use of hormone treatment intermittently in combination with immunotherapy. *Eur J Cancer*, 31A (6), 859–860; Rana, A. and others, 1995. A case for synchronous reduction of testicular androgen, adrenal androgen and prolactin for the treatment of advanced carcinoma of the prostate. *Eur J Cancer*, 31A (6), 871–875.

50. Hinuma, S. and others, 1998. A prolactin-releasing peptide in the brain. *Nature*, 393 (6682), 272–276.

51. Smith, S.S. and others, 1986. Presence of luteinising hormone-releasing hormone (LHRH) in milk. Endocrinol Exp., 20 (2–3), 147–153; Koldovsky, O., 1989. Search for the role of milk borne biologically active peptides for the suckling. J.Nutr., 119 (11), 1543–1551; Nair, R.M. and others, 1987. Studies on LHRH and physiological fluid amino acids in human colostreum and milk. *Endocrinolologia Experimentalis*, 21 (1), 23–30.

52. White, M.E. and others, 1986. Milk progesterone concentrations following simultaneous administration of buserelin and cloprostenol in cattle with

normal corporal lutea. *Canadian Journal of Veterinery Research*, 50 (2), 285–286; Dinsmore, R.P. and others, 1989. Effect of gonadotropin-releasing hormone on clinical response and fertility in cows with cystyic ovaries, as related to milk progesterone concentration and days after partarition. Journal of the American Veterinary Medical Association, 195 (3), 327–330.

53. Berseth, C.I. and others, 1990. Postpartum changes in pattern of gastrointestinal regulatory peptides in human milk. *Am J Clin Nutr*, 51 (6), 985–990.

54. Berseth, C.I. and others, 1990. Postpartum changes in pattern of gastrointestinal regulatory peptides in human milk. *Am J Clin Nutr*, 51 (6), 985–990.

55. Flood, J.F. and others, 1991. Increased food intake by neuropeptide Y is due to an increased motivation to eat. *Peptides*, 12 (6), 1329–1332.

56. Amarant, T. and others, 1982. Luteinising hormone-releasing hormone and thyrotropin-releasing hormone in human and bovine milk. *European Journal of Biochemistry*, 127 (3), 647–650; Baram, T. and others, 1977. Gonadotropin-releasing hormone in milk. *Science*, 198 (4314), 300–302.

57. Koike, K. and others, 1997. The pituitary folliculo-stellate cell line TtT/GF augments basal and TRH-induced prolactin secretion by GH3 cells. *Life Sci*, 61 (25), 2491–2497; Tyson, J.E. and others, 1975. The influence of prolactine secretion on human lactation. *J Clin Endocrinol Metab*, 40 (5), 764–773.

58. Grochowska, R. and others, 1999. Stimulated growth hormone (GH) release in Friesian cattle with respect to GH genotypes. *Reproduction Nutrition Development*, 39 (2), 171–180; Bourne, R.A. and others, 1977. Serum growth hormone concentrations after growth hormone or thyroid-releasing hormone in cows. *Journal of Dairy Science*, 60 (10), 1629–1635.

59. Chomczinsky, P. and others, 1993. Stimulatory effect of thyroid hormone on growth hormone gene expression in a human pituitary cell line. *J Clin Endocrinol Metab*, 77 (1), 281–285; Reynolds, A.M., 1991. The effects of chronic exposure to supraphysiological concentrations of 3,5,3/triiodo-L-thyronine (T3) on cultured GC cells. *Journal of Cellular. Physiology*, 149 (3), 544–547.

60. Tenore, A. and others, 1980. Thyroidal response to peroral TSH in suckling and weaned rats. *American Journal of Physiology*, 238 (5), E428–430.

61. Slebodzinski, A.B. and others, 1998. Triiodothyronine (T3), insulin and characteristics of 5/-monodiodinase (5/-MD) in mare's milk from partarition to 21 days post-partum. *Reproduction Nutrition Development*, 38 (3), 235–244.

62. Fujimoto, N. and others, 1997. Upregulation of the estrogen receptor by triiodothyronine in rat pituitary cell lines. *Journal of Steroid Biochemistry and Molecular Biology*, 61 (1–2), 79–85.

63. Koldovsky, O., 1989. Search for the role of milk borne biologically active peptides for the suckling. *J Nutr*, 119 (11), 1543–1551; Buts, J.P., 1998. Bioactive factors in milk. (in French.) *Arch Pediatr*, 5 (3), 298–306.

64. Faulkner, A., 1998. Insulin-like growth factor concentrations in milk and plasma after growth hormone treatment. *Biochemical Society Transactions*, 26 (4), S386; Baldini, E. and others, 1994. In vivo cytokinetic effects of recombinant human growth hormone (rhGH) in patients with advanced

breast carcinoma. *Journal of Biological Regulators and Homeostatic Agents*, 8 (4), 113–116; Scheven, B.A. and others, 1991. Effects of recombinant human insulin-like growth factor-1 and -2 (IGF) and growth hormone (GH) on the growth of normal adult human osteoblast-like cells and human osteogenic sarcoma cells. *Growth Regulation*, 1 (4), 160–167; Hodate, K. and others, 1990. Plasma growth hormone, insuline-like growth factor-1, and milk production response to exogenous human growth hormone-releasing factor analogs in dairy cows. *Endocrinologia Japonica*, 37 (2), 261–273.

65. Koldovsky, O., 1989. Search for the role of milk borne biologically active peptides for the suckling. *J Nutr*, 119 (11), 1543–1551; Buts, J.P., 1998. Bioactive factors in milk. (in French.) *Arch Pediatr*, 5 (3), 298–306.

66. Westrom, B.R. and others, 1987. Levels of immunoreactive insulin, neurotensin, and bombesin in porcine colostreum and milk. *J Pediatr Gastroenterol Nutr*, 6 (3), 460–465; Ehman, R. and others, 1985. Bombesin, neurotensin and pro-gamma-melanotropin in immunoreactants in human milk. *Regulatory Peptides*, 10 (2–3), 99–105.

67. Shutt, D.A. and others, 1985. Comparison of total and free cortisol in bovine serum and milk colostreum. *J Dairy Sci*, 68 (7), 1832–1834.

68. Vaarala, O. and others, 1998. Cow milk feeding induces antibodies to insulin in children – a link between cow milk and insulin-dependent diabetes mellitus? *Scandinavian Journal of Immunology* 47 (2), 131–135; Slebodzinsky, A.B. and others, 1998. Triiodothyronine (T3), insulin and characteristics of 5'-monodiodinase (5'-MD) in mare's milk from partarition to 21 days post-partum. *Reprod Nutr Dev*, 38 (3), 235–244; Westrom, B.R. and others, 1987. Levels of immunoreactive insulin, neurotensin, and bombesin in porcine colostreum and milk. *J Pediatr Gastroenterol Nutr*, 6 (3), 460–465.

69. Ferrando, T. and others, 1990. Beta-endorphin-like and alpha-MSH-like immunoreactivities in human milk. *Life Sci*, 47 (7), 633–635.

70. http://www.13.waisays.com/cancer2.htm; Newcomb, P.A. and Egan, K.M., 2006. Dairy food and ovarian cancer risk. *The Lancet*, March 2006, 797–799; Stang, A. and others, 2006. Adolescent milk fat and galactose consumption and testicular germ cell cancer. *Cancer Epidemiology and Biomarkers Prevention*, 15, 2189–2195.

71. Maruuchi, T. and others, 1998. Effects of gonadotropin-releasing hormone agonist on rat ovarian adenocarcinoma cell lines in vitro and in vivo. *Japanese Journal of Cancer Research*, 89 (9), 977–983; Kuroda, H. and others, 1998. Human chorionic gonadotrophin (hCG) inhibits cisplatin-induced apoptosis in ovarian cancer cells: possibe role of up-regulation of IGF-1 by hCG. *Int J Cancer*, 76 (4), 571–578; Kurbacher, C.M. and others, 1995. Influence of luteinising hormone on cell growth and CA 125 secretion of primary epithelial ovarian carcinomas in vitro. *Tumour Biology*, 16 (6), 374–384; Manetta, A. and others, 1995. Inhibition of growth of human ovarian cancer in nude mice by luteinising hormone-releasing hormone antagonist Cetrorelix (SB-75). *Fertility and Sterility*, 63 (2), 282–287.

72. Reiter, E. and others, 1999. Effects of pituitary hormones on the prostate. *Prostate*, 38 (2), 159–165; Lamharzi, N. and others, 1998. Luteinising

hormone-releasing hormone (LH-RH) antagonist Cetrorelix inhibits growth of DU-145 human androgen-independent prostate carcinoma in nude mice and suppresses the levels and mRNA expression of IGF-2 in tumors. *Regulatory Peptides.*, 77 (1–3), 185–192; Jungwirth, A. and others, 1997. Luteinising hormone-releasing hormone (LH-RH) antagonist Cetrorelix (SB-75) and bombesin antagonist RC-3940-2 inhibit the growth of androgen-independent PC-3 prostate cancer in nude mice. *Prostate*, 32 (3), 164–172; Maezawa, H. and others, 1997. Potentiating effect of buserelin acetate, an LHRH agonist, on the proliferation of ventral prostatic epithelial cells in testosterone-treated castrated rats. *Int J Urol*, 4 (4), 411–416; Hsing, A.W. and others, 1993. Serological precursors of cancer serum hormones and risk of subsequent prostate cancer. *Cancer Epidemiol Biomarkers Prev*, 2 (1), 27–32; Garde, S. and others, 1993. Effect of prostatic inhibiting peptide on prostate cancer cell growth in vitro and in vivo. *Prostate*, 7 (2), 183–194.

73. Bosland, M.C., 1996. Hormonal factors in carcinogenesis of the prostate and testis in humans and in animal models. *Progress in Clinical and Biological Research*, 394, 309–352.

74. Chapman, S. and others, 1992. Changes in adult cigarette consumption per head in 128 countries, 1986–1990. *Tobacco Control*, 1, 281–284.

75. http://www.who.int

76. Chapman, S. and others, 1992. Changes in adult cigarette consumption per head in 128 countries, 1986–1990. *Tobacco Control*, 1, 281–284.

77. http://www.who.int

78. http://www.13.waisays.com/cancer2.htm

79. Underwood, L.E., D'Ercole, J.A. and Van Wyk, J.J., 1980. Somatomedin-C and the assessment of growth. *Ped Clin N Amer*, 27, 4, 771–782, and Perdue, J.F., 1984. Chemistry, structure and function of insulin-like growth factors and their receptors: a review. *Can J Biochem Cell Bio*, 62, 1237–1245.

80. http://vvv.com/healthnews/milk.html

81. Pollack, Michael, 2003. Cancer, aging and IGF physiology. Meeting of the Royal Society of Medicine in London in October 2003, entitled 'Biology of IGF-I: its interaction with insulin in health and malignant states'.

82. Lonning, Per Eystein, 2003. IGF-I and breast cancer. Meeting of the Royal Society of Medicine in London in October 2003, entitled 'Biology of IGF-I: its interaction with insulin in health and malignant states'.

83. Yee, Doug, 2003. Targeting the IGF system for anti-tumour therapy. Meeting of the Royal Society of Medicine in London in October 2003, entitled 'Biology of IGF-I: its interaction with insulin in health and malignant states'.

84. Pollack, Michael, 2003. Cancer, aging and IGF physiology. Meeting of the Royal Society of Medicine in London in October 2003, entitled 'Biology of IGF-I: its interaction with insulin in health and malignant states'.

85. Holly, Jeff, 1998. Insulin-like growth factor-1 and new opportunities for cancer prevention. *Lancet*, 351, 9113, 9 May, 1373–1375.

86. Chan, J.M., Stampfer, M.J., Giovannucci, E. and others, 1998. Plasma insulin-like growth factor-I and prostate cancer risk: a prospective study.

Science, 279, 563–566; Harman, S.M., Metter, E.J., Blackman, M.R., Landis, P.K. and Carter, H.B., 2000. Serum levels of insulin-type growth factor 1 (IGF-I), IGF II, IGF-binding protein-3, and prostate-specific antigen as predictors of clinical prostate cancer. *J Clin Endocrinol Metab*, 85, 4258–4265; Stattin, P and nine others, 2000. Plasma insulin-like growth factor-I insulin-like growth-binding proteins, and prostate cancer risk: a prospective study. *J Natl Cancer Inst*, 92, 1910–1917; Chokkalingam, A.P. and 12 others, 2001. Insulin-like growth factors and prostate cancer: a population-based case-control study in China. *Cancer Epidemiol Biomarkers Prev*, 10, 421–427; Chan, J.M., Stampfer, M.J., Ma, J. and others, 2002. Insulin-like growth factor-I (IGF-I) and IGF binding protein-3 as predictors of advanced-stage prostate cancer. *J Natl Cancer Inst*, 94, 1099–1106; Mantzoros, C.S., Tzonou, A., Signorello, L.B. and others, 1997. Insulin-like growth factor 1 in relation to prostate cancer and benign prostatic hyperplasia. *British Journal of Cancer*, 76, 1115–1118; Wolk, A., Mantzoros, C.S., Andersson, S.O. and others, 1998. Insulin-like growth factor 1 and prostate cancer risk: a population-based, case-control study. *J Natl Cancer Inst*, 90, 911–915; Holly, J.M.P., Gunnell, D.J. and Davey Smith., G, 1999. Growth hormone, IGF-I and cancer. Less intervention. Less intervention to avoid cancer? More intervention to prevent cancer. *J Endocrinol*, 162, 321–330.

87. Yu, H. and others, 1999. Plasma levels of IGF-I and lung cancer risk. *Journal of the National Cancer Institute*, 91, 151–156.

88. Ma, J. and others, 2001. Milk intake, circulating levels of IGF-I and risk of colorectal cancer in men. *Journal of the National Cancer Institute*, 93 (17), 1330–1336.

89. LeRoith, D and others, 1995. The role of the IGF-I receptor in cancer. *Annals of the New York Academy of Sciences*, 766, 402–408; Butler, J., 2006. *White lies*. Vegetarian and Vegan Foundation.

90. Campbell, T. Colin, Campbell, Thomas M. II, Robbins, John and Lyman Howard, 2006. *The China Study: The Most Comprehensive Study of Nutrition Ever Conducted and the Startling Implications for Diet, Weight Loss and Long-term Health*. Benbella Books.

91. Bradford Hill, A., 1965. The environment and disease: association or causation? *Proceedings of the Royal Society of Medicine*, 58 295–300.

92. Holly, J.M.P., Gunnell, D.J. and Davey Smith, G., 1999. Growth hormone, IGF-I and cancer. Less intervention. Less intervention to avoid cancer? More intervention to prevent cancer. *J Endocrinol*, 162, 321–330.

93. Robbins, John, 1987. *A Diet for a New America*. Stillpoint Publishing.

94. www.dhn.csiro.au/crctissue.html

95. Xian, C., 1995. Degradation of IGF-1 in the Adult Rat Gastrointestinal Tract is limited by a Specific Antiserum of the Dietary Protein Casein. *Journal of Endocrinology*, 146, 2, 1 August, 215; Thornburg, W. and others, 1984. Gastrointestinal absorption of epidermal growth factor in suckling rats. *American Journal of Physiology*, 246, G80–G85.

96. The European Commission. Health and Consumer Protection. Scientific Committee on Veterinary Measures relating to Public Health – Outcome of discussions. http://europa.eu.int/comm/dg24/health/sc/scv/out19_en.html

97. Allen, N.E., and others, 2000. Hormones and Diet: Low Insulin-like Growth Factor-1 but Normal Bioavailable Androgens in Vegan Men. *Brit J Canc*, 83 (1), 95–97.

98. Steinman, G., 2006. Can the chance of having twins be modified by diet? *The Lancet*, 367 (9521), 1461–1462.

99. Norat and others, 2007. Diet, serum IGF-1 and IGF-BP3 in European women. *European Journal of Clinical Nutrition*, 61, 91–98.

100. The European Commission. Health and Consumer Protection. Scientific Committee on Veterinary Measures relating to Public Health – Outcome of discussions. http://europa.eu.int/comm/dg24/health/sc/scv/out19_en.html

101. Heaney, R.P. and others, 1999. Dietary changes favourably affect bone remodelling in older adults, *Journal of the American Dietetic Association*, 99 (10), 1228–1233.

102. Gunnell, D.L. and 10 others, 2003. Are diet – prostate-cancer associations mediated by the IGF axis? A cross-sectional analysis of diet, IGF-I and IGFBP-3 in healthy middle-aged men. *British Journal of Cancer*, 88, 1682–1686.

103. World Cancer Research Fund, 1997. *Food, nutrition and the prevention of cancer: a global perspective*. Washington, DC: American Institute of Cancer Research.

104. Allen, N.E., Appleby, P.N., Davey, G.K. and Key, T.J., 2000. Hormones and diet: low insulin-like growth factor-I but normal bioavailable androgens in vegan men. *Br J Cancer*, 83, 95–97.

105. Yaker, S. and others, 2005. The role of the growth hormone/IGF axis in tumour growth and progression: lessons from animal models. *Cytokine and Growth Factor Reviews*, 16 (4–5), 407–420; Butler, J., 2006. *White lies*. Vegetarian and Vegan Foundation.

106. Mannisto, S. and others, 1999. Diet and the risk of breast cancer in a case control study: does the threat of disease have an influence on recall bias? *Journal of Clinical Epidemiology*, 52 (5), 429–439; Outwater, J.L. and others, 1997. Dairy products and breast cancer: the IGF-1, estrogen and bGH hypothesis. *Medical Hypotheses*, 48 (6), 453–461; Gaard, M. and others, 1995. Dietary fat and the risk of breast cancer: a prospective study of 25,892 Norwegian women. *Int J Cancer*, 63 (1), 13–17; Decarli, A. and others, 1986. Environmental factors and cancer mortality in Italy: correlational exercise. *Oncology*, 43 (2), 116–126; Rose, D.P. and others, 1986. International comparisons of mortality rates for cancer of the breast, ovary, prostate, and colon, and per capita food consumption. *Cancer*, 58 (11), 2363–2371; Shimada, A. and others, Ecological approach to the eating habits and the cancer mortality of Brazilian people. (in het japans.) *Gan No Rinsho*, 32 (6), 631–640; La Vecchia, C. and others, 1986. Age at first birth, dietary practises and breast cancer mortality in various Italian regions. *Oncology*, 43 (1), 1–6; Talamini, R. and others, 1984. Social factors, diet and breast cancer in a northern Italian population. *Br J Cancer*, 49 (6), 723–729.

107. Rose, D.P. and others, 1986. International comparisons of mortality rates for cancer of the breast, ovary, prostate, and colon, and per capita food consumption. *Cancer*, 58 (11), 2363–2371.

108. Schuurman, A.G. and others, 1999. Animal products, calcium and protein and prostate cancer risk in The Netherlands Cohort Study. *Br J Cancer*, 80 (7), 1107–1113; Giovannucci, E., 1999. Nutritional factors in human cancers. Advances in Experimental Medicine and Biology, 472, 29–42; Giovanucci, E., 1998. Dietary influences of 1,25(OH)2 vitamin D in relation to prostate cancer: a hypothesis. *Cancer Causes and Control*, 9 (6), 567–582; Willet, W.C., 1997. Nutrition and Cancer. *Salud Publica de Mexico*, 39 (4), 298–309; De Stefani, E. and others, 1995. Tobacco, alcohol, diet and risk of prostate cancer. *Tumori*, 81 (5), 315–320; Le Marchand, L. and others, 1994. Animal fat consumption and prostate cancer: a prospective study in Hawaii. *Epidemiology*, 5 (3), 276–282; Talamini, R. and others, 1992. Diet and prostate cancer: a case control study in northern Italy. *Nutrition and Cancer*, 18 (3), 277–286; La Vecchia, C. and others, 1991. Dairy products and the risk of prostatic cancer. *Oncology*, 48 (5), 406–410; Mettlin, C. and others, 1989. Beta-carotene and animal fats and their relationship to prostate cancer risk. A case control study. *Cancer*, 64 (3), 605–612; Snowdon, D.A., 1988. Animal product consumption and mortality because of all causes combined, coronary heart disease, stroke, diabetes, and cancer in Seventh-day Adventists. *Am J Clin Nutr*, 48 (3 Suppl.), 739–748; Talamini, R. and others, 1986. Nutrition, social factors, and prostate cancer in a northern Italian population. *Br J Cancer*, 53 (6), 817–821; Rose, D.P. and others, 1986. International comparisons of mortality rates for cancer of the breast, ovary, prostate, and colon, and per capita food consumption. *Cancer*, 58 (11), 2263–2271.

109. Newby, J.A. and Howard, 2006. *Environmental influences in cancer aetiology*, 2006, 1–59.

110. Butler, J., 2006. *White lies*. Vegetarian and Vegan Foundation.

111. Butler, J., 2006. *White lies*. Vegetarian and Vegan Foundation.

112. Lawrence R., 1994. *Breastfeeding – A Guide to the Medical Profession*, Fourth edition. Mossby.

113. Holly, J.M.P., Gunnell, D.J. and Davey Smith, G., 1999. Growth hormone, IGF-I and cancer. Less intervention to avoid cancer? More intervention to prevent cancer? *J Endocrinol*, 162, 321–330.

114. Giudice, L.A., 1992. Insulin-like growth factors and ovarian follicular development. *Endocrine Reviews*, 13, 641–669.

115. Westley, B.R. and May, F.E.B., 1994. Role of insulin-like growth factors in steroid modulated proliferation. *Journal of Steroid Biochemistry and Molecular Biology*, 51, 1–9; Marcelli, M., Haidacher, S.J., Plymate, S.R. and Birnbaum, R.S., 1995. Altered growth and insulin-like growth factor-binding protein-3 production in PC-3 prostate carcinoma cells stably transfected with a constitutively active androgen receptor complementary deoxyribonucleic acid. *Endocrinology*, 136, 1040–1048.

116. Holly, J.M.P., Gunnell, D.J. and Davey Smith, G., 1999. Growth hormone, IGF-I and cancer. Less intervention to avoid cancer? More intervention to prevent cancer? *J Endocrinol*, 162, 321–330.

117. Bernstein, l. and Ross, R.K., 1993. Endogenous hormones and breast cancer risk. *Epidemiol Res*, 15, 48–65; Pike, M.C. and others, 1993,

Estrogens, progestogens, normal breast proliferation and breast cancer risk. Epidemiol Reviews, 15, 17–35.

118. Bocchinfuso, W.F. and others, 2000. Induction of mammary gland development in estrogen receptor-alpha knockout mice. Endocrinology, 141, 2983–2994; Attwood, C.S. and others, 2000. Progesterone induces side-branching of the ductal epithelium in the mammary glands of prepubertal mice. J Endocrinology, 167, 39–52.

119. Campbell, T. Colin, Campbell, Thomas M. II, Robbins, John and Lyman Howard, 2006. *The China Study: The Most Comprehensive Study of Nutrition Ever Conducted and the Startling Implications for Diet, Weight Loss and Long-term Health.* Benbella Books.

120. www.breakthrough.org.uk

121. Campbell, T. Colin, Campbell, Thomas M. II, Robbins, John and Lyman Howard, 2006. *The China Study: The Most Comprehensive Study of Nutrition Ever Conducted and the Startling Implications for Diet, Weight Loss and Long-term Health.* Benbella Books.

122. Cramer, D.W. and others, 1989. Galactose consumption and metabolism in relation to the risk of ovarian cancer. *Lancet*, 2, 66–71.

123. Fairfield and others, 2004. A prospective study of dietary lactose and ovarian cancer. *Int J of Cancer*, 110 (2), 271–277.

124. Larsson, S.C. and others, 2004. Milk and lactose intakes and ovarian cancer risk. in the Swedish Mammography Cohort. *Amer J Clinical Nutrition*, 80 (5), 1353–1357.

125. Larsson, S.C. and others, 2005. Milk, milk products and lactose intake and ovarian cancer risk: a meta analysis of epidemiological studies. *Int J of Cancer*.

126. Ganmaa, D. and Sato, A., 2005. Possible role of female sex hormones in milk from pregnant cows in the development of breast, ovarian and corpus uteri cancers. *Medical Hypotheses*, 65 (6), 1028–1037.

127. Hartman, S. and others, 1998. Natural occurrence of steroid hormones in food. *Food Chemistry*, 62, 7–20; Butler, J., 2006. *White lies.* Vegetarian and Vegan Foundation.

128. Plant, Jane and Tidey, Gill, 2005. *Eating for Better Health.* Virgin Books.

129. Bahna, S.L., 1987. Milk allergy in infancy. *Ann Allergy*, 59, 131.

130. Dunea, G., 1982. Beyond the Etheric. *BMJ*, 285, 428–429.

131. Kretchmer, N., 1981. The Significance of lactose intolerance. In: Paige, D.M. and Bayless, T.M., Editors., *Lactose Digestion: Clinical and nutritional implications.* Johns Hopkins University Press.

132. http://www.fda.gov/fdac/features/2001/401_food.html

133. http://www.ifst.org/hottop19.htm

134. Taylor, S L, 1992. Chemistry and detection of food allergens. *Food Technology*, 46 (5), 146–152.

135. Saarinen, K.N. and others, 2005. Clinical course and prognosis of cow's milk allergy are dependent on milk-specific IgE status. *Journal of Allergy and Clinical Immunology*, 116 (4), 869–875.

136. http://www.ifst.org/hottop19.htm

137. Martin, Peter, 2002. Milk: Nectar or poison? *Sunday Times Magazine*, July 21, 2002.

138. Thorsdottir, I. and Ramel, A., 2003. Dietary intake of 10- to 16-year-old children and adolescents in Central and Northern Europe and association with the incidence of type-1 diabetes. *Annals of Nutrition and Metabolism*, 47 (6), 267–275.

139. Campbell, T. Colin, Campbell, Thomas M. II, Robbins, John and Lyman Howard, 2006. *The China Study: The Most Comprehensive Study of Nutrition Ever Conducted and the Startling Implications for Diet, Weight Loss and Long-term Health.* Benbella Books.

140. TB bacteria found in treated milk. *Sunday Times*, 20 February, 2000.

141. Bull, T.J. and others, 2003. Detection and verification of *Mycobacterium avium* subsp. *paratuberculosis* in fresh ileocolonic mucosal biopsy specimens from individuals with and without Crohn's disease. *Journal of Clinical Microbiology*, 41 (7), 2915–2923.

142. Millar, D. and others, 1996. IS900 PCR to detect *Mycobacterium paratuberculosis* in retail supplies of whole pasteurized cows' milk in England and Wales. *Applied and Environmental Microbiology*, 62 (9), 3446–3452.

143. Pickup, R.W. and others, 2005. MAP in the catchment area and water of the River Taff in South Wales, UK and its potential relationship to clustering of Crohn's disease cases in the city of Cardiff. *Applied and Environmental Microbiology*, 71 (4), 2130–2139.

144. FSA/SE, 2001. Task force on E.coli 0157. www.food.gov.uk/multimedia/pdfs/ecolitaskfinreport.pdf

145. Butler, J., 2006. *White lies*. Vegetarian and Vegan Foundation.

146. Plant, Jane and Tidey, Gill, 2003. *Understanding, Preventing and Overcoming Osteoporosis.* London: Virgin Books

147. Robbins, John, 1987. *A Diet for a New America*. Stillpoint Publishing.

148. Hegsted D.M., 1986. Calcium and osteoporosis. J Nutr, 116, 2316–2319.

149. Campbell, T. Colin, Campbell, Thomas M. II, Robbins, John and Lyman Howard, 2006. *The China Study: The Most Comprehensive Study of Nutrition Ever Conducted and the Startling Implications for Diet, Weight Loss and Long-term Health.* Benbella Books.

150. Ademamowo, C.A. and others, 2005. High-school dietary dairy intake and teenage acne. *Journal of the American Academy of Dermatology*, 52 (2), 207–214.

151. Butler, J., 2006. *White lies*. Vegetarian and Vegan Foundation.

152. Toohey, M.L. and others, 1998. Cardiovascular disease risk factors are lower in African-American vegans compared to lacto-ovo-vegetarians. *Journal of the American College of Nutrition*, 17 (5), 425–434.

153. Park, M. and others, 2005. Consumption of milk and calcium in mid-life and the future risk of Parkinson disease. *Neurology*, 64, 1047–1051.

UPDATE TO CHAPTER FIVE

1. World Cancer Research Fund and American Institute for Cancer Research. 1997. *Food, Nutrition and the Prevention of Cancer: a Global Perspective.* Washington DC: American Institute for Cancer Research. (http://www.aicr.org/report2.htm)

2. http://www.pcrm.org/health/Dairy_and_Prostate_Cancer/d_p_article.html

3. Plant, Jane and Tidey, Gill, 2002. *The Plant Programme*. Paperback edition. Virgin Books; Plant, Jane and Tidey, Gill, 2003. *Understanding, Preventing and Overcoming Osteporosis*. Virgin Books; Plant, Jane, 2004, updated 2007. *Prostate Cancer: Understand, Prevent and Overcome*. Virgin Books; Plant, Jane and Tidey, Gill, 2005. *Eating for Better Health*. Virgin Books.

4. Smith-Warner, S.A. and Giovannucci, E., 1999. Fruit and vegetable intake and cancer. In: Heber, D., Blackburn, G.L. and Go, V.L.W., editors. *Nutritional oncology*. San Diego: Academic Press. 153–183.

5. American Institute for Cancer Research, 2000. Press Release (August 31, 2000) from the AICR Annual Research Conference 2000: New Methods in Clinical Trials Lending New Insights on Diet-cancer Connection, Expert Says.

6. National Cattlemen's Beef Association, 1999. Conjugated Linoleic Acid and Dietary Beef – An Update. *Beef Facts: Nutrition*, Series No. FS/N 016.

7. Ip, C., Scimeca, J.A. and Thompson, H.J, 1994. Conjugated linoleic acid. A powerful anticarcinogen from animal fat sources. *Cancer*, 74, 1050–1054.

8. Steinhart, Carol, 1996. Conjugated Linoleic Acid: The Good News about Animal Fat. *Journal of Chemical Education*, 73, A302. (http://jchemed.chem.wisc.edu/Journal/Issues/1996/Dec/absA302.html)

9. Campbell, T.C. and Junshi, C., 1994. Diet and chronic degenerative disease perspectives from China. *American Journal of Clinical Nutrition*, 59 (Suppl.), 11,535–11,615.

10. Bernstein, L. and Ross, R.K., 1993. Endogenous hormones and breast cancer risk. *Epidemiol Reviews*, 15, 48–65; Pike and others, 1993. Estrogens, progestogens, normal breast proliferation and breast cancer risk. *Epidemiol reviews*, 15, 17–35.

11. Prentice. R. and others, 1990. Dietary fat reduction and plasma oestrodial concentration in healthy postmenopausal women. J Natl Cancer Inst, 82, 129–134.

12. Waxman, Jonathan, 2001. *The Prostate Cancer Book*. London: Vermillion.

13. Campbell, T. Colin, Campbell, Thomas M. II, Robbins, John and Lyman Howard, 2006. *The China Study: The Most Comprehensive Study of Nutrition Ever Conducted and the Startling Implications for Diet, Weight Loss and Long-term Health*. Benbella Books.

14. Ornish, D and others, 2005. Intensive lifestyle changes may affect the progression of prostate cancer. *Journal of Urology*, 174 (3), 1065–1069.

15. Waxman, Jonathan, 2001. *The Prostate Cancer Book*. London: Vermillion.

16. Campbell, T. Colin, Campbell, Thomas M. II, Robbins, John and Lyman Howard, 2006. *The China Study: The Most Comprehensive Study of Nutrition Ever Conducted and the Startling Implications for Diet, Weight Loss and Long-term Health*. Benbella Books.

17. Plant, Jane and Tidey, Gill, 2005. *Eating for Better Health*. Virgin Books. See also, Campbell, T. Colin, Campbell, Thomas M. II, Robbins, John and Lyman Howard, 2006. *The China Study: The Most Comprehensive Study of Nutrition Ever Conducted and the Startling Implications for Diet, Weight Loss and Long-term Health*. Benbella Books; Robbins, John, 1987. *A Diet for a New America*. Stillpoint Publishing.

18. Newby, J.A. and Howard, C.V., 2006. Environmental influences in cancer aetiology. *Journal of Nutritional and Environmental Medicine*, 2006, 1–59.

19. Campbell, T.C. and Junshi, C., 1994. Diet and chronic degenerative disease perspectives from China. *American Journal of Clinical Nutrition*, 59 (Suppl.), 11,535–11,615.

20. *Food Chemical News*, April 29, 1996.

21. Kurzer, M.S. and Xu, X., 1999. Dietary Phytoestrogens. *Annual Reviews of Nutrition*, 17, 353–381.

22. Adlercreutz, H., 1995. Phyto-oestrogens: Epidemiology and a Possible Role in Cancer Protection. *Environmental Health Perspectives*,103 (Supppl 7), 103–112; Adlercreutz, H., Mazur, W., Bartels, P., Elomaa, V.-V., Watanabe, S., Wähälä, K., Landström, M., Lundin, E., Bergh, A., Damber, J.-E., Åman, P., Widmark, A., Johansson, A., Zhang, J.-X. and Hallmans, G., 2000. Phyto-oestrogens and Prostate Disease. *J Nutr*, 130, 658S–659S.

23. http://www.ifst.org/hottop34.htm

24. Adlercreutz, H., Mazur, W., Bartels, P., Elomaa, V.-V., Watanabe, S., Wähälä, K., Landström, M., Lundin, E., Bergh, A., Damber, J.-E., Åman, P., Widmark, A., Johansson, A., Zhang, J.-X. and Hallmans, G., 2000. Phyto-oestrogens and Prostate Disease. *J Nutr*, 130, 658S–659S.

25. Zhou, J.-R., Gugger, E.T., Tanaka, T., Guo, Y., Blackburn, G.L. and Clinton, S.K., 1999. Soy-bean phytochemicals inhibit the growth of transplantable human prostate carcinoma and tumor angiogenesis in mice. *J Nutr*, 129, 1628–1635; Davis, J.N., Singh, B., Bhuiyan, M. and Sarkar, F.H., 1998. Genistein-induced upregulation of p21WAF1, downregulation of cyclin B, and induction of apoptosis in prostate cancer cells. *Nutr Cancer*, 32, 123–131; The Royal Society, 2000. Endocrine-disrupting chemicals. *Document* 06/00. The Royal Society; Setchell, K.D.R., 1998. Phyto-oestrogens: the biochemistry, physiology and implications for human health of soy isoflavones. *Nutrition*, 68, 1333S–1346S.

26. Glenville, Marilyn, 2003. *The New Natural Alternatives to HRT*. Second edition. Kyle Cathie.

27. Campbell, T. Colin, Campbell, Thomas M. II, Robbins, John and Lyman Howard, 2006. *The China Study: The Most Comprehensive Study of Nutrition Ever Conducted and the Startling Implications for Diet, Weight Loss and Long-term Health*. Benbella Books.

28. Glenville, Marilyn, 2003. *The New Natural Alternatives to HRT*. Second edition. Kyle Cathie.

29. Robbins, John, 1987. *A Diet for a New America*. Stillpoint Publishing; Kradjian, R.M., 1994. *Save Yourself from Breast Cancer*. New York: Berkley Books; McDougall, John, 2000. *The McDougall Program for Women*; Lee, John R., 1999. *Natural Progesterone*. Second revised edition. Jon Carpenter; Plant, Jane and Tidey, Gill, 2003. *Understanding, preventing and overcoming osteoporosis*. Virgin Books; Fox, Douglas, 2001. Hard cheese. *New Scientist*, 15 December 2001, 42–45.

30. http://wayne.unl.edu/00aprilcolumn.htm

31. Martin, Peter, 2002. Milk: Nectar or Poison? *Sunday Times Magazine*, July 21, 2002, 46–54.

32. Website of the American Cancer Society, http://www.cancer.org/docroot/ eto/content/eto_5_3x_soybean.asp?siteare a=&viewmode=print

33. Gottlieb, Scott, 2003. Men should eat nine servings of fruit and vegetables a day. *BMJ*, 326, 1003.

34. UK Ministry of Agriculture, Fisheries and Food advice as reported in the *Sunday Times*, 1999.

35. Willet, W.C., 1994. Micronutrients and cancer risk. *Am J Clin Nutr*, 59, (suppl), 1162S–5S. See also: Willett, Walter C., Colditz, Graham A. and Mueller, Nancy A., 1996. Strategies for Minimising Cancer Risk. *Scientific American*, Special Issue, What you need to know about Cancer, September, 275, 3, 88–95.

36. Huang, M.-T., Asawa T., Ho C.-T., Rosen R.T., eds, 1994. *Food phytochemicals for cancer prevention I – fruits and vegetables*. Washington, DC: American Chemical Society; Ho, C.-T., Osawa, T., Huang, M.-T. and Rosen, R.T., eds, 1994. *Food phytochemicals for cancer prevention II – teas, spices, herbs*. Washington, DC: American Chemical Society; American Institute for Cancer Research, ed., 1996. *Dietary phytochemicals in cancer prevention and treatment*. New York: Plenum Press; Liu, R.H. and Espinosa, A., 2000. Bio-active Compounds from Fruits and Vegetables in the Prevention of Cancer. In: *Agriculture in the New Century: Managing Bio-Resources and Bio-Diversity*, National Taiwan University, Taipei, Taiwan, 53–59.

37. Greenwald, Peter, 2002. Cancer chemoprevention. *BMJ*, 324, 714–718.

38. Alpha-Tocopherol Beta-Carotene Cancer Prevention Study Group, Heinonen, O.P., Huttunen, J.K. and Albanes, D., 1994. The effect of vitamin E and beta-carotene on the incidence of lung cancer and other cancers in male smokers. *N Engl J Med*, 330, 1029–35; Omenn, G.S., Goodman, G.E., Thornquist, M.D., Balmes, J., Cullen, M.R. and Glass, A., 1996. Effects of a combination of beta carotene and vitamin A on lung cancer and cardiovascular disease. *N Engl J Med*, 334, 1150–1155.

39. Ursell, Amanda, 2007. Eat a rainbow to stay healthy. *The Times* (T2), 6 February 2007.

40. Gunnell, D L and 10 others, 2003. Are diet – prostate-cancer associations mediated by the IGF axis? A cross-sectional analysis of diet, IGF-I and IGFBP-3 in healthy middle-aged men. *British Journal of Cancer*, 88, 1682–1686.

41. Mucci, L.A. and six others, 2001. Are dietary influences on the risk of prostate cancer mediated through the insulin-like growth factor system. *BJU Int*, 87, 814–820.

42. http://www.flax.com.fda

43. http://info.cancerresearchuk.org/healthyliving/dietandhealthyeating/th eepicstudy

44. *Am J Epidemiol*, 1994, 139 (11), s37.

45. Inside Story. *Which?* April 2002, 4.

46. Lu, C. and others, 2006. Organic diets significantly lower children's dietary exposure to organophosphorus pesticides. *Environmental Health Perspectives*, 114 (2), 260–263.

47. Doll, R. and Peto, R., 1981. *The causes of cancer: quantitative estimates of avoidable risks of cancer in the United States today*. New York: Oxford University Press.

48. Boseley, Sarah, 2006. Expert revered for painstaking work that proved link between smoking and cancer. *Guardian*, 8 December, 2006.

49. Colborn, T.T., 1993. Developmental effects of endocrine-disrupting chemicals in wildlife and humans. *Environmental Health Perspectives*, 101 (5), 378–384.

50. McKinlay, R. and others, in press. Endocrine-disrupting pesticides: implications for risk assessment.

51. Royal Commission on Environmental Pollution, 2005. *Special report, crop spraying and health of residents and bystanders*.

52. Mittelstaedt, Martin, 2002. Data point to breast-cancer risk. *Globe and Mail*, 22 November 2002, A5.

53. McMichael, A.J., 1993. *Planetary Overload – Global Environmental Change and the Health of the Species*. Cambridge University Press.

54. Royal Commission on Environmental Pollution, 2002. *A Short Report on the Environmental Effects of Civil Aircraft in Flight*. Royal Commission on Environmental Pollution.

55. Bristow, Amanda, 2002. *Which?*, April 2002, 22–23.

56. Campbell, T. Colin, Campbell, Thomas M. II, 2006. *The China Study*. Benbella Books; McDougall, J. and others, 1995. Rapid reduction of serum cholesterol and blood pressure by a twelve-day, very low fat, strictly vegetarian diet. *J Am Coll Nutr*, 14, 491–496.

57. *ICON*, September 2002.

58. http://www.eurocbc.org/page641.html; http://www.ciwf.co.uk/Trust/FF/farm_facts_fish_farming.htm

59. Cho, E. and others, 2006. Red meat intake and risk of breast cancer among premenopausal women. *Archives of International Medicine*, 166, 2253–2259.

60. http://info.cancerresearchuk.org/healthyliving/dietandhealthyeating/theepicstudy

61. *JAMA*, 1985, 254 (3), 356–357.

62. http://www.prostatepointers.org/cmyers/pf0696.html

63. http://info.cancerresearchuk.org/healthyliving/dietandhealthyeating/theepicstudy

64. *J Nat Cancer Inst*, 1994, 86 (18), 1409–1415.

65. *Am J Epidem*, 1994, 139 (11), S37.

66. http://www.prostatepointers.org/cmyers/pf0696.html; *American Heart Association Cookbook*, fifth edition, 1995. New York: Times Books, Random House; Pritikin, Nathan, 1979. *The Pritikin Program for Diet and Exercise*. New York: Bantam Books; Ornish, D., 1990. *Dr Dean Ornish's Program for Reversing Heart Disease*. New York: Ballantyne Books.

67. Van de Weyer, Courtney, 2005. Changing diets, changing minds. Sustain.

68. www.annieappleseedproject.org/nutgenprotin.html

69. Van de Weyer, Courtney, 2005. Changing diets, changing minds. Sustain.

70. Trichopoulos, Dimitrios, Li, Frederick P. and Hunter, David J., 1996. What Causes Cancer? *Scientific American*, Special Issue, What you need to know about Cancer, September, 275, 3, 80–85.

71. Djamgoz, M.B.A. and Isbilen, B., 2006. Dietary compounds as anti-cancer agents: a preliminary evaluation of ion channels and membrane excitability as possible target mechanisms. *The Lancet*.

72. http://www.findarticles.com/cf_0/m0FKA/5_62/62702338/p1/article.jhtml? term = turmeric%2C + Liz + Brown

73. Steinmetz, K.A. and Potter, J.D, 1991. Vegetables, fruit, and cancer, II. Mechanisms. *Cancer Causes Control*, 2, 427–442; Lam, L.K.T., Zhang, J., Hasegawa, S. and others, 1994. Inhibition of chemically induced carcinogenesis by citrus liminoids. In: Huang, M-T., Asawa, T., Ho, C-T. and Rosen, R.T., eds. *Food phytochemicals for cancer prevention, I – fruits and vegetables*. Washington, DC: American Chemical Society, pp. 209–219; Zheng, G,Q., Zhang, J., Kenney, P.M. and Lam, L.K.T., 1994 Stimulation of glutathione S-transferase and inhibition of carcinogenesis in mice by celery seed oil constituents. In: Huang, M.-T., Asawa, T., Ho, C.-T. and Rosen, R.T., eds. *Food phytochemicals for cancer prevention, I – fruits and vegetables*. Washington, DC: American Chemical Society, pp. 230–238.

74. Nakatani, N, 1994. Chemistry of antioxidants from Labiatae herbs. In: Ho, C.-T., Osawa, T., Huang, M.-T. and Rosen, R.T., eds. *Food phytochemicals for cancer prevention, II – teas, spices, herbs*. Washington, DC: American Chemical Society, pp. 144–153.

75. Ho, C.-T., Ferraro, T., Chen, Q and others, 1994. Phytochemicals in teas and rosemary and their cancer-preventive properties. In: Ho, C.-T., Osawa, T., Huang, M.-T. and Rosen, R.T., eds. *Food phytochemicals for cancer prevention, II – teas, spices, herbs*. Washington, DC: American Chemical Society, pp. 2–19.

76. Kikuzaki, H. and Nakatani, N, 1993. Antioxidant effects of some ginger constituents. *Journal of Food Science*, 58, 1407–1410.

77. Zheng, G.Q., Kenney, P.M. and Lam, L.K.T., 1993. Potential anticarcinogenic natural products isolated from lemongrass oil and galanga root oil. *Journal of Agricultural and Food Chemistry*, 41, 153–156; Zheng, G.Q., Kenney, P.M. and Lam, L.K.T., 1992. Anethofuran, carvone, and limonene: potential cancer chemopreventive agents from dill weed oil and caraway oil. *Planta Medica*, 58, 338–341; Zheng, G.Q., Kenney, P.M., Zhang, J. and others, 1993. Chemoprevention of benzo[a]pyrene-induced forestomach cancer in mice by natural phthalides from celery seed oil. *Nutr Cancer*, 19, 77–86; Zheng, G.Q., Kenney, P.M. and Lam, L.K.T., 1992. Sesquiterpenes from clove (Eugenia caryophyllata) as potential anticarcinogenic agents. *Journal of Natural Products*, 55, 999–1003; Zheng, G.Q., Kenney, P.M. and Lam, L.K.T., 1992. Myristicin: a potential cancer chemopreventive agent from parsley leaf oil. *J Agric Food Chem*, 40, 107–110.

78. http://www.pcrm.org/health/Dairy_and_Prostate_Cancer/d_p_article.html; World Cancer Research Fund and American Institute for Cancer Reseach. 1997. *Food, Nutrition and the Prevention of Cancer: a global perspective*. Washington DC: American Institute for Cancer Research. (http://www.aicr.org/report2.htm)

79. *Journal of the American Diabetic Association*, May 2001; http://www.wadsworth.com/nutrition_d/special_features/news/nutu1201.ht ml.

80. Thompson, L.U., 1994. Antioxidants and hormone-mediated health benefits of whole grains. *Critical Reviews in Food Science and Nutrition*, 34, 473–497.

81. Thompson, L.U., 1992. Potential health benefits of whole grains and their components. *Contemp Nutr*, 17 (6), 1–2.

82. Elson, C.E. and Yu, S.G., 1994. The chemoprevention of cancer by mevalonate-derived constituents of fruits and vegetables. *J Nutr*, 124, 607–614.

83. Elson, C.E. and Yu, S.G., 1994. The chemoprevention of cancer by mevalonate-derived constituents of fruits and vegetables. *J Nutr*, 124, 607–614.

84. Fox, Douglas, 2002. Bread to blame for plague of pimples. *New Scientist*, 7 December 2002.

85. http://www.dorway.com/badnews.html

86. http://www.stevia.net; http://www.holisticmed.com/sweet/

87. Pesticide residues found in Indian bottled water. 2003. *BMJ*, 326, 352.

88. http://www.annieappleseedproject.org/nutgenprotin.html, reporting on a conference on nutritional genomics and proteomics in cancer prevention in September 2002, at the USNIH, Bethesda.

89. Why tea is not so good for you after all. *The Times*, 9 January 2007.

90. www.diagnose-me.com

91. http://research.kib.ki.se/e-uven/public/51419.html

92. ENDS Report.

93. http://www.vegansociety.com/html/info/info28.html

94. http://www.vegansociety.com

95. Royal College of Physicians, 2002. Nutrition and patients: a doctor's responsibility.

96. http://www.pcrm.org/health/Dairy_and_Prostate_Cancer/d_p_article.html

97. www.mdanderson.org/departments/nutrition/display.cfm?id=51f759d8-98b2-11d5-813300508b603a14&method=displayfull&pn=51f7589e-98b2-11d5-813300508b603a14

UPDATE TO CHAPTER SIX

1. Berger, Abi, 2002. Science commentary: What does zinc do? *BMJ*, 325, 1062–1063.

2. Hambridge, K. M., Casey, C. E. and Krebs, N. F., 1986. Zinc, In: *Trace Elements in Human and Animal Nutrition*, Fifth Edition, Mertz, W., Ed. Academic Press, Inc, London.

3. Medical Report: Prostate Cancer. *ICON*, 2002, 1 (5), 8–10.

4. McCusker, R.H., 1998. Controlling Insulin-Like Growth Factor Activity and the Modulation of Insulin-Like Growth Factor Binding Protein and Receptor Binding. *J Dairy Sci*, 81, 1790–1800.

5. Josefson, Deborah, 2002. Popping a multivitamin daily can keep disease at bay. *BMJ*, 324, 1544.

6. Van de Weyer, C., 2005. *Changing diets, changing minds*. Sustain.

7. Van de Weyer, C., 2005. *Changing diets, changing minds*. Sustain.

8. *The Lancet*, 1976, 880–881.

9. Johnson, C., 1999, Environmental controls in iodine deficiency disorders (IDD), *Earthworks*, 9 November, p. 3, British Geological Survey.

10. Greenwald, Peter, 1996. Chemoprevention of cancer. *Scientific American*, September 1996, 96–99.

11. Olivotto, Ivo, Hoffer, Abram and Lesperance, Mary, 2002. In *Breast Cancer Research and Treatment*, http://www.nlm.nih.gov/medlineplus/news/fullstory_10706.html

12. Bender, David A., 2002. Daily doses of multivitamin tablets. *BMJ*, 325, 173–174.

13. *Annals of Internal Medicine*, July 1, 2003; http://www.nlm.nih.gov/medlineplus/news/fullstory_13210.html

14. Kmietowicz, Zosia, 2003. Food watchdog warns against high doses of vitamins and minerals. *BMJ*, 326, 1001.

15. http://www.nlm.nih.gov/medlineplus/news/fullstory_13219.html

16. Gluud, C., 2007. *Journal of the American Medical Association*, 297, 842; *see also* Can vitamin supplements do more harm than good? *New Scientist*, v28, February 2007, 6.

17. Oakley, Godfrey P., 2002. Delaying folic acid fortification of flour. *BMJ*, 324, 1348–1349.

18. Reynolds, Edward, 2002. Fortification of flour with folic acid. BMJ, 324, 918.

19. Feldman, David, 2002. Pathways of Vitamin D Action to Inhibit Prostate Cancer Cell Growth. www.annieappleseedproject.org/nutgenprotin.html

20. Campbell, T.C. and Campbell, T.M., 2006. *The China Study*. Benbella Books.

21. http://bioscience.igh.cnrs.fr/2001/v6/d/hansen/2.asp

22. Seol, J.G. and five others, 1998. Telomerase activity in acute myelogenous leukemia: clinical and biological implications. *Br J Haematology*, 100, 156–165; Savoysky, E. and seven others, 1996. Down-regulation of telomerase activity is an early event in the differentiation in HL-60 cells. *Biochem Biophys Res Commun*, 226, 329–334; Albanell, J. and five others, 1996. Telomerase activity is repressed during differentiation of maturation-sensitive but not resistant human tumor cell lines. *Cancer Res*, 56, 1503–1508.

23. Campbell, T. Colin, Campbell, Thomas M. II, Robbins, John and Lyman Howard, 2006. *The China Study: The Most Comprehensive Study of Nutrition Ever Conducted and the Startling Implications for Diet, Weight Loss and Long-term Health.* Benbella Books.

24. Barretto, A.M., Schwartz, G.G., Woofruff, R. and Cramer, S.C., 2000. 5-hydroxyvitamin D-3, the prohormone of 1,25-dihydroxyvitamin D-3, inhibits the proliferation of primary prostatic epithelial cells. *Cancer Epidemiology Biomarkers & Prevention*, 9, 3, 265–270.

25. http://www.rense.com/general/dair.htm

26. Spallholz, J.E., Stewart, J.R., 1989. Advances in the role of minerals in immunobiology. Center for Food and Nutrition, Texas Tech University, Lubbock 79409. *Biol Trace Elem Res Mar*, 19 (3) 129–151.

27. *Gynecologic*, 2004, 93, 320–327.

28. Redbook, April, 1989, v172, n6, p. 96 (5).

29. Niki, E., Noguchi, N, Tsuchihashi, H. and others, 1995. Interaction among vitamin C, vitamin E and beta-carotene. *Am J Clin Nutr*, 62 (Suppl), 1322S–1326S.

30. Craig, Winston J., 2002. Phytochemicals: Guardians of Our Health, http://www.andrews.edu/NUFS/phyto.html, 03/12/02.

31. *New Scientist*, August 2006.

32. Anon, 2003. Growing problems: Endocrine disruptors under the spotlight. *ENDS Report*, 336, 20–23.

33. Vikse, R. and others, 1999. Heterocyclic amines in cooked meat. *Tidsskr Nor Laegeforen*, 119 (1), 45–49.

34. Skog, K. and others, 1997. Polar and non-polar heterocyclic amines in cooked fish and meat products and their corresponding pan residues. *Food Chemical Toxicology*, 35 (6), 555–565.

35. *BMJ*, 325, 1250.

36. *JAMA*, 1985, 254 (3), 356–357.

37. JIFSTAN/NCFST Acrylamide in Food Workshop, 1989. White paper for Working Group 5: Risk Communication. National Research Council, National Academy of Sciences (NRC-NAS). *Improving Risk Communication*. National Academy Press, Washington DC.

38. Fleck, Fiona, 2002. Experts launch action on staple foods. *BMJ*, 325, 120; Anon, 2002. Acrylamide clues found in Asparagine. *ICON*, 1 (6), 24.

39. website of the US Environmental Protection Agency, http://www.epa.gov/ttn/atw/hlthef/acrylami.html

40. http://ntp-server.niehs.nih.gov/htdocs/Chem_H&S/NTP_Chem7/Radian79-06-1.html

41. http://www.nsc.org/library/chemical/Acrylami.htm

42. Anon, 1997. Acrylamide. Toxic Air Contaminant Identification. List Summaries – ARB/SSD/SES. September 1997.

43. Advisory Committee on Hazardous Substances. *Sixth Annual Report* (2001–2002). Department for Environment, Food and Rural Affairs; The Royal Commission on Environmental Pollution, 2003. Chemicals in products: safeguarding the environment and human health. *Report* 24.

44. website of the US Environmental Protection Agency, http://www.epa.gov/ttn/atw/hlthef/acrylami.html

45. http://ntp-server.niehs.nih.gov/htdocs/Chem_H&S/NTP_Chem7/Radian79-06-1.html

46. http://www.foodstandards.gov.uk/multimedia/webpage/acrylamide_study_fa q

47. www.cancerresearchuk.org

48. White, Craig A. and Macleod, Una, 2002. ABC of psychological medicine: Cancer. *BMJ*, 325, 377–380.

49. Walsh, Kiri, King, Michael, Jones, Louise, Tookman, Adrian and Blizzard, Robert, 2002. Spiritual beliefs may affect outcome of bereavement: prospective study. *BMJ*, 324, 1551–1554.

50. White, Craig A. and Macleod, Una, 2002. ABC of psychological medicine: Cancer. *BMJ*, 325, 377–380.

51. White, Craig A. and Macleod, Una, 2002. ABC of psychological medicine: Cancer. *BMJ*, 325, 377–380.

52. White, Craig A. and Macleod, Una, 2002. ABC of psychological medicine: Cancer. *BMJ*, 325, 377–380.

53. Petticrew, Mark, Bell, Ruth and Hunter, Duncan, 2002. Influence of psychological coping on survival and recurrence in people with cancer: systematic review. *BMJ*, 325, 1066–1069.

54. Graham, J, Ramirez, A, Love, S, Richards, M and Burgess, C. 2002. Stressful life experiences and risk of relapse of breast cancer: observational cohort study. *BMJ* 324, 1420-1422.

55. Beales, D., 2004. Beyond mind-body dualism: implications for patient care. *Journal of Holistic Healthcare*, 1 (3).

56. Ernst, Edzard (ed.), 2001. *The desktop guide to complementary and alternative medicine*. Mosby.

57. King, Michael and five others, 2002. Effectiveness of teaching general practitioners skills in brief cognitive behaviour therapy to treat patients with depression: randomised controlled trial. *BMJ*, 324, 947.

58. http://www.nccn.org/patient_gls/_english/_prostate/

59. *European Journal of Cancer*, 2003, 39, 1562–1567; quoted in *BMJ*, 327, 402.

60. Plant, Jane and Stephenson, Janet, in preparation. *Breakthrough Anxiety and Depression*.

61. Bartram, Thomas, 1998. *Bartram's Encyclopedia of Herbal Medicine.* London: Robinson.

62. Miller, G H. 1996. Can Active or Passive Smoking Increase Breast Cancer Mortality? *Cancer Detect Prevent* 20 (5).

63. Mayor, Susan. 2002. Pregnancy and early smoking increases breast cancer risk. *BMJ*, 325, 12 October 2002, 793.

64. *Cancer Epidemiology, Biomarkers and Prevention*, July 2003; http://www.nlm.nih.gov/medlineplus/news/fullstory_13352.html

65. Plant, Jane and Tidey, Gill, 2003. *Understanding, preventing and overcoming osteoporosis*. Virgin Books.

66. Goodman-Gruen, D. and Barrett-Connor, E., 1997. Epidemiology of insulin-like growth factor-I in elderly men and women. The Rancho Bernardo Study. *American Journal of Epidemiology*, 145, 970–976; Kaklamani, V.G., Linos, A., Kaklamani, E., Markaki, I. and Mantzoros, C., 1999. Age, sex, and smoking are predictors of circulating insulin-like growth factor 1 and insulin-like growth factor-binding protein 3. *Journal of Clinical Oncology*, 17, 813–817.

67. Colborn, T., Dumanoski, D. and Myers, J.P., 1996. *Our Stolen Futures*, Dutton, Penguin Books, USA.

68. The Environment Agency, March 2000. *Endocrine-disrupting substances in the environment: The Environment Agency's Strategy*, The Environment Agency, Bristol, UK.

69. Miller, W.R. and Sharpe, R.M., 1998. Environmental oestrogens and human reproductive cancers. *Endocrine-Related Cancer*, 5, 69–96; Plant, J.A. and Davis, D.L., 2003. Breast and prostate cancer: sources and pathways of endocrine-disrupting chemicals (EDCs). In *Geology and Health*. Skinner, H.C.W. and Berger, A.R. (editors). OUP. 95–99.

70. McKinlay, R. and others, in press. Endocrine disrupting pesticides: implications for risk assessment.

71. Toppari, J., Larsen, J.C., Christiansen, P., Giwercman, A., Grandjean, P., Guillette, L.J., Jr, Jégou, B., Jensen, T.K., Jouannet, P., Keiding, N.,

Leffers, H., McLachlan, J.A., Meyer, O., Müller, J., Rajpert-De Meyts, E., Scheike, T., Sharpe, R.M., Sumpter, J.S. and Skakkebaek, N. E., 1996. Male reproductive health and environmental xenoestrogens. *Environmental Health Perspectives*, 104, 741–803.

72. www.cancersupportinternational.com

73. The Royal Commission on Environmental Pollution, 2003. Chemicals in products: safeguarding the environment and human health. *Report* 24; Annual Reports of the (UK) Chemical Stakeholders Forum, 2002, and The Advisory Committee on Hazardous Substances, 2002; Miller, W.R. and Sharpe, R.M., 1998. Environmental oestrogens and human reproductive cancers. *Endocrine-Related Cancer*, 5, 69–96.

74. Charlier, C.C.J., 2002. Determination of organochlorine pesticide residues in the blood of healthy individuals. *Clinical Chemistry and Laboratory Medicine*, 44, 361–364; WWF, 2003. *UK national biomonitoring survey*. WWF.

75. MDuffie, H.H., 2005. Host factors and genetic susceptibility: a paradigm of the conundrum of pesticide exposure and cancer associations. *Reviews on Environmental Health*, 20 (2), 77–101.

76. Mathur, V., 2002. Breast cancer incidence and exposure to pesticides among women originating from Jaipur. *Environment International*, 28 (5), 331–336; Starek, A., 2003. Estrogen and organochlorine xenoestrogens and breast cancer risk. *International Journal of Occupational Medicine and Environmental Health*, 16 (2), 113–124.

77. Frigo, D.E., 2004. Mechanism of AP-1-mediated gene expression by select organochlorines through the p38 MAPK pathway. *Carcinogenesis*, 25 (Feb), 249–261; Lewis, J.S. and others, 2005. Differential effects of 16-hydroxyestrone and 2-methoxyestradiol on cyclin D1 involving the transcription factor ATF-2 in MCF-7 breast cancer cells. *Journal of Molecular Endocrinology*, 34, 91–105; Tessier, D.D., 2001. Increased ErbB-2 tyrosine kinase activity, MAPK phosporylation, and cell proliferation in the prostate cancer cell line LNCaP following treatment by select pesticides. *Toxicological Sciences*, 60 (1), 38–43.

78. Swan S.H. and others, 2005. Decrease in anogenital distance among male infants with prenatal phthalate exposure. *Environmental Health Perspectives*, 113, (8).

79. Kawauchi, H., 2002. Identification of growth hormone in the sea lamprey, an extant representative of a group of the most ancient vertebrates. *Endocrinology*, 143 (12), 4916–4921; Park, J.I., 2005. Conservation of the heterodimeric glycoprotein hormone subunit family proteins and the LGR signalling system from nematodes to humans. *Endocrine Journal*, 26 (3), 267–276.

80. *Environmental Endocrine Disruptors: A Handbook of Property Data*, John Wiley and Sons.

81. Edwards, T.T., 2006. Reproductive dysgenesis in wildlife: a comparative view. *International Journal of Andrology*, 29 (1), 109–121; Guillette, L.L., 1999. Plasma steroid concentrations and male phallus size in juvenile alligators from seven Florida lakes. *General and Comparative Endocrinology*, 116 (3), 356–372.

82. Colborn, T., Dumanoski, D. and Myers, J.P., 1996. *Our Stolen Futures*, Dutton, Penguin Books, USA.

83. Webb, S.F., 2000. Risk assessment approaches for Pharmaceuticals. In: International Seminar: Pharmaceuticals in the Environment, Technological Institute, Section on Environmental Technology, Brussels, 2000.

84. Kolpin, D.A., Furlong, E.T., Meyer, M.T., Thurman, E.M., Zaugg, S.D., Barber, L.B. and Buxton, H.T., 2002. Pharmaceuticals, Hormones, and Other Organic Wastewater Contaminants in US Streams, 1999–2000: A National Reconnaissance. *Environmental Science & Technology*, 36, 1202–1211.

85. McQuillan, D., Mullany, J., Parker, J., Mills, D., Sherrell, K. and Chapman, T.H., 2000. Drug Residues in Ambient Water: Initial Surveillance in New Mexico, USA. December 2000 Progress Report, http://www.nmenv.state.nm.us/gwb/drugs.html; Morelli, J., 2000. Are Our Medicines Tainting the Environment? http://webmd.lycos.com/content/article/25/1728_58159?

86. McQuillan, D., Mullany, J., Parker, J., Mills, D., Sherrell, K. and Chapman, T.H., 2000. Drug Residues in Ambient Water: Initial Surveillance in New Mexico, USA. December 2000 Progress Report, http://www.nmenv.state.nm.us/gwb/drugs.html

87. The Royal Commission on Environmental Pollution, 2003. Chemicals in products: safeguarding the environment and human health. *Report* 24.

88. Hamburger Umwelt Institute, 1997. Poor Design Practices – gaseous emissions form complex products.

89. Brown, S.K. and Cheng, M., 2000. Volatile Organic Compounds (VOCs) in New Car Interiors. Presented at the 15th International Clean Air & Environment Conference Sydney, 26–30 November 2000.

90. http://www.le.ac.uk/ieh

91. Clapp, R.W. and others, 2005. *Environmental and occupational causes of cancer*. The Lowell Centre for Sustainable Production, University of Massachusetts Lowell.

92. The Globe and Mail, November 22, 2002, page A5. Data point to breast-cancer risk. By Martin Mittelstaedt.

93. Newby, J.A. and Howard, C.V., 2006. Environmental influences in cancer aetiology. Journal of Nutritional and Environmental Medicine, 2006, 1–59.

94. Clapp, R.W. and others, 2005. *Environmental and occupational causes of cancer*. The Lowell Centre for Sustainable Production, University of Massachusetts Lowell.

95. Birnbaum, L.S. and Fenton, S.E., 2003. Cancer and developmental exposure to endocrine disruptors. *Environmental Health Perspectives*, 11 (4), 389–395.

96. www.obgyn.net/newsrx/womens_health-Colorectal_Cancer-20001214-7.asp

97. http://info.cancerresearchuk.org/healthyliving/dietandhealthyeating/theepicstudy

98. www.ucdmc.ucdavis.edu/ucdhs/health/a-z/06BreastCancer/doc06lowerisk.ht ml

99. Epidem, 1994, 23 (6), 1133–1136.

100. Spurgeon, D., 2006. Vitamin D is associated with a lower risk of cancer. *BMJ*, 332, 70.

101. Miller, W.R. and Sharpe, R.M., 1998. Environmental oestrogens and human reproductive cancers. *Endocrine-Related Cancer*, 5, 69–96.

102. http://cis.nci.nih.gov/fact/3_13.htm

103. Gottlieb, Scott. 2002. Study supports evidence on oral contraception and breast cancer. *BMJ*, 325, 6 July 2002, 8.

104. Writing Group for the Women's Health Initiative Investigators. 2002. Risks and Benefits of Estrogen Plus Progestin in Healthy Postmenopausal Women. *Journal of the American Medical Association*, 288, No 3.

105. Collaborative Group on Hormonal Factors in Breast Cancer, 1997. Breast cancer and hormone replacement therapy. *Lancet*, 350, 1047–1059.

106. Schairer, C., Lubin, J., Troisi, R., and others, 2000. Menopausal estrogen and estrogen-progestin replacement therapy and breast cancer risk. *JAMA*, 283 (4), 485–491.

107. www.nih.gov/news/pr/nov2002/nichd-29.htm

108. Ross, R.K., Paganini-Hill, A., Wan, P.C. and others, 2000. Effective hormone replacement therapy on breast cancer risk: estrogen versus estrogen plus progestin. *J Natl Cancer Inst*, 92, 328–332. Schairer, C., Lubin, J., Troisi, R. and others. 2000. Menopausal estrogen and estrogen-progestin replacement therapy and breast cancer risk. *JAMA*, 283 (4), 485–491.

109. *The Times*, 15 December 2006.

110. Ernst, E (editor), 2001. *The Desktop Guide to Complementary and Alternative Medicine: an evidence based approach*. Mosby.

111. Lee, John R, 1999. *Natural Progesterone*. Second revised edition. Jon Carpenter.

112. Cowan, L.D., Gordis, L., Tonascia, J.A. and Jones, G.S., 1981. Breast cancer incidence in women with a history of progesterone deficiency. *Am J Epidemiology*, 114, 209–217.

113. Hrushesky, W.J.M., 1996. Breast cancer, timing of surgery, and the menstrual cycle: call for prospective trial. *J Women's Health*, 5, 555–566.

114. Mohr, P.E., Wang, D.Y., Gregory, W.M., Richards, M.A. and Fentiman, I.S., 1996. Serum progesterone and prognosis in operable breast cancer. *British J Cancer*, 73, 1552–1555.

115. Butler, J., 2006. *White lies*. Vegetarian and Vegan Foundation.

116. Dibble, S.L. and others, 2002. Risk factors for ovarian cancer; lesbian and heterosexual women. *Oncol Nursing Forum*, 29 (1), E1–7.

117. Ives, A. and Semmens, J., 2007. Pregnancy after breast cancer: population based study. *BMJ*, 334, 194.

118. www.cancer.org/docroot/cri/content/cri_2_4_5x_what_happens_after_treat ment_5.asp?sitearea=cr

119. http://www.cancer.org/docroot/cri/content/cri_2_6x_can_having_an_abort ion_cause_or_contribute_to_breast_cancer.asp

120. http://www.cancer.org/docroot/cri/content/cri_2_6x_can_having_an_abort ion_cause_or_contribute_to_breast_cancer.asp

121. www.cspinet.org/new/200206251.html

UPDATE TO CHAPTER SEVEN

1. Campbell, T. Colin, Campbell, Thomas M. II, Robbins, John and Lyman Howard, 2006. *The China Study: The Most Comprehensive Study of Nutrition Ever Conducted and the Startling Implications for Diet, Weight Loss and Long-term Health*. Benbella Books.

2. Kannel W.B. and others, 1961. Factors of risk in the development of coronary heart disease – six year follow up experience. *Anna. Internal medi.*, 55.

3. Campbell, T. Colin, Campbell, Thomas M. II, Robbins, John and Lyman Howard, 2006. *The China Study: The Most Comprehensive Study of Nutrition Ever Conducted and the Startling Implications for Diet, Weight Loss and Long-term Health*. Benbella Books.

4. Campbell, T.C. and Junshi, C., 1994. Diet and chronic degenerative disease perspectives from China. *American Journal of Clinical Nutrition*, 59 (Suppl.), 11,535–11,615.

5. Marwick, Charles, 2003. Food industry obfuscates healthy eating message. *BMJ*, 327, 121.

6. Campbell, T. Colin, Campbell, Thomas M. II, Robbins, John and Lyman Howard, 2006. *The China Study: The Most Comprehensive Study of Nutrition Ever Conducted and the Startling Implications for Diet, Weight Loss and Long-term Health*. Benbella Books.

7. Schlosser, Eric, 2002. *Fast Food Nation*. Penguin Books.

8. Martin, Peter, 2002. Milk: Nectar or Poison? *Sunday Times Magazine*, 21 July 2002, 46–54.

9. Mercer, Chris, 2007. EU unveils milk shake-up plans. www.foodnavigator.com

10. http://www.cafod.org.uk

11. Butler, J., 2006. *White lies*. Vegetarian and Vegan Foundation.

12. Anon, 2003. UK supports exclusive breast feeding for six months. *BMJ*, 326, 1052.

13. Laurens, Claire, 2003. Baby milk company fined for advertising direct to consumers. *BMJ*, 327, 307.

14. Butler, J., 2006. *White lies*. Vegetarian and Vegan Foundation.

15. Atkins, P.J., 2005. Fattening children or fattening farmers? School milk in Britain, 1921–1941. *Economic H-58*.

16. http://www.nationaldairycouncil.org

17. Kradjian, R.M., 1994. *Save Yourself from Breast Cancer*. Berkley Books, New York.

18. Martin, Peter, 2002. Milk: Nectar or Poison? *Sunday Times Magazine*, 21 July 2002, 46–54.

19. Outwater, J.L. and others, 1997. Dairy Products and Breast Cancer: the IGF-1, estrogen and bGH hypothesis. *Med Hypotheses*, 48, 453–461.

20. European Commission, Scientific Committee on Vetinerary Measures relating to Public Health. 1999. Report on Public Health Aspects of the Use of Bovine Somatotropin, 15–16 March.

21. Yu, H. and Rohan, T., 2002. Role of the insulin-like growth factor family in cancer development and progression. *J Natl Cancer Inst*, 92, 1472–1489.

22. http://www.milksucks.com/osteo.html

23. New, S.A. and Francis, R.M., 2003. *Science in Parliament*, 60 (4), 21.

24. Plant, Jane and Tidey, Gill, 2004. *Science in Parliament*, 61 (1), 28.

25. Kradjian, R.M., 1994. *Save Yourself from Breast Cancer*. Berkley Books, New York.

26. New, S.A. and Francis, R.M., 2004. *Science in Parliament*, 61 (3), 21.

27. Robbins, John, 1987. *A Diet for a New America*. Stillpoint.

28. www.foodnavigator.com

29. Parry, Vivienne, 2007. It's udder confusion. *The Times (Body and Soul)*, 20 January 2007.

30. Butler, Justine, 2007. Second opinion. *The Times (Body and Soul)*, 27 January 2007.

31. *ICON*, 2006, issue 4.

32. Bristow, A., 2002. Organic processed food. *Which?* April 2002, 22–23.

33. Martin, Peter, 2002. Milk: Nectar or Poison? *Sunday Times Magazine*, 21 July 2002, 46–54.

34. Bristow, A., 2002. Organic processed food. *Which?* April 2002, 22–23.

35. Inside Story. *Which?* April 2002, 4.

36. Clapp, R.W., Howe, K.H. and Jacobs, M.M., 2005. Environmental and occupational causes of cancer. www.sustainableproduction.org

37. Plant, J.A., Turner, K.T. and Highley, D.E., 1998. Minerals and the environment. Proceedings of Minerals '98 Conference, June 1998; Republished in the *Mineralogical Society Bulletin*, No.119, July 1998, 3–11; *Mineral Planning* 77, December 1998, 3–8; *IM&M Journal*, December 1998, 1, 12, 331–336.

38. Kushi L.H. and others, 2007. Lifestyle factors and survival in women with breast cancer. *The Journal of Nutrition*, Special supplement; Intern. Research conf. on food, nutrition and cancer, 236S–242S.

39. Getz, Linn, Sigurdsson, Johann A. and Hetlevik, Irene, 2003. Is opportunistic disease prevention in the consultation ethically justifiable? *BMJ*, 327, 498.

40. Research muddled by political pressures. *The Times (Public Agenda)*, 19 August 2003.

41. Chaturvedi, P., 2003. Medical community may be partly responsible for cancer misery. *BMJ*, 326, 1146.

42. Kmietowicz, Zosia, 2002. Research spending on cancers doesn't match their death rates. *BMJ*, 325, 920.

43. Smith, Richard, 2003. Do patients need to read research? *BMJ*, 326, 1307.

44. Smith, Richard, 2003. Do patients need to read research? *BMJ*, 326. 1307.

45. Corrie, Pippa, Shaw, Justin and Harris, Roy, 2003. Rate limiting factors in recruitment of patients to clinical trials in cancer research: descriptive study. *BMJ*, 327, 320–321.

46. Wald, Nicholas J. and Morris, Joan K., 2003. Teleoanalysis: combining data from different types of study. *BMJ*, 327, 616–618.

47. *The Times* (Public Agenda), 6 March 2007.

48. Smith, Richard, 2003. Editor's choice: The screening industry. *BMJ*, 326, 26 April 2003.

49. Lechin, Fuard and others, 2002. *Neurocircuitry and Neuroautonomic Disorders*. Karger.

50. Gottlieb, Scott, 2003. US drug sales continue to rise. *BMJ*, 326, 518.
51. Gottlieb, Scott, 2002. Drug companies maintain 'astounding' profits. *BMJ*, 324, 1054.
52. Kjaergard, Lise L. and Als-Nielsen, Bodil, 2002. Association between competing interests and authors' conclusions: epidemiological study of randomised clinical trials published in the *BMJ*. *BMJ*, 325, 249–252.
53. Eaton, Lynn, 2003. Readers want transparency in link between doctors and drug firms. *BMJ*, 326, 1352.
54. Mayor, Susan, 2002. Researchers claim clinical trials are reported with misleading statistics. *BMJ*, 324, 1353.
55. *JAMA*, 2003, 389, 454–465, quoted by Hopkins Tanne, Janice, 2003. Industry is deeply involved in funding US research. *BMJ*, 326, 179.
56. Tonks, Alison, 2002. Authors of guidelines have strong links with drugs industry. *BMJ*, 324, 383.
57. Spurgeon, David, 2002. Doctors accept $50 a time to listen to drug representatives. BMJ, 324, 1113.
58. Gottlieb, Scott, 2003. A fifth of Americans contact their doctor as a result of direct to consumer drug advertising. *BMJ*, 325, 854.
59. BMJ, 2003. Drug companies want to inform patients. *BMJ*, 326, 1286.
60. Watson, Rory, 2003. EU health ministers reject proposal for limited direct to consumer advertising. *BMJ*, 326, 1284.
61. Watson, R., 2006. Cancer group denies company funding will influence its agenda. *BMJ*, 333, 874.
62. Mayor, Susan, 2002. GMC issues new guidance on clinical research. *BMJ*, 324, 384.
63. Marwick, Charles, 2002. US tackles drug company gifts to doctors. *BMJ*, 325, 795.
64. Mosconi, Paola, 2003. Declaration of competing interests is rare in Italian breast cancer associations. *BMJ*, 327, 344.
65. Herxheimer, A., 2003. Relationships between the pharmaceutical industry and patients' organisations. *BMJ*, 326, 1208–1210.
66. Hirst, J., 2003. Charities and patient groups should declare interests. *BMJ*, 326, 1211.
67. Clark, Jocalyn, 2003. A hot flush for Big Pharma. *BMJ*, 327, 400.
68. Writing Group for the Women's Health Initiative Investigators, 2002. Risks and benefits of estrogen plus progestin in healthy postmenopausal women. *JAMA*, 288, 321–333.
69. *The Times*, 15 December 2006.
70. Moynihan, Ray, 2003. US seniors group attacks pharmaceutical industry 'fronts'. *BMJ*, 326, 351.
71. Cho, E. and others, 2006. Red meat intake and risk of breast cancer among premenopausal women. *Archives of International Medicine*, 166, 2253–2259.
72. Lenzer, Jeanne, 2002. The operation was a success (but the patient died). *BMJ*, 325, 664.
73. Moynihan, Ray, 2003. Blurring the boundaries. *BMJ*, 326, 1094.
74. The selling of a wonder drug. *The Guardian*, 29 March 2006.
75. http://en.wikipedia.org/wiki/Trastuzumab.

76. Barrett, A. and others, 2006. How much will Herceptin really cost? *BMJ*, 333, 118–120.

77. Bartlett, Christopher, Sterne, Jonathan and Egger, Matthias, 2002. What is newsworthy? Longitudinal study of the reporting of medical research in two British newspapers. *BMJ*, 325, 81.

78. Several versions of the poem, of which this is an extract, may be found on the internet; for example, http://www.madnessmansion.com/!!jimkc/txt/ambulanc.txt; http://www.public.asu.edu/!!tadams2/Quotes/Ambulance

79. www.cancersupportinternational.com

80. Campbell, T. Colin, Campbell, Thomas M. II, Robbins, John and Lyman Howard, 2006. *The China Study: The Most Comprehensive Study of Nutrition Ever Conducted and the Startling Implications for Diet, Weight Loss and Long-term Health.* Benbella Books.

81. Robbins, John, 1987. *A Diet for a New America*. Stillpoint.

82. Butler, J., 2006. *White lies*. Vegetarian and Vegan Foundation.

FURTHER READING

Blauer, Stephen, 1989. *The Juicing Book*, New York, Avery Publishing Group, 176p.

Bremness, Lesley, 1990. *World of Herbs*, London, Ebury Press, 176p.

Conil, Christopher and Jean, 1993. *New Tofu Recipes*, W. Foulsham and Co Ltd, USA.

Lamont, Heather, 1988. *The Gourmet Vegan*, London, Victor Gollancz, 160p.

Jaffrey, Madhur, 1981. *Eastern Vegetarian Cooking*, London, Arrow Books, 544p.

Pert, CB, 1997. *Molecules of Emotion: Why you Feel the Way you Feel*, London, Simon & Schuster.

Ramsay, Ray,1994. *Easy Thai Cooking*, Wellingborough, J B Fairfax Press, 80p.

Shurtleff, William and Aoyagi, Akiko, 1975. *The Book of Tofu: Food for Mankind*, Autumn Press, USA.

So Yan-Kit, 1992. *Classic Food of China*, London, Macmillan, 400p.

Thorson Editorial Board, 1989. *The Complete Raw Juice Therapy*, London, Thorsons, HarperCollins, 128p.

Wheater, Caroline, 1993. *Juicing for Health*, London, Thorsons, HarperCollins, 256p.

Recommended Reading from the Bristol Cancer Help Centre

Daniel, R, 2000. *Living with Cancer*, London, Robinson.

Sen, J, 1996. *Healing Foods Cookbook*, London, Thorsons, HarperCollins.

Index